Acknowledgment

The author wishes to gratefully acknowledge Dr. Ken O'Neill and Warren White for asking her to write their clinic's history and then patiently enduring the two-and-a-half year process; Norma Turner, Virginia "Ginny" Stover, Sheryl Paloucek, Carolyn Philip, and Dr. Dennis Hensley at Taylor University for researching, editing, proofreading, and advising the manuscript in its various stages; Lakeland Marketing & Communications Department, including Cindy Myers for layout and design and Laura Bailey for line editing; and the 60-plus past and current members, staff, family, and friends of Southwestern Medical Clinic who shared stories and dug up their old photos, clippings, and memories to chronicle some of the most momentous mountaintops of their lives. What a blessing this project has been. Thank you all.

Introduction

God works amid both triumph and disaster, and His plans are not always our plans. But for the faithful, His providence is evident. That's the story of Southwestern Medical Clinic (SWMC). It is a saga of challenge, victory, grace, surprises, lessons learned, prayers answered, lives changed, and goals surpassed. However, it is also a tale of personal sacrifice, humble service, and godly obedience.

The purpose of this book is to share stories that provide evidence of God's hand on the clinic over the years. From its earliest beginnings in tiny, rural Berrien County Hospital to its survival and surprising growth even after the hospital closed, God worked through the clinic. From their heady triumphs after miraculous surgeries to their gut-wrenching losses, SWMC physicians could see the hand of God. The following pages present an honest account of the successes and setbacks, heroics and heartbreaks, triumphs and tragedies that make up the legacy of SWMC.

As is so often the case, a great ministry found its origins in humble circumstances.

A student at Wheaton College in Illinois in the 1950s, Weldon Cooke believed God was calling him to the mission field, and he was eager to go. Subsequent years spent in medical school only heightened Dr. Cooke's desire to become a medical missionary in some distant land. Interested in a spectrum of training, he took practicums and residencies everywhere from Chicago's busy Cook County Hospital to tiny Berrien County Hospital, which still grew its own produce and raised its own cattle. These experiences, he reasoned, would certainly shape him into a broadminded and rugged missionary surgeon.

Then everything fell apart. His family suffered a shattering medical diagnosis. His wife did not want to live overseas. Dr. Cooke found himself strongly called to missions but unable to go.

Heartsick, Dr. Cooke did not ditch his dream altogether. He looked for the right way.

On numerous occasions God has altered the plans and directions of His servants, sending them in directions they had not anticipated, yet which, ultimately, proved to be of greater service to God than their original ideas. Dr. Cooke buried himself in work, trusting the Lord for new opportunities of service.

At rural Berrien County Hospital, where he returned to lead as medical director, Dr. Cooke realized the benefits of training missions-minded physicians in surgery while they staffed the hospital. Then Dr. Cooke formulated the concept of starting a clinic specifically with missionary physicians. There was no precedent for Southwestern Medical Clinic. It was birthed by his newly morphed dream of somehow supporting other medical missionaries, aiding in their callings to the field, if he couldn't go himself.

Eventually, the clinic officially incorporated as one of the world's first multispecialty mission-minded clinics. SWMC needed structure, organization, and focus. They hired Don Gast to come in as chief administrator.

The members of SWMC were committed to their callings to missions, to highest professional standards, and, along the way, to each other. These men and women would deny they were heroes, but they believed they were part of a plan greater than themselves. They were mavericks, hired and organized by mavericks and, ultimately, working for the Almighty maverick healer. In thanksgiving and faith, they prayed about everything. They cared about each other.

When adversity struck — when other area doctors became unhappy with the hospital's relations with the clinic, or SWMC faced shortages of staff and funds, or there was a sudden departure of leadership — God's providence would always make a way.

SWMC doctors had a hand in Christian service that transcended their small clinic. They served with the tri-county health department, worked in migrant clinics and local hospitals, and went out on short- and long-term mission trips worldwide. They helped change state laws and promoted the collaborative climate of doctors across the U.S. and around the world. They advanced medicine in Berrien County in the areas of long-term care, obstetrics, and surgical procedures; then, later, subspecialization, a hospitalist program, and computerized medical records.

Expanding the ministry, they also improved medical treatments dramatically in the Congo, South Africa, Zimbabwe, Rwanda, Kenya, the United Arab Emirates, Sierra Leone, Haiti, Ecuador, Brazil, Borneo, and Asia. They became involved in national governments to affect policy changes with regard to medicine, medical services, and practices. They were leaders in the great vaccination drives, including inoculating the majority of the population of Haiti. They built and continue to build churches and clinics, and they built or greatly improved and expanded bush hospitals. They have developed and continue to develop medical schools and put together respected international medical training programs. They organize and plan short-term mission trips for their families and friends, other colleagues, and medical students. At times of disaster, they embark on emergency mission trips. They believe in training nationals so that work can continue to advance after they leave. Their influence ripples exponentially around the world.

Through it all—changes in structure, reimbursement, policy, practice, and culture—Southwestern Medical Clinic has flexed, grown, and advanced. At its core, however, it is inflexible. The clinic has always maintained its values and its calling. For this, God has blessed the clinic and its physicians. Here are the stories of God's providential hand at work in and through His Southwestern Medical Clinic.

Contents

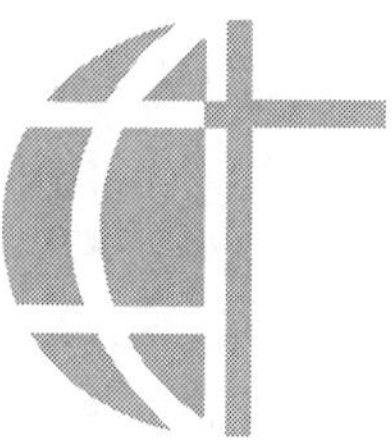

Chapter 1

How It All Started

Chapter 1

How It All Started

The summer of 1960 changed Dr. Roland Stephens' life. That summer marked transitions and progress worldwide: America's new 50-star flag slapped in a Philadelphia breeze. Young Cassius Clay boxed his way around Rome's seven hills for an Olympic gold medal. Wilson Greatbatch's new invention, the cardiac pacemaker, was beating inside patients for the first time.

But nothing excited young Dr. Stephens more than Africa. Revolutions redrew the African map on a weekly basis. Mali and Senegal, then Somaliland, gained independence, then the Central African Republic and Congo. By the end of the year Nigeria, Mauretania, Togo, Chad, and the Ivory Coast chiseled new, independent boundaries across the continent.

Dr. Stephens wanted to go. A Christian physician just completing his residency, he felt called to medical missions. For him, each new country beckoned with opportunities to save lives and serve Christ. But he wasn't quite ready.

He knew he needed more practical experience before embarking on a one-man medical adventure in the rough terrains. One day, poring over the Christian Medical Society's monthly newsletters, a small print ad caught his eye: Learn surgery at a rural county hospital to prepare for the mission field. Dr. Stephens picked up the phone. Berrien County Hospital's ebullient, young, medical director, Dr. Weldon Cooke, urged him to visit.

Dr. Stephens and his wife, Kathy, drove out to take a look. Located midway between the three little towns of Eau Claire, Berrien Center, and Berrien Springs, Michigan, the hospital stood like a lone sentry in the hills. At the end of a long, shady drive set far back from Dean's Hill Road stood a three-story hospital connected to an older, four-story infirmary. Barns and a water tower poked up behind the hospital. The surrounding waist-high cornfield was owned by the county infirmary, but leased at that time to a local farmer.

Instead of parking out front in the visitors' lot, they pulled around behind the hospital. While Dr. Stephens entered the hospital for a tour and interview with Dr. Cooke, Kathy waited in the car. An old barn towered atop a knoll behind the hospital. Until recently the barn had kept cows for the county infirmary's farm. That summer day it housed felines. While Dr. Stephens became acquainted with the hospital and its staff, Kathy befriended about a hundred cats of all sizes.

The Stephenses moved to Berrien County that summer. Dr. Stephens and Dr. Cooke enjoyed a complementary, as well as a complimentary, professional relationship. Dr. Cooke had spent a residency in a veterans' hospital with male patients, whereas Dr. Stephens had served many gynecological patients and studied urology. Dr. Stephens taught Dr. Cooke how to do hysterectomies and other gynecological surgeries, and Dr. Cooke taught him orthopedics. They respected and learned from each other.

Other doctors Dr. Stephens met that summer included Dr. Charles Patton, as well as Dr. Cooke's sister, Dr. Almarose Cooke. Dr. Almarose Cooke worked intermittently with them in between missions appointments to Honduras and later to Rhodesia. Dr. Charlie Patton left for Brazil with Mission Aviation Fellowship (MAF) around 1961.

Within a year or so, Dr. Wayne Meyers, Dr. Douglas H. Taylor, and Dr. Wendell Geary joined the pre-clinic. Like Dr. Cooke himself, they all worked for and received their salaries from Berrien County. Many only stopped at the county hospital for one year to learn surgery from Dr. Cooke while gathering support to go overseas. Drs. Meyers and Geary never returned to the staff after leaving for their mission assignments, although they both visited and stayed in touch. Dr. Doug Taylor did remain affiliated with SWMC while serving full time at Mosvold Provincial Hospital in Ingwavuma, South Africa, until 1989.

Unlike many of the doctors, Dr. Taylor came to Berrien County Hospital with missionary experience. He'd already spent a decade at Mosvold with The Evangelical Alliance Mission (TEAM). Willing to share many missionary stories, he arrived in late 1961, two or three months before the Stephenses left for Rhodesia, and found an eager audience for his tales. He and his family moved into the big house the Stephenses were vacating in Eau Claire. The Stephens family downsized into a smaller home close to the hospital to prepare for their transition overseas.

Dr. Taylor was the older brother of Kenneth N. Taylor, the compiler of The Living Bible and founder of Tyndale Publishing House. Ken Taylor founded Tyndale in 1962, right around the time Dr. Taylor arrived at Berrien County Hospital.

Despite his decades-long connection with the hospital and, as it formed and grew, Southwestern Medical Clinic, Dr. Taylor did not seek leadership positions. He spent most of his time in the operating room. He wanted to learn as many surgical skills as Dr. Cooke was able to teach. He was not inexperienced. The first resident medical officer at Mosvold, Dr. Taylor had been instrumental in expanding that facility. He started medical training for nationals and opened two satellite clinics, to which he dropped medical supplies via airplane starting in 1954. He came to Berrien County Hospital for renewal and expert training.

Many people left tracks in Berrien County Hospital's halls. Some tracks were pint-sized. Dr. Roland Stephens's young son Dan explored the hospital's nooks and crannies. Clattering down into the basement one day, Dan discovered a laboratory crawling with Dr. Meyers' white mice. A brilliant researcher, Dr. Meyers once gave his mice some drug and all their tails fell off.

For a boy like Dan, the hospital teemed with history and fascinations. Scampering up the front steps and ducking under the "1936" inscription above the double doors, he slipped inside. In the cool vestibule, families waited in little chairs while a woman rattled papers behind the reception window.

Perhaps waiting for an opportunity to finagle his way through the east door, the boy might have paused to read all the names inscribed on the bronze plaques in the vestibule. The plaques, high on the east wall past the reception window, documented the Berrien County Board of Supervisors and other men. Reading slowly, he might have stumbled on names such as John Warman, Chairman, and the special committee made up of Clarence W. Bartz, E. Willis Emerson, Martin Kretchman, and Theodore Katzbach.

If he paused in the vestibule, Dan would have heard quiet voices waft from under the administrator's office door. Mr. Richard Chaudoir served as hospital administrator from 1959-1964, and had also been and would again later be the pharmacist. Most days Dan hurried through the east door to the staff hall. On the left, in the medical library, he might have snacked on a leftover doughnut from the doctors' breakfast meeting.

Beyond the library the boardroom echoed of weighty discussions. While imposing to a small boy, the surprisingly diminutive room was dominated by a table, not oversized, and a humble fireplace. If the room was empty, Dan kept going down the hall.

The next door opened into three offices, including one of Medical Director Dr. Cooke. Across the hall more offices tumbled over each other, bustling with activity. A telephone rang, and someone answered crisply, "Berrien County Hospital. How may I help you?"

But perhaps Dan didn't turn down the east hall. From the vestibule, patient wings stretched south and west, filled with folks waiting to tell a boy a joke or share a box of chocolates. In addition, south of the vestibule, elevator doors snapped open and shut like an eager, secret-sharing mouth.

At the west end of the three-story 1936 structure, a diagonal hallway led to the drafty, four-story 1903 infirmary. In the 1960s, up to 60 long-term patients lived here in large wards on upper floors: for treatment of tuberculosis and other chronic diseases.

Dan's father, Dr. Roland "Rolly" Stephens, came down with hepatitis A in 1961. He spent a month at home. Dr. Almarose Cooke brought over his charts for him to work on while he was in bed. Kathy didn't show symptoms of hepatitis until the end of the year, at a most inopportune time, when the family was on its way to the ship for Africa. They canceled their boat trip and flew to Rhodesia one month later when she was well, in January 1962.

Like the Stephens family, most doctors did not stay at Berrien County Hospital for long. As doctors soaked up surgical techniques and flew away for their overseas missions, Dr. Cooke madly sought more doctors. Throughout the next few years, Dr. Carroll Loomis (ca. 1961-1963), Dr. Norbert Anderson (1962-1963), Dr. William R. McCurry (summer 1963), Dr. Jim Verlee (1963-1964), Dr. John Bennett (ca. 1963-1964), Dr. Paul H. Brown (ca. 1964-1971), and others came and went.

Many experienced the small-world reality of medical missions. Even if they never returned to Berrien County, they ran across each other in odd corners of the globe. Dr. John Bennett worked with Dr. Taylor at Mosvold. Through Dr. Taylor, he met Dr. Roland Stephens in Africa. After Dr. Bennett's first wife died, he later married one of Dr. Stephens' field secretaries.

Meanwhile, Dr. Cooke transformed quiet Berrien County Hospital into an unlikely medical missions hub in rural middle-America. For years, county leaders discussed their little hospital's viability. Dr. Cooke was widely credited in local newspapers and the hospital's historical documents for keeping it open.

Dr. Cooke and his swinging door of bright, young doctors perked up the hospital. The hospital changed its name from Berrien County Hospital and

Infirmary to Berrien General Hospital. Dr. Cooke had positioned the hospital for regional attention.

Through his and his doctors' hard work, quality care, and keen sense of necessary improvements, the hospital once snubbed by some locals became a source of community pride and a destination for the sick or injured countywide and beyond. It attracted patients from as far away as Sturgis and northern Indiana.

The hospital built a new, single-story 250-bed wing. On October 24, 1963, the long-term infirmary patients moved out of their drafty old wards into the sparkling addition. The pride of the hospital, it was southwestern Michigan's only hospital-based long-term care unit.

However, a subsequent inspection turned ugly. On January 1, 1964, the state threatened to cancel the hospital's health permit. Michigan ordered plans for a sewage system to be submitted by February 1. In cold sweats, Dr. Cooke, his doctors, and staff worked through that dark, icy month. On January 31, 1964, the hospital and its architects submitted plans just in time.

On May 21, 1964, they officially dedicated their new facility. The St. Joseph News Palladium described the unit as a "monument to men who dreamed and dared to do something about that dream."

The doctors prayed and dreamed in the little board room and worked hard to achieve the callings they felt on their lives. As seasons and years marched on, something that would be called Southwestern Medical Clinic began to imbed itself in the doctors' hearts and minds.

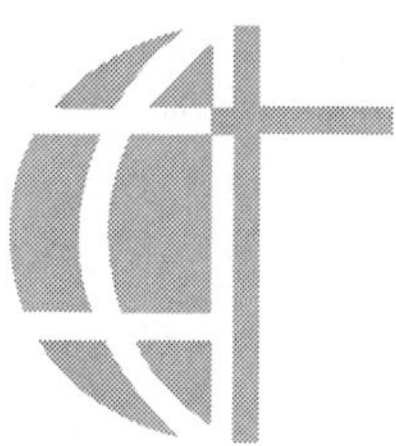

Chapter 2

Signing the Papers

Chapter 2

Signing the Papers

After completing his surgical residency in 1965 and making long-term plans to go to the mission field, Dr. Robert W. Wesche continued to page monthly through the Christian Medical Society newsletter. In one particular issue there was an intriguing advertisement similar to the one Dr. Stephens had seen five years earlier. As Dr. Wesche recalls, the ad offered an option for doctors "looking for something to do before going on the mission field."

Dr. Wesche liked the idea of a mission-minded group. He met Dr. Weldon Cooke, whom he immediately considered brilliant. Dr. Cooke introduced Dr. Wesche to his sister, Dr. Almarose Cooke, who was preparing to leave permanently for the mission field later that year. He also met Dr. Charlie Patton, back briefly from Brazil and described as "the first alumnus to return to the hospital where he spent one year from 1959-1960." He also met Dr. Herb Atkinson, and possibly Dr. Burt Sutherland.

Dr. Wesche joined, thinking the opportunity would be a very brief stint, a "short-term stop" before heading out to the field. While working at Berrien General Hospital, Dr. Wesche completed his board exams. In 1966, he and his wife, Dora, adopted their daughter. The Wesches actually spent two years at pre-SWMC before leaving for their first two-year period at Tenwek Hospital in Bomet, Kenya, through World Gospel Mission.

Dr. Wesche's "brief stint" became a decades-long relationship. In 1969, he was installed as the second full time doctor at Tenwek Hospital. From then on he typically cycled two years at Tenwek, then a year at SWMC until he retired in 1990's.

Becoming a sort of quasi-SWMC satellite, nicknamed "Location 25," Tenwek Hospital played a prominent role in SWMC history. Many SWMC doctors invested years in Tenwek. But none was as instrumental in the Kenyan hospital's success as Dr. Wesche. According to the hospital's website, Dr. Wesche treated "everything from spear wounds to bowel obstructions." Tirelessly, he toiled continuous days and nights in that OR deep in Africa.

God's providential hand blessed and expanded the places where Dr. Wesche worked. During Dr. Wesche's career, Tenwek grew from a 50-bed rural hospital manned by just himself and one other physician to a complex with more than 300 beds. Southwestern Medical Clinic incorporated and grew from four or five physicians to more than 50 by 1998.

Even after retiring in 1998, Dr. Wesche and his wife returned to Tenwek on numerous occasions, usually for three to six months. Tenwek will not forget Dr. Wesche. In 2005, Tenwek's directors named its new surgical complex in honor of him.

SWMC was instrumental in the growth of Tenwek Hospital because SWMC allowed Dr. Wesche to focus on Tenwek while maintaining his continuing education and the details of American citizenship. Other doctors, some with years of previous missionary experience like Dr. Taylor, came to work under Dr. Cooke for those same reasons.

In the summer of 1965 a young red-haired man named Dr. James L. Wierman spent three hot months at Berrien County Hospital, rubbing elbows with Dr. Cooke, Dr. Sutherland, and possibly Dr. Wesche. He was still a medical student. He recalled of that experience, "Dr. Cooke was a great teacher for a young physician. I enjoyed it immensely. So much, in fact, that my mother had to call to remind me to come home to visit in July."

Dr. Wierman left in September for an internship; worked as a family practitioner from 1968-1969; married Denise Borst, a nurse he had met at Berrien General Hospital; spent a year in Haiti; came home for a residency; then worked again at Berrien General Hospital from 1973-1978. In 1978 he set up his solo practice in Dowagiac, Michigan.

In 1966, five doctors served under Dr. Cooke: Dr. Wesche, Dr. Robert I. Crawford, Dr. Robert S. Schindler, Dr. Robert A. Chapman, and Dr. Eugene R. Stockdale. The hospital's 1966 annual report noted:

> *Since 1959 our medical staff has been composed entirely of medical missionaries on furlough, or missionary candidates, who upon completion of their year will be going to the foreign field. It must be emphasized, however, that each of the physicians at Berrien General Hospital is a licensed physician and surgeon in the state of Michigan and of varied medical background having an unusual dedication to medicine and to their [sic] patients.*

The staff doctors kept the hospital's two operating rooms occupied. In 1966 they performed 959 operations, ranging from tonsillectomies to embolectomies. That year also saw the arrival of Medicare, and with it swept in a whole series of confusions, reimbursement delays, and mountains of paperwork.

Dr. Roland Stephens and his family returned in June of 1967. Dr. Crawford left as they arrived. Dr. Burton M. Sutherland, Dr. Harold Mason, Dr. Eugene Stockdale, and Dr. Herb Atkinson worked with Dr. Cooke in those days.

Meanwhile, the doctors built an outpatient clinic clientele, seeing patients behind privacy curtains in the emergency room. They worked their appointments around emergencies that came in. Clinic patients checked in upstairs and placed in an ER space. When someone was brought in by ambulance, he or she was put into an adjoining ER space. This situation only worked because there were a couple of doctors on the premises all the time. As every doctor rotated nights and weekends in the emergency room, Berrien General Hospital had the first 24-hour ER in Berrien County.

The ER was frequently "bedlam," as Dr. Atkinson described it. Other times, the doctors found a few moments to swap stories. Someone later told Dr. Janet Frey about Dr. Roland Stephens, the aggressive and fearless surgeon serving in Rhodesia. One day, they said, he was working in the ER and somebody came in suffering of a heart attack and had a cardiac arrest. Dr. Stephens whipped out his knife, opened the man up and performed internal cardiac massage. To everyone's relief, the technique was a success. No more intense drama could be found in any ER anywhere.

Decades later Dr. Roland Stephens can neither confirm nor deny the story. He wrote that if the event occurred, it was "probably in 1960 or 1961 before external cardiac massage was popular. If a cardiac arrest occurred, it was felt that internal cardiac massage was the only hope of saving a person's life; hence, it would not surprise me if this was my action, but I do not remember the specific incident. I have done a good many internal cardiac massages over the years and a number have been successful."

Such is the case for these fellows who performed so many daring medical feats, they blur over the decades into one long wrestling match to save lives... both physical and spiritual.

Another wrestling match of sorts became a motivator in the SWMC's incorporation.

Before SWMC was incorporated, physicians were actually employees of the county. They received a salary and worked only out of Berrien General Hospital, a county-owned facility. When they began seeing patients in the ER on the side, other area physicians and some county people grew upset, resentful of them practicing and competing with other local doctors for patients, while all their overhead was paid for by the county. Discussions ensued between the county and Dr. Cooke. Pressure mounted to come up with a solution and temper the community unrest.

Dr. Cooke and the others put their heads together over coffee and doughnuts in the library; over coffee and sandwiches in between clinic and ER patients; and over coffee and crackers in the wee hours after surgery. They began formulating ideas about a more organized physician group. Dr. Sutherland applauded the Wheaton study-break vision that Dr. Cooke and Dr. Atkinson shared. Dr. Sutherland stressed that as a group, the doctors could do better than to simply work for Berrien General Hospital. He saw a greater potential impact in an independent physicians' group working out of other area hospitals as well, such as Mercy Hospital in Benton Harbor, Memorial Hospital in St. Joseph, Lee Memorial Hospital in Dowagiac, and Pawating Hospital in Niles.

The discussion soon led to action. Dr. Cooke had papers drawn up to form a multispecialty physicians group known as "Berrien Medical Clinic, P.C." On June 28, 1968, Drs. Weldon J. Cooke, Burton M. Sutherland, Harold A. Mason, Roland R. Stephens, and Douglas H. Taylor signed the articles of incorporation notarized by Richard Chaudoir. Drs. Cooke, Sutherland, and Mason formed the first board of directors.

Little changed immediately. The signers continued to toil many hours at Berrien General Hospital. Even following the formalities of incorporation as a separate entity, they still faced antagonism from the local physicians and others. But word got around about these caring, highly skilled doctors' private practice. Patients flowed in and life was very busy.

At the time of incorporation, Dr. Cooke, still hospital medical director, did daily rounds and knew the charts of all the patients – his and all the others, too. He was a patient's doctor, and that rarely left little time for him to manage a clinic. The group had to start collecting for its services instead of just earning salaries through the county. They hired their first staff member, Virginia "Ginny" Stover, in 1968, as financial secretary. Ginny and her husband had known Dr. Cooke and his wife, Fran, since Dr. Cooke's first years interning at Berrien County Hospital in the 1950s. Ginny stayed until retirement on January 31, 1990. When first hired, she only worked one day each week.

As the son of two Wheaton professors, Dr. Cooke taught and learned by asking iconoclastic and challenging questions. He kept the staff sharp. At times he could be exasperating. He insisted that meetings start on time, but frequently rushed in late, demanding a summary and asking devil's advocate questions about all they'd already discussed. Meetings were known to last until 11:30 p.m. Nevertheless, most people admired him and thought him to be brilliant. Ginny Stover believed Dr. Cooke wanted everyone to think issues and solutions through at every level before plowing into a second-best solution.

On August 23, 1969, Dr. Cooke as corporation president and Dr. Sutherland as corporation secretary signed a document changing Berrien Medical Clinic, P.C.'s name to Southwestern Medical Clinic, P.C. Richard Chaudoir notarized the papers and sent them to P.O. Drawer 3, Lansing, along with the five dollar filing fee.

The staff of the Southwestern Medical Clinic at the time of incorporation included Don Gast, Susan Gast, Irene Berger, Sally Firman, Lela Harper, Millie Hoadley, Jean Kistler, Lieron "Lee" Morales, Ernestine Wilkes, Ruth Ann Stover, Ginny Stover, and Beverly Stover.

Bev Stover, a shirttail cousin of Ginny, started working for Southwestern Medical Clinic in 1970 and 40 years later was the "longest-years-working" employee. One of her original duties was typing all medical diagnoses on yellow punch tape. The long strings of tape were unwieldy and prone to damage. To type the diagnoses, Bev first had to decipher the physicians' handwriting. Dr. Cooke's handwriting was especially clear. After a while Bev could read all the others.

To stay afloat, the clinic and the hospital ran a taut operation. If someone needed a pencil, storeroom supervisor Hazel Bennett asked for the used stub. The hospital and the clinic gladly accepted hand-me-down equipment and office furniture from Borgess Hospital in Kalamazoo and others. The hospital auxiliary appreciated every volunteer, including Dr. Sutherland's wife, Jane, who volunteered tirelessly from 1966 until 1971, when the Sutherlands moved to California.

Adding more part-time and full time staff, overcrowding ensued. Dr. Roland Stephens returned in 1973 after five years in Rhodesia. Dr. Stephens lived in Dowagiac and divided his time among Lee Memorial Hospital, Berrien General, and Pawating Hospital in Niles for a year before returning to Rhodesia.

In August of 1978, because of the war in Rhodesia-Zimbabwe, the mission hospital was temporarily closed, very much against Dr. Stephens' wishes. The mission's home office ordered the evacuation and closure of the hospital. Disappointed, Dr. Stephens and his family returned to SWMC, where he worked for the next 16 years. In a church photo he sported a narrow bow tie and clean-cut hair parted on the left. He displayed a strong jaw and a modest smile. His wife and four sons were shown sitting serenely around him, bearing no sign of the anxiety they must have experienced while fleeing Rhodesia just months before.

Each time Dr. Stephens returned from Africa, the clinic had grown and expanded. He befriended many doctors, especially fellow surgeons, including Dr. Wesche. Both men loved their work, Africa, and the Divine Healer. For one year they traded places: Dr. Wesche filled in for Dr. Stephens at SWMC while he filled in for Dr. Wesche at Tenwek Hospital. They maintained a close friendship for the rest of their lives. As of this book's writing, Dr. Stephens still works full time at Karanda Hospital in Zimbabwe, as he has for the last half-decade, and Dr. Wesche returns regularly to fill in short-term at Tenwek.

Doctors like Weldon Cooke, Bob Wesche, and Roland Stephens were high-energy then and remain high-energy, working long after typical retirement age. In 2010, at his beloved Karanda Hospital, Dr. Stephens (age 80) may have broken a world record for performing eight C-sections in one day. These doctors still refuse to slow down. They pay no attention to their own limitations, so focused they are on the work God has led them to do.

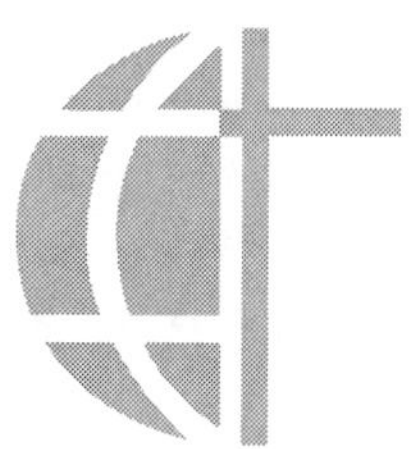

Chapter 3

Unlikely Missionary, God-Appointed

Chapter 3

Unlikely Missionary, God-Appointed

God's hand cradled SWMC decades before the clinic incorporated. When He created little Herbie Atkinson and put him in a poor evangelist's family in inner-city Philadelphia, the Lord must have had SWMC in mind.

When Herbie was three years old his father died of appendicitis. Because of this, God appointed a church minister to act as pseudo-father. About age nine, concerned about what his dad's death had meant, Herb asked his mother questions about salvation. She answered them and he accepted Christ. His mother was a good woman, but often ill, so Herb spent a lot of his time in the streets. Childhood in Philly taught Herb numerous hard lessons, but God oversaw the long view of this tough kid's life.

Already knowing Herb's future, God brought a missionary to Herb's church when he was about 13 years old. This pastor came up from South America, the Amazon area, and encouraged Herb to serve God in any way he could. Herb's life changed. He rededicated his life to Christ, determined to "grab hold of the heavy end of the log" and serve the Lord. He decided to be the man of the house. He got a job in a grocery store.

Upon graduating from high school, Herb attained a scholarship to Wheaton College in Illinois. This was the opportunity of a lifetime. But he didn't have any idea how to get there when the semester started. One of his Sunday school teachers worked as a ticket agent and got him a one-way ticket to Wheaton. Another friend gave him luggage. Herb climbed on the train with $11 in his pocket. God was teaching him about faith and Christian kinship.

At Wheaton, Herb ran against Bob Schindler for class president, wondering how to beat gregarious, larger-than-life Bob. Creative inspiration finally hit. Herb convinced a professor-aviator to take him up on a one-hour flight. High above Wheaton College, he dropped campaign pamphlets. So close to The Windy City, a stiff breeze picked up, and instead of them landing on the campus, Herb's pamphlets blew all over the city of Chicago. He still won the election, but he narrowly escaped a summons for littering.

As president, Herb met some of the guys on the Wheaton student council. Future martyr Jim Elliot and Dave Howard were among them.

Already on fire for missions, they remained accountability partners for Herb even beyond the years at Wheaton – in fact, all the way through medical school. Herb attended a church planting conference in Urbana with them as well. He looked ahead to see the value of training in church planting, wherever in the world he might be called.

Medical missions was a huge topic on Christian college campuses in the 1950s. As Herb remembered it, he and his buddies, including Weldon Cooke and Bob Schindler, developed a vision for a medical missionary clinic during study breaks. They put their heads together, trying to figure out how to make it all work.

Graduating from Wheaton in 1952, Herb could only afford to apply to one medical school. Several of his former professors at Wheaton were teaching at the University of Illinois medical school in Urbana. He made an appointment to visit the medical school. During his appointment, one of his former professors just happened to walk through the office. He hailed Herb cordially. The University of Illinois interviewing professor asked Herb's former professor about him, and the man gave Herb a glowing recommendation. Herb was always certain he got into medical school because of that man's words.

So it was then, that when Dr. Herbert Andrew Atkinson graduated from the University of Illinois at Urbana Medical School in 1956, he packed up his young family and moved to Zaire. All of Africa was politically unstable. Zaire changed names frequently. "Every time we went back, the country's name had changed," Dr. Atkinson joked. The Democratic Republic of the Congo, for all intents and purposes, seemed to be in the middle of nowhere, and Dr. Atkinson's hospital, the Africa Inland Mission, was the only medical facility in the region. A bundle of energy, Dr. Atkinson taught third-year medical students how to do hernia surgery. He helped build little churches. The nationals taught him how to mix mud for bricks and put up thatched roofs. Some of the nationals became the closest friends of Dr. Atkinson and his family.

During their first furlough, the Atkinsons returned to Wheaton for additional training. At that time Dr. Atkinson looked up some of his old friends and learned about the county hospital where his old classmate, Dr. Cooke, was teaching surgery to missionaries.

Upon returning to Africa, they found Zaire in flux. The deadly rebellion soon descended on the little hospital. Under great anxiety, Dr. Atkinson's wife, Frieda, delivered a stillborn, full-term son, Peter. They buried him in the forest. They had barely laid down their shovels when the rebels came for them. Cramming what they could into three suitcases, they ran for their lives.

Once back in the States, Dr. Atkinson called Berrien General Hospital. "It looks like we're going to need some time to recoup," he said. "Could you use the likes of me?"

"Come on, come on," Dr. Cooke told him.

When the Atkinsons arrived in Berrien County in 1965, still in the fog of grief and shock, another surprise awaited them. Dr. Cooke's wife, Fran, and the others had chosen a little house for the Atkinsons on Lake Chapin, furnished it with a stocked refrigerator, silverware, dishes, and even curtains. They'd made the beds. The downstairs came equipped with a washing machine and dryer.

"Right away Herb was put to work, and that was a wonderful thing," Frieda said.

Dr. Atkinson didn't always sport a white tuft of a beard. A nurse anesthetist, Myrt Brazington, was so amused by his youngness, she called him Dr. Kiddo. "Are you going to help with the surgeries, Dr. Kiddo?"

Dr. Cooke, Dr. Atkinson, and the others working there at the time saw great needs at little Berrien General Hospital. They planned an intensive care unit with pie-shaped rooms coming off it, and a new chronic care unit, since the infirmary was woefully outdated and inadequate. Dr. Cooke negotiated with the county and sent Dr. Atkinson out to raise money. It was a big challenge.

In a video recording not long before his death, Dr. Atkinson recalled, "You just can't imagine. Berrien County just jumped aboard in no time flat… The Lord provided out of nowhere for us to make a hospital. We always put our hands to the wheel. We had a big ER, a square room with two rooms on each side of the room, eight rooms to use. We could yell across the ER to help each other — no confidentiality. It was absolute bedlam. We grew along with it. You wouldn't think of practicing medicine in the U.S. that way today… The Lord was with us. His hand was in it all the way."

They stayed at SWMC a year that first time, in 1965. Their daughter Essie was born, and not long after, they felt pulled to return to Africa. Friends feared for them and begged them not to go back. Other missionaries and their families had been beheaded. The government still rocked with instability. One pastor said, "How could you think of going back there after that other doctor and his wife and children were all slaughtered?"

The Atkinson family had been reading in The Living Bible, "With these weapons we will be able to capture rebels and change them into men whose hearts' desire is obedience to Christ." (II Cor. 10:5b) They saw this verse as a personal directive from God. They packed their suitcases and diaper bags and headed back.

Dr. Atkinson made less than $300 a month out on the field. Sometimes discouragement set in. He would turn to Frieda, rub his eyes ruefully and moan, "Here I have all this education, all this training, and I can't even provide for my family." However, the Lord provided in many ways, and the Atkinsons were blessed with friends and support on both continents. Dr. Atkinson reflected of his SWMC colleagues later:

> *All these guys had a real heart for missions, a heart for each other. These early docs were a bunch of independents fighting a hostile world. We all came to Southwestern [Medical Clinic] with ideas not always compatible with each other, but we learned to support each other despite minor disagreements. The turnover was less as years went by.*
>
> *We had to listen to each other. We had problems being pliable. We all thought we knew the right thing for us and the right thing for the other guy. Docs came back for furloughs and retraining, and we learned to listen to each other and just pray about it. We learned not to hold our dreams inside, but to share with each other what we wanted to do, and sure enough, within a year, you were doing it.*

They also put into place a novel concept in medicine at the time: They learned to grab the phone and talk with partners of different specialties. The pliability that seeped into the clinic became almost tangible.

They considered each other brothers. Their wives and children became like extended family. On weekends off, several doctors would pack up their sons and go hunting or fishing. They threw together picnics and birthday parties. The Atkinsons became "Uncle Herb" and "Aunt Frieda." There were many reasons to sink roots into Berrien County and just stay, yet God called them back to The Dark Continent.

Before long, the Atkinsons returned to Zaire. They sent their two boys to Kenya to boarding school. In order to get there, the boys had to fly in a small missionary airplane. They had to travel over Uganda, a troubled country, where planes were often targets of gunfire. Dr. Atkinson and Frieda were looking for word about them more than a thousand miles away.

On the way back home, the plane had to detour into Rwanda and make an unplanned landing. Somehow in the mess, the boys' passports were taken from them. Standing there bewildered and afraid, the boys watched tractors making long ditches. The rebels were digging massive graves. The missionary pilot approached the wild-eyed rebels and said, "You can't take these passports away from these kids."

Unbelievably, their passports were given back to them. They were able to return to Zaire and their parents. Amid the hubbub, their older son, David, injured his spine. The Atkinsons were advised to send Frieda with David back to the states.

Frieda said, "David's father is in medicine. David deserves to be with his father. I don't think we should go."

They spent several unhappy hours in discussion. In the end, they decided to pack up and come home as a family. Right away, the SWMC took Dr. Atkinson back on staff.

Almost immediately Dr. Atkinson began showing symptoms of a severe illness. The final diagnosis: liver problems that would haunt him the rest of his life. Because of his compromised liver, he was unable to take antimalarial medicine and never returned full time to Africa again. Realizing such was his future, he asked the SWMC administrator, Don Gast, to help them find a house.

He recalled, "I didn't have a driver's license, and we had no money for equity, nothing. So, Don Gast takes us over to the bank. I've probably got a plaid shirt and jeans on, all I had left. I must've looked a wreck."

But Don was unabashed. He talked to the bank president. "We want money for a down payment on a house, and we want it today."

"We got our house on Don's signature," Dr. Atkinson recalled. "Don made that possible."

Frieda helped her husband at the clinic for 12 years. She could empathize with the heartbreaking cases. About half of Dr. Atkinson's practice was unwed mothers. Frieda asked him, "How do I approach this?"

He said, "Treat them all the same – with loving concern. If they are unwed mothers, they're probably terrified that we're going to condemn them."

Dr. Atkinson and Frieda praised them for coming to SWMC and saving their babies. They offered to help the mothers keep their babies or put them up for adoption, whatever help they wanted. Many came to the Lord. Two of the Atkinsons' grandchildren were adoptees from that practice.

In the early 1970s the clinic practiced mostly in Berrien General Hospital. A great deal of the work was treating the migrants who were working as seasonal temps on the local farms. The migrants spread word to all their coworkers about the kind, quality care they received at Berrien General. The clinic did not become financially stabilized by treating patients who couldn't pay. SWMC didn't have good health insurance or malpractice insurance coverage. But the Lord made provisions again and again.

One case stands out in Frieda's memory. A patient was nearing full-term and everything was going along fine. Then a visiting nurse at the clinic, overzealous of vaccines, gave the mother a vaccine, only thinking about the ramifications later. The husband said he was going to sue the clinic for $3 million dollars. The lawyers at the hospital advised Dr. Atkinson to cause an abortion, or he and the clinic would be paying for it the rest of their lives. Of course, Dr. Atkinson wouldn't consider that option. He prayed hard. The woman went to see a communicable disease specialist in Chicago. It was a dark time at the clinic.

In Chicago, the specialist said to the woman, "Who is your doctor? He must be a fine man, because he's right, you don't need an abortion. The baby was not harmed."

The baby was born on time at Berrien General Hospital, healthy and happy. One of his middle names was Herb.

Along with running a busy family practice, Dr. Atkinson served in leadership at Southwestern Medical Clinic. In fact, his colleagues knew he wouldn't turn down a position if he was needed. In 1977, they acted on this knowledge. Dr. Cooke wrote about it in his Christmas letter that year:

We made Herb Chief of Staff this year. Actually, he was the only one who couldn't enter a protest, being absent from medical staff meeting during election time. (Let me tell you, he hasn't missed a meeting — ANY meeting — since!) Herb is easy to identify these days by the circles around his eyes; his OB practice has been keeping him at the hospital three and four days at a time. He invested in a CB radio this year, and now whenever he makes a mad dash for a delivery, the police listen for him and head for the other end of the county.

Even though Dr. Atkinson felt out of his element and didn't believe it was his gift, he served as chief of staff at Berrien General for several years between 1977-1983. He was a beloved leader. He also served as secretary of the board from 1983-1985 and vice president from 1986-1988. His name shows up on boards off and on after that. In addition, he served as chairman of the Credentials and Ethics Committee for the Berrien County Medical Society.

Looking back at the clinic's history, from the Wheaton vision on through the decades, more than 200 physicians later, Dr. Atkinson shared his insights just before his death in 2009. "People are the success of the clinic. I marvel at it. The Lord did it. I'm thanking the Lord it's happened… You try to put the Lord first. 'He who honors Me I will honor.'"

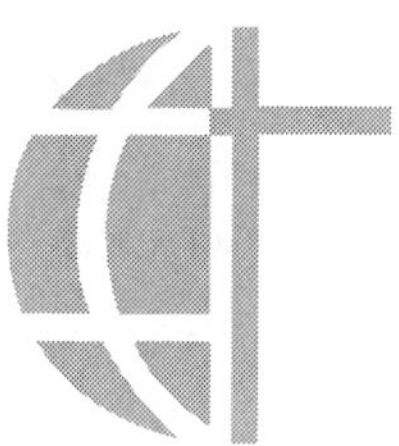

Chapter 4

SWMC's First Administrator

Chapter 4

SWMC's First Administrator

Don Gast attended Wheaton College with Weldon Cooke, Herb Atkinson, and Bob Schindler, and he avidly listened as they excitedly planned for their futures abroad. However, his goal was not to be a medical missionary. He was studying business management. He was going to go back home to Baroda and inherit his father's well-established hardware store.

For nearly 20 years Don worked faithfully at his father's hardware store, earning a plumbing license and becoming one of the first licensed electricians in the state. Then, out of the blue, his father sold the store and kept the earnings for his retirement. Don found a job in the hardware department of Sears.

Right around this same time, Dr. Cooke and the others at Southwestern Medical Clinic realized they needed to make some significant role changes. New billing procedures, as well as the success and growth of both Berrien General Hospital and Southwestern Medical Clinic, had increased Dr. Cooke's and the other physicians' and staff's already staggering workloads. They needed help.

They began to recognize that they should find an administrator. Don Gast's name came up. They looked around at each other and figured he would be their ideal prospect. Don possessed all the qualities for the job, but years had passed since all their Wheaton dreams. Don was poised for a lucrative career, they believed, as a Sears executive. Their clinic was working out of a busy, tiny, outdated building. They didn't even know where they could fit an administrator's desk. Dr. Atkinson recalled:

> *We idiots, we went and invited him to come with us. We offered him a broom closet at Berrien General Hospital – literally the thing was a broom closet – and could give him a fraction of the salary that Sears was going to pay him. And Don, something just caught him and he said, 'Okay, guys, I'm coming,' much to our surprise. I don't think we seriously thought he ever*

would do it. But we misunderstood Don; we underestimated him by a yardstick…"

Don Gast officially joined Southwestern Medical Clinic on January 1, 1972. Prior to that, he recalled:

I said I would come help get them started. I would work for one month and help them get things set up. At the end of the month, we hadn't done anything; hadn't touched the mountain of work, so I agreed to come aboard a little longer. In the meantime, I was recruited by Sears Roebuck to go through their management program. After I was here for three months, I had to go back and talk to Sears. They said, 'Okay, you want more money, we'll give you more money and you can start in another month. Work there one more month and come to Sears.'

When I decided I was going to work at the clinic, I gave up the opportunity. I would've been a lot better off financially. In fact, my salary and options would've been four times what this was.

What made me stay here was [the people]. The three greatest people who'd affected my life were Dr. Wesche, and Dr. Schindler, and Dr. Atkinson, and here they were all together, asking me to stay. They convinced me that it was something unusual. I still was never going to stay permanently, but the more I met the other missionaries as they came back, the more it touched me. They were quite unique and they had [great financial] need and they worked in missions, and it affected me, so I was able to enjoy [my contributions as administrator to their efforts].

Another big factor to keep me at SW was the news about the five missionaries in South America [Nate Saint, Jim Elliot, and Ed McCully from Wheaton and their two other missionary friends who became martyrs in Ecuador in 1956]. I knew those people personally, and I felt that I needed to respond: I can take that road, as well. I then decided I would work here to try to build it up as a place for missionaries to come and go. Everybody here, all the people, they worked because they were committed to the Lord and to the missionaries. It just kept going. It never ended.

Technically, John Taylor, an acting accountant for SWMC, hired Don. John worked out of an accounting firm in South Bend and came to Berrien one day a week. More than a decade later, when John left his accounting firm, Don hired him in a role reversal that still makes Don chuckle.

When John hired him, Don was assigned to be "Dr. Cooke's right-hand man." By all accounts — and such accounts are extensive — Don carried out this job description to the letter. He became not only Dr. Cooke's right hand, but both arms and legs, running around behind the scenes to arrange countless details. His one-month stay grew to six months, and after that he could see he had plenty to do at SWMC for as long as he wanted to stay.

Throughout the years, Three Oaks Bank needled Don with an open job offer. They saw the excellent job he was doing at SWMC and wanted him on their team. He recalls:

They told me that if I ever wanted to come work with them… they would guarantee a VP position after five years, and maybe in ten years be the president of the bank. I kept turning them down, and I fought with that, because… I would've had some money and lived a lot different. They called me a dozen times.

His reasoning for staying each time was the same.

The doctors and all the staff were committed to this program. It was the only organization I knew that every person who worked here had given their lives to this, and I felt then that's what I should do too. I should fit in here and do the work I could to make it go, and to build this program, this vision. It grew all over.

The missionaries went all over the world, and in the meanwhile I can stay here and do what I can and work with everybody else. It took a lot of hours, weekends. It took everything to make it go. And every person was working those kinds of hours. They all worked more than I'd ever seen anywhere else, to make it work so that those missionaries could come home and go out.

Dr. Atkinson referred to the quote, "'An institution is the length and shadow of a man,' or maybe several men." He credited Dr. Weldon Cooke for getting SWMC started. And he credited Don Gast with giving SWMC its soul. "He had a heart for people, really reached out to our employees," Dr. Atkinson said. "You need help, you run to Don Gast; you're going to get some help."

It seems everyone who has ever worked with the clinic has a Don Gast story. From the most revered medical missionaries to the lowliest co-op student, employees felt cared for and attended to. Here are two behind-the-scenes stories that typify this man who became the heart of the clinic:

Debbie Crane was hired by Don and steadily moved up the ranks. She started as a receptionist, part of a team. When clinical moved to the old juvenile center building, she moved up to insurance, then to administrative assistant, and finally to accounts coordinator.

Not long after Debbie started with SWMC, her little Escort wagon went bad. She commuted from Niles to work and needed transportation. As a single mother with a young son, money was tight, and she couldn't afford to have the car fixed on the weekend. In tears, she approached Don. When he learned of her predicament, he didn't even hesitate. "Use it as long as you need it," he said, as he handed Debbie the keys to the company car.

Now billing department supervisor, Mindi Sirk was hired as a high school co-op student at 6:30 a.m. on a Saturday in 1990. Roused out of bed by a ringing phone, she remembers how Don offered her the job if she could start on Monday. She said "yes" and fell back asleep. When she woke up later, half-wondering if she'd dreamed the telephone conversation, she told her mother, "I think I have a job."

When Mindi and her husband were newlyweds, they found themselves house-poor with no furniture. Don learned of their situation. Gears turning, he said, "Wesche is storing all this furniture – hasn't used it in years. I'm sure he doesn't need it anymore."

Mindi perked up. So Don called Dr. Wesche in Africa and talked him out of his living room set, and the Sirks moved it into their house and kept it ever since.

People said "yes" to Don Gast's requests, knowing it went both ways. Someday he'd be asking someone else for a favor to help them out.

Outside the clinic, people didn't always say "yes." In 1972, a bond to improve facilities at Berrien General Hospital was defeated by public vote. This was a blow. The doctors had worked very hard to upgrade the hospital staff's skills and all the patient care. In order to advance, the woefully outdated physical facility needed attention. They couldn't understand why the community didn't support it.

Don, Dr. Cooke, and others appealed to the county supervisors. In September of 1972, the Board of Supervisors approved $300,000 for capital improvements. They originally planned for a new obstetrics section, clearly seeing the need. Later, the supervisors decided to build a new surgery section as well. But it took nearly two years to break ground.

Don Gast's first 18 months as administrator were difficult, as evidenced by an end-of-the-fiscal-year letter still retained in the clinic's archives:

July 3, 1973

Dear Cookie, Bob, and Dewain:

Often words cannot express the thoughts and wishes of a person, but I would like to attempt to express my feeling and desires in relation to the Southwestern Medical Clinic.

This past year has had its ups and downs, times of rewards and times of disappointment, and yet I can't help but feel that we can profit much by the conditions which we experienced. We must use this as a learning experience and advance with new expectations and goals for the coming year.

Some of the activities for which we can be thankful were: the ability of Dr. Schindler and Dr. Drake to return to the mission field; the short-term involvement of Bob and Dewain; the retaining of Berrien General Hospital as a complete acute hospital; the gifts received from outside groups for new equipment; the additional monies made available to the hospital by the county; helping in the support of the light bearers; our opportunity in helping hundreds of needy patients both in their physical and spiritual needs; the ability of each of us to give personally to the Lord's work made possible by our income from the clinic; the physical recovery of Helene; the new doctors coming to join our group; and many more numerous day to day blessings to come.

My personal prayer is, 'Thank you, Lord, for this past year, and provide me with strength and direction to meet the challenge of each coming day. Give me added enthusiasm, the ability to utilize my time wisely, make us conscious of our responsibility in representing Christ to all those to whom we come in contact by our actions and words."

As a part of the directing and administrative staff, I ask the Lord to give us the desire and patience to 'pray together' and work together as a team, to be thoughtful and considerate of each other, and to be a source of spiritual and physical encouragement to each other.

I am looking forward to this year with great expectation. It's a real thrill for me to be a part of this, the Southwestern Medical Clinic.

With this, I am willing to accept an increase of my salary to $15,000 a year. Thank you.

The clinic paid Don Gast's salary, but the county was still paying the doctors' salaries for their hospital work. This lasted until 1975, when the clinic separated physically and financially from Berrien County, although the hospital continued to hire SWMC doctors.

Don saw Dr. Cooke ("Cookie") from a unique perspective as a friend and as an administrator. He saw that Dr. Cooke used abrasiveness to make things happen at the hospital, the clinic, and in the community. Whereas Dr. Cooke's strong tactics were sometimes an irritation to doctors, he deeply cared for them and agonized over their preparations for the future. To broaden their experience, all the doctors had to work in the ER. All had to make hospital rounds. All were exposed to being the sole doctor on call to be responsible for everything in the hospital.

"On the mission field, [Dr. Cooke knew they would have to] do the same thing," Don Gast reasoned.

Through Dr. Cooke's efforts, SWMC helped Berrien General Hospital open the first 24-hour ER in Berrien County and also the county's first birth department. Dr. Atkinson and Dr. Cooke once laid down all the first things SWMC had done in the county. They came up with the list under duress sometime around 1980. At that time some local doctors coordinated to try to close the hospital down. They didn't think it was necessary to have a tiny rural hospital with all the shiny, new, big hospitals in the area. The county began to listen to this noise.

A public meeting was organized. In a big sweat Dr. Atkinson put it all together, and Dr. Cooke spoke vehemently describing the influence of the hospital on the whole area and listing all the firsts that Berrien General Hospital had implemented: first 24-hour emergency room, first birthing center, first hospital in the area to allow fathers in the delivery room, first in the county with a poison control center. Doctors from both SWMC and the community gave strong pitches for the hospital, and several people gave their testimony that they'd been cured at the clinic. They hired a bus, and a busload came from Benton Harbor to the meeting to support the hospital.

After the meeting, the county changed its mind and agreed the hospital was necessary. The area doctors started to work together, and attention was brought to SWMC doctors. As a result, other hospitals accepted SWMC doctors into their doors. Looking back, the crisis directly influenced the spread of SWMC beyond Berrien General Hospital.

Another of SWMC's firsts included being the first organization in the state where medical doctors (MDs) and doctors of osteopathic medicine (DOs) worked together. Back then, cultural differences divided these separately trained physicians. In the broader realm, MDs and DOs didn't see eye to eye. But Don Gast believed SWMC should "put our clinic wealth together." So, he talked to Lansing legislators in an effort to help change laws so that MDs and DOs could work side by side. Until that point, DOs could not share the same privileges.

"We had so many good DOs, I took the responsibility to push that through," Don recalled. "It was important not only for Southwestern, but also for the whole community that these doctors should work together."

This revolutionary concept was essential in a clinic staffed by doctors with one foot in Berrien General and the other foot on another continent. In order for the clinic to operate, it was less "working together" than surviving together. Often physicians left — or arrived — on a moment's notice. More than once Don received a telephone call in the night that a doctor and his family had been evacuated out of a mission post and were sitting in an airport. Don jumped into his car, sped through the darkened countryside, loaded up the family, and brought them home to his basement.

In the morning, Don figured out where to plug in their war-torn but beloved colleague.

If a doctor came back from the field, they made every effort to put him into his area of specialization. If he was a surgeon, he'd be added to the clinic for surgeons. That's how the clinic expanded — when a doctor came with specialties, if there was no space for him, a space would be created for him.

Expansion was also driven by growth. Don Gast saw the community's need for good physicians, and he intended to fill that need through SWMC. Don networked on mission fields and medical schools. At first there was no formal recruiting, just those little advertisements in the Christian Medical Society newsletter and word of mouth.

In Virginia Stover's view:

> *The Lord just seemed to send these doctors here. Don had a big job, finding out when the doctors came home [from mission fields] and finding a place for them to work and live. Each doctor needed different continuing education, and he took it upon himself to help figure out where each would go. When someone was leaving, he had to find a replacement. It had to be a higher power making this run smoothly.*

It didn't always feel smooth. But even the larger medical community seemed to sense the clinic's running power, whether or not it sensed the source of that power. The larger medical community learned during those years to call on the SWMC whenever there was a need. At least once a week the SWMC doctors met as a group, and it was not uncommon to be presented with a dilemma. One week the migrant clinic was begging for a doctor. Another week it was public health or something else. The doctors looked around the table trying to find someone who could help. Often schedules were impossibly full.

"Well, they need an answer by the end of the month," Dr. Cooke would say. "We'd better pray."

They'd bow their heads during the meeting, and they'd pray about it other times during the month. At the last minute before the deadline, Don Gast would come running in with news about a doctor coming home imminently from the field or a new doctor wanting to come.

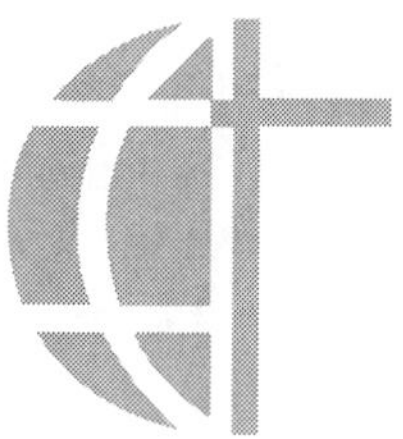

Chapter 5

One Who Came with a Smile

Chapter 5

One Who Came with a Smile

For many who knew him, Dr. Robert S. Schindler's booming bass voice, "I'm here, let's move!" and his infectious laugh still seem to echo in the back halls of the former Berrien General Hospital.

In the larger realm Dr. Schindler's influence on Liberian medicine and also on American and international professional physicians remains evident years after his death in August 2002. He lived large for Christ his Savior.

Bob Schindler attended Wheaton College for three years along with Herb Atkinson, Weldon "Cookie" Cooke, and Don Gast. As a student back in 1954, he joined the CMDA, then the Christian Medical and Dental Society. Transferring to New York University, he earned his medical degree in 1958 from New York Medical College and then returned to the Midwest to intern at Saginaw General Hospital on the east side of Michigan.

In 1962, Dr. Schindler and his wife, Marian, moved to the emerging capitol of Monrovia, Liberia, West Africa, as missionaries with Sudan Interior Mission (SIM). Dr. Schindler opened a clinic in a room at the local carpenter shop and built a lively friendship with the operators of the local Christian radio station, ELWA. Within a year, plans for a hospital were underway. Marian Schindler designed a modern, 35-bed structure that capitalized on the tropical breezes blowing in from the Atlantic Ocean, in view from the hospital. ELWA Hospital opened in 1965. It quickly became one of Liberia's leading hospitals, with Dr. Schindler, as founder and director, the key player.

Kenneth Y. Best, founder of Liberia's first daily newspaper in 1981, and named by the International Press Institute as one of the world's top 60 world press freedom heroes, was a longtime friend of Dr. Schindler. His recollection is:

> *I have known Dr. Schindler for nearly 40 years. We first met in 1965. As a young reporter in the Press and Publications Bureau of then the Department (now Ministry) of Information and Cultural Affairs, I had been assigned to cover the formal opening of the ELWA Hospital in*

Paynesville, near Monrovia, which Dr. Schindler founded. We struck a friendship that lasted a lifetime.

Little did I know at the time that I, too, would soon be under Dr. Schindler's surgical knife. Several months later, I felt a pain in my lower abdomen, and went to see this great physician and surgeon, who had already gained a considerable reputation in the country and around West Africa. After a brief examination, he told me the pain came from a hernia, which had to be removed. A few days later, he performed the surgery, and thanks to the excellent surgeon he was, I have never felt that kind of pain since. Until this day, every doctor who has examined me has said Dr. Schindler did a superb job.

Dr. Schindler… reached out to some who were bruised. He told me that he once gave a lift in his car to his good friend and my uncle, Albert Porte. Mr. Porte was an agitator with the pen, who was always at loggerheads with the powers that were over something he had written. Dr. Schindler told me that a day later, to his surprise, he received a phone call from one of the powerful men in government. The voice said, 'Doctor Schindler, you have to be careful who you invite to ride in your car.'

He asked the caller, 'What do you mean?'

The caller replied, 'Yesterday we spotted Albert Porte in your car.'

Dr. Schindler told me that he straightaway told the caller, 'I give rides to whomever I want in my car.' And that was the end of the conversation. Clearly, Dr. Schindler was not in politics—that is not why he went to Liberia. But he discussed many times with me the glaring injustices he saw in the country, and how he longed for a more just society. But though not a politician, he did his share through the two things he knew best—the spiritual and medical ministries. Even during the civil war, Dr. Schindler returned periodically to lend a helping hand at the hospital, which had received more than its share of the bombing and looting…

Dr. Schindler was the light in darkness in a country that was riddled with ignorance, poverty, and disease, where scarce or misallocated government resources could not match the astounding health needs of the population.

Still learning missionary medicine himself, Dr. Schindler taught nationals everything he knew. From 1966-1967, he worked under Dr. Cooke at Berrien County Hospital and often talked about "helping found the SWMC." He returned to Liberia afterward with new skills and renewed energy.

ELWA Hospital soon gained a reputation as one of the best hospitals in northern Africa. Top government officials and leading citizens in Liberia and beyond sought services with Dr. Schindler. His dedication to the people was not overlooked. On June 26, 1971, in a ceremony at the presidential mansion, Liberian President Tolbert bestowed Dr. Schindler with the country's highest honor: the Knight Great Band, Humane Order of African Redemption. "It was the last official act of President Tolbert," Dr. Schindler explained in an article in the Niles Star. "He died in July following surgery in a London hospital."

Just before Christmas 1971, the Schindlers were in the U.S. when they received a trans-Atlantic phone call that sent them quickly packing. Incoming Liberian President William R. Tolbert, Jr. had invited them to his inauguration. Other distinguished Americans at the inauguration included Mrs. Richard Nixon and the Reverend Billy Graham. Rev. Graham visited the Schindlers at ELWA at that time as well.

By 1974, the hospital had grown to 45 beds. It was the favored hospital in the region and attracted many patients of fame and notoriety. No matter the patient or the prognosis, Dr. Schindler did his best to help him or her.

One difficult case that Dr. Schindler was unable to share with his SWMC colleagues was documented years later in a book by CIA expert Ted Gup. In the middle of the night on November 23, 1974, a CIA agent was clubbed over the head during a break-in at his house. Though disoriented, he did not immediately lose consciousness, so he did not go to the hospital that night.

By morning, his wife and friends insisted he seek medical treatment. They went to ELWA. Dr. Schindler diagnosed a subarachnoid hemorrhage, a deep brain bleed. It was serious. The CIA readied a plane to transfer the agent to a hospital in Germany, but without first reducing the swelling in his brain, he would certainly not survive the flight. This sort of injury was beyond Dr. Schindler's expertise.

Gup explained, "The closest neurosurgeon was in Abidjan, hundreds of miles away. The hospital, while the best the region had to offer, did not even have a single working telephone." Nevertheless, it was necessary to try to save the man's life.

Via short-wave, a neurosurgeon at Bethesda Hospital in Maryland talked Dr. Schindler through the delicate surgery. Gup wrote:

> *The radio link was open and families in [the CIA community] clustered early that morning around radio sets on their porches, listening as a doctor an ocean away gave surgical instructions on how to operate on the agent's brain. They sat in rapt silence, six and eight to a group, their ears to the over-and-out radio. The conversation detailed Dr. Schindler's struggle to save him. The bleeding was deep in the base of the brain. Things were not going well. "I am losing him, I am losing him," they heard Dr. Schindler say. Then there was a prolonged silence. "He is gone," said Dr. Schindler.*

People sometimes asked Dr. Schindler how he found the willpower to go on, day after day, month after month, the only doctor at the hospital. He had a ready answer. "When I feel tired, I ask myself, 'Did Christ die for this person?' and the answer has always been 'yes.' That gives me the strength to do my best."

Dr. Schindler built the hospital on miracles. Each piece of equipment was provided in a special way. Many patients who arrived with poor prognoses left healed. The stories of ELWA Hospital inspired SWMC colleagues, and their stories inspired him as well. As Liberia descended into political chaos in 1975, Dr. Schindler left Liberia after 13 years as director of ELWA Hospital, never to return full time. He made SWMC his new mission and naturally accepted leadership roles.

In his 1977 Christmas letter, Dr. Cooke wrote about Dr. Schindler's indispensability:

> *We made Bob Chief of Surgery this year (just to let him down easy after the weighty position as Chief of Staff last year). He seems to be bearing up under the change. He spent the summer back at ELWA Hospital in Liberia with his family and returned looking tanned and relaxed. We're glad to have him back on the OR crew.*

Dr. Schindler had a skeleton in his closet. He hung the skeleton in the diminutive closet behind the library door in the 1936 building. The skeleton was useful in referencing bone structure, but it also came out on other, unexpected occasions. Dr. Schindler once said there are "four things you need to be a part of this group: flexibility, flexibility, flexibility, and a sense of humor!"

Dr. Schindler's gregarious nature made him an informal spokesman for SWMC. During an interview with Herald-Palladium reporter Ginger Hanchey, he described the clinic this way:

> *[SWMC] is the only functioning multispecialty clinic in the United States and around the world that has such a program… [SWMC] really was the vision of the founder, Weldon Cooke. Dr. Cooke, father of the local ophthalmologist David Cooke, had this dream of running Berrien General Hospital, having college friends of his going overseas as missionaries and hiring them when they came back.*

Ginger Hanchey further summarized:

> *The idea of the clinic is to provide a place for physicians serving in missions to return to, whether short-term or on a more permanent basis, where they can see patients, update their skills and have the opportunity to advance their training. The clinic also supplies a means of support for those serving in the missions. They have career missionaries who they consider a part of their group.*

"When missionaries return to the states 'for whatever reason,' we make space for them. We don't consider if we need someone," Dr. Schindler explained. When doctors return from mission work, the other doctors give them an office and divide the workload with them, giving their missionary physicians a home base.

Schindler recalled working with five other physicians in his early days at SWMC. "Now we have 45 to 50 physicians, plus 15 allied health personnel. We've gone from a Mom and Pop operation to a sophisticated operation," he said.

He said this within a few years after the clinic had incorporated. While he was overseas, the clinic moved out of the ER and began to open branch clinics, or satellites. In 1975, when he returned for a third time from ELWA, he helped open offices in Bridgman and Berrien Center.

Good-natured and professionally respected, Dr. Schindler found leadership opportunities everywhere. He served as president of the International Christian Medical and Dental Association (ICMDA, 1998), as well as national president of the Christian Medical and Dental Association (CMDA, 1985-1987). From 1983-1988 Dr. Schindler was a member of CMDA's Board of Trustees. He and wife Marian launched and administrated the CMDA's Commission on International Medical Educational Affairs (COIMEA, ca. 1987-2000). In 1996, CMDA presented Dr. Schindler with its Servant of Christ Award, an annual honor bestowed upon one physician across the U.S. He served locally on the board of directors of Lakeland Regional Health System and the Berrien County Cancer Service. In 1995 he was one of 17 physicians in Michigan to receive a community service award by the state medical society.

With these and numerous other accomplishments, Dr. Schindler said that his highest privilege in life was serving the Lord. Relationships with patients, colleagues, and others gave him opportunities to share Christ. He also had a great singing voice. He had sung with a Word of Life quartet during graduate school in New York and from then on sang at many occasions, including SWMC Christmas parties.

Past director of finances Carol Gonnerman Jewell remembered one of the most wrenching events for which Dr. Schindler was asked to sing. The only child of a local pastor was murdered during a robbery at a grocery store, and Dr. Schindler was asked to sing at the funeral. When he was practicing, Dr. Schindler told Carol he could not get through the song. His son, John, was about the same age as the boy. He was concerned he would not be able to sing properly at the service. That day he stood and sang from the heart, "Because He Lives, I Can Face Tomorrow." Every eye was damp in the congregation, but Dr. Schindler's voice did not falter.

Dr. Schindler even sang at no fewer than two events after his death. Here is how he did it: One day by request, still in his scrubs, he drove to his church sanctuary and sang "How Great Thou Art," and one of the church sound technicians recorded it.

The recording was played years later on August 30, 2002, at his own funeral. Later, when Ginny Stover's husband Jim passed away, Ginny remembered that Jim had requested Dr. Schindler should sing at his funeral. Ginny called Marian and asked if she could use the tape for Jim's funeral, and it was kindly arranged.

Dr. Schindler once made a comment about SWMC that sums up the serendipitous success of the clinic from initial Wheaton dreams through the many decades. The comment also could be said about Dr. Schindler himself. He said, "We could never have designed, never planned this kind of thing, could never have foreseen the impact around the world."

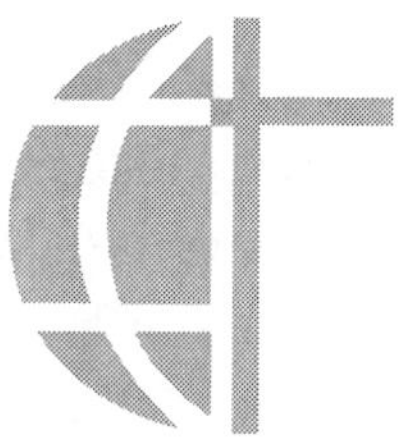

Chapter 6

Train or Stay in Berrien Center

Chapter 6

Train or Stay in Berrien Center

Dr. Charles Rhodes came to study under Dr. Cooke in 1969, just in time to hear about the clinic's name change from Berrien Medical Clinic to Southwestern Medical Clinic. He knew at the time that he was going to be part of something special.

Home from Ippy Hospital in Central African Republic, where he'd been the only acting surgeon since 1964, he was in the states for a year doing a residency under Dr. Cooke. Dr. Cooke served as preceptor so Dr. Rhodes could qualify to pass his boards in surgery and become a fellow of the American College of Surgeons. Dr. Rhodes had learned about the ministry of Dr. Cooke through Dr. Roland Stephens, who had graduated from the University of Michigan a few years before Dr. Rhodes. Dr. Rhodes had also known Dr. Harold Mason as they served together in Central African Republic. Dr. Mason was leaving Berrien General Hospital the year the Rhodeses came.

Berrien General Hospital made a practice of treating migrants and the indigent pretty much gratis, without any subsidy from the government. By billing for their surgeries at the hospital, and taking low salaries, they were able nearly to cover what they were doing for people who today would be on Medicaid.

On weekends the doctor on call covered the hospital, handling the ER, deliveries, emergency surgery, internal medicine, and pediatrics – anything coming through the door. "Basically, it was excellent training for the mission field," Dr. Rhodes recalled. "That's why the training program was so well received and so sought-after by missionary physicians. Not only could we come get experience under men like Dr. Cooke and Dr. Wesche, but another thing Dr. Cooke insisted on was that we get further training to update our medical knowledge. He insisted we make time to take courses. He always had one specialist or another come out to the hospital, orthopods, urologists, and other specialties – so that Berrien General became a teaching institution."

Dr. Schindler's skeleton often came out of the closet. While teaching spinal blocks and such, or if someone had a question about anatomy or bone structure, the skeleton dutifully illustrated.

Dr. Cooke's radically instructional environment spawned several SWMC doctors' future careers. One specifically seemed God-ordained. Dr. Richard Roach left SWMC to become an associate professor at a Michigan State University extension in Kalamazoo. For a while Dr. Roach formed and edited a magazine called The Scan, designed to help missionary doctors learn the latest developments in medicine. He'd scan medical literature, medical journals, and compile his findings in concise, easy-to-understand monthly issues. Dr. Rhodes eagerly subscribed and subsequently credited Dr. Roach's magazine with helping him introduce some of the latest medicines, technology, and procedures to Ippy Hospital. One of those procedures was a new, 10-minute test to diagnose tuberculosis without the need for an x-ray. This one piece of information transformed the way Dr. Rhodes and his bush staff diagnosed TB.

Dr. Schindler took a short course in laparoscopic cholecystectomy and demonstrated it, the first doctor to introduce that technique in southwestern Michigan. Dr. John Spriegel, at Tenwek Hospital in Kenya when not at SWMC, availed himself to Dr. Rhodes any time. Dr. Wesche also taught Dr. Rhodes techniques. The SWMC physicians generously shared their knowledge with all in decades when, culturally, doctors of different specialties did not associate with each other.

They'd take things they learned at SWMC and apply them in difficult situations on the mission field. Dr. Al Snyder taught his SWMC colleagues what he knew about the emergency use of blood. He shared how to scoop leaked blood from body cavities, sterilize it, and pour it back into a vein through a filter.

Back then, blood was hard to come by, but they didn't have to worry about HIV. Dr. Rhodes joked that Ippy had a walking blood bank: All Ippy staff and missionaries were typed. When necessary, a staff member with the right blood type sat and donated the needed blood, and when used, it was still warm from the donor.

Knowing Dr. Snyder's technique helped Dr. Rhodes save many lives. One time the wife of a deacon was brought to Dr. Rhodes in shock, with a ruptured ectopic pregnancy. She was quickly bleeding out. Dr. Rhodes couldn't spend any time to look for somebody with the same blood type. It happened to be his own blood type, so he lay down and gave a pint of his blood before he operated. He also scooped her blood out of her abdomen and reused it as well.

"We got involved in more ways than one," Dr. Rhodes joked.

By 1977, according to Dr. Cooke's Christmas letter, Ippy Hospital was crammed, above capacity by 50 percent, in part due to a measles epidemic. The staggering workload at least partly pushed new medical policies; allowing, first, African nationals to be trained and, second, dispensaries to be built that could be run by nationals.

Dr. Rhodes had heard all about the Atkinson family being forced out of war-torn Congo. The same thing happened in Central African Republic in 1996. In Dr. Rhodes' absence, the native midwives and nurses kept the hospitals running. Several years later missionary doctors could return short-term for a month to teach techniques. Dr. Rhodes was encouraged to see the continuation of the nationals' training, but he said, "It's hard to get people to go out there into the fourth world. It's not like Kenya, I'll tell ya. We weren't quite at the end of the world, but you could see it from there."

Dr. Rhodes further said:

SWMC is unique. In those days, SWMC was the only one in the country of its kind...Southwestern was an ideal situation to come home to. We were able to buy our first home during one of those furloughs. It worked out very well for us. When I retired from the mission field, I continued on in a migrant clinic and other things SWMC provided. Christ came to the world and He was a light, and the light shined in the darkness, and the darkness didn't overcome it. I think Southwestern has been a light shining in the darkness.

Dr. Rhodes helped open the offices in Stevensville, Berrien Springs, and Bridgman. Each time SWMC expanded, it raised the funds beforehand so there would be no going into debt. Dr. Rhodes said, "The Lord has really blessed. Yes, we've stubbed our toes along the way, but God has blessed Southwestern with almost a worldwide impact."

Dr. Rhodes listed a few of the things he's aware that God has done in Africa directly or indirectly because of SWMC:

At the peak in the Central African Republic, Ippy Hospital and six satellite dispensaries flourished in the wilderness and initiated upward of 600 churches. These churches, in turn, opened a Bible school. Now, completely independent of missionaries since 1996, the nationals have established another new Bible school. One of the dispensaries is becoming a hospital, with 25 new babies delivered monthly.

"That's the fruit of our labor, to see others follow on, and they have had the same vision to train others and multiply the evangelistic and medical outreach. It's thrilling to see how God is working," Dr. Rhodes said.

Southwestern had a significant impact financially, by providing for big needs, medically with supplies, and spiritually with countless hours of prayer over the decades. Southwestern doctors also impacted by sharing knowledge, vision, and encouragement.

One of SWMC's written goals was duplication. Across Africa, a surgical training program is even now forming, approved by the American College of Surgeons. Several hospitals staffed by SWMC physicians are spearheading the effort, including Tenwek Hospital in Kenya, a hospital in Togo, one in Nigeria, and another in Cameroon. Part of the inspiration for this on-Africa training was that Dr. Mason sent a man to the states for medical school with the expectation that the man would return home to be in charge of the ministry. The man married an American woman and stayed in the U.S.

Training at a somewhat less formal level has been happening at SWMC-staffed hospitals in Africa for several decades. Dr. Wesche was an early educator at Tenwek in the late 1960s. Dr. Spriegel has established a family practice residency at Tenwek. Dr. Rick Bardin is training Cameroonians in internal medicine. Southwestern continues to have influence on the medical training of Africans, and this spills over into evangelism, establishing churches, and setting up clinics.

Southwestern has also shared its wealth of experience and knowledge with other physicians hoping to set up similar multispecialty missions-minded clinics. Don Gast was involved in helping a clinic open on the U.S. west coast. They came to SWMC to see SWMC's model firsthand. Other Christian physicians have learned SWMC's way of doing things and transferred the model in various ways across the U.S. It all started with Southwestern, and Dr. Rhodes is forever grateful to have been part of it.

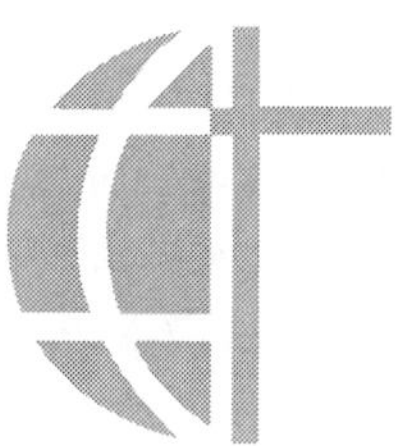

Chapter 7

Early Ecuador

Chapter 7

Early Ecuador

Dr. William Douce took the long road to Saraguro and an even longer road to SWMC.

When Bill Douce graduated from high school in rural Ohio, he had no idea what he wanted to do. At the time, he worked on his dad's farm and immersed himself in the New Testament. One day, sent to the back pasture to get the horses, he took respite on a tree stump to pray. God told him in an almost audible voice, "I want you to be a missionary, a medical missionary. A doctor."

Bill hadn't planned to go to college and didn't know anyone who was a doctor. About his father's reaction Bill said, "There was no one more surprised. He said if that was what I wanted to do, he would help some if he could, but the war had started and he knew that I would soon be drafted."

In the Army, Bill served as a surgical technician. He drove an ambulance, assisted in some surgeries, and gained experience he knew he would use later. When he arrived back home, he went to Asbury College, where he met Ilene. They married, full of hopes and dreams for the future, but Bill couldn't get into medical school. This bewildered him because he was certain of his calling. His pastor advised, "If you're going out to cut wood, the best time you can spend first is sharpening your axe."

Bill got a job as a lab technician, and this experience proved invaluable later in Saraguro. Eventually, he did get into medical school and graduated. Dr. Eugene Erny of Oriental Mission Society (OMS) contacted young Dr. Douce about opening an urban medical clinic in Guayaquil, Ecuador. The Douces began the arduous process. They learned Spanish in Costa Rica. Dr. Douce took courses, wrote a thesis, and completed examinations in Spanish to obtain an Ecuadorian medical license. They raised funds and prayer support.

During the Douces' deputation, the world was rocked by the news of the five missionaries killed by the Auca Indians in Ecuador. Suddenly everyone was talking about the need for rural missions in Ecuador. OMS's plans began to morph. OMS surveyed the Saraguros, who had no doctor and had never been evangelized by Protestants. The Douces agreed to open the first rural clinic in that area.

In 1957, they arrived in the mountain village of Saraguro (population fewer than 4,000) and lived above their little clinic. Ilene had studied Christian education, and had no plans to do any sort of nursing, even after marrying Bill and preparing for the mission field. But she quickly saw her husband's need for an assistant. Necessity motivated her to learn by his side.

As Protestant missionaries in a remote village populated by superstitious Incas and tribal Catholics, they were hated, mistrusted, and once nearly thrown out of town by rioters. They often wondered if they would be alive in the morning. Yet they saw more patients weekly in their little remote clinic than most of his medical school classmates saw in a month. As the only physician in the area, Dr. Douce was on 24-hour call, seven days a week.

A boy, Luis Antonio Vacacela, used to hang around the clinic, and Dr. Douce befriended him. Dr. Douce could see the boy was intelligent. He encouraged Luis and helped him become one of the first Saraguros to graduate from the medical school in Cuenca. After graduating, Dr. Luis Vacacela returned to Saraguro to serve as a dentist to his hometown.

Meanwhile, in the mid-1960s, Mr. Hal L. Kime and his wife, Nancy, taught in the American School in Guayaquil. During their vacation time they came to help in Dr. Douce's clinic for three months. They were a big help to the Douces, and they enjoyed it. After the Kimes finished their two-year teaching contract, Hal applied to medical school in the U.S. and got in.

In 1969, just out of his internship, Dr. Kime came to SWMC looking for further training. He stayed with SWMC for several years until 1972, when he and Nancy left to serve in Saraguro while the Douces were on furlough. Working alone in an isolated mountainous region, Dr. Kime considered the training he had received under Dr. Cooke invaluable. "I always felt SWMC was God's place for us from the first day we were there," Dr. Kime wrote. "I used hundreds or more times the extra training I got there."

When the Douces returned, the Kimes stayed four more years in Saraguro, and even after that returned for many short-term stays. The Douces credit Dr. Kime for introducing them to SWMC. Upon his recommendation, they came to SWMC in 1973.

Twice, Dr. Kime returned to SWMC when on furlough. During his furlough in 1979, he moved closer to his childhood roots in the western U.S. Dr. Kime still goes back to clinics in Cuenca and the hospital in Shell.

Dr. Bill Douce remembers one special thing from his initial interview at Berrien Center. His father, who drove with him from Ohio, was a pretty good judge of character. He said Dr. Silvernale looked like an honest man.

The Douces' original motive in going to SWMC was that it was a place to plug in temporarily in order to stay updated on medicine. It was also a place to work while home on furlough. At the outset, they never dreamed their ties to SWMC would be lifelong.

From 1973 to 1992, Dr. Bill Douce worked intermittently at SWMC while on furloughs from Ecuador. He'd spend four or five years in Ecuador, then one year on furlough at SWMC. There were "always new faces" every time he returned to SWMC, Dr. Douce recalled. The clinic "kept growing. It felt like another mission. It was a joy." At SWMC, he witnessed to patients the same as he did in Ecuador — a practice encouraged by SWMC.

SWMC gave the Douces finances and time off to attend conferences. SWMC also assisted in keeping up licensure and malpractice insurance. It also provided invaluable career boosts by offering job shadowing of physicians in other specialties and on-the-job training and updating.

One staple of the clinic was the Berrien Center Bible Meetings, held weekly for about an hour. Nearly half the doctors on staff regularly attended the meetings; some attended irregularly as they could or felt led to. Typically, about 15 doctors attended per week.

Doctors took turns around the table giving a devotional message or testimony. Discussion was always lively, both about the devotional and about any interpersonal or other issues. The meetings harmonized and united the staff. Often, at these or other specially held meetings, a doctor would be asked to give a report about a mission field from which he'd recently returned. Dr. Douce always found reports about Tenwek Hospital in Kenya interesting. SWMC encouraged physicians to visit each other on the field. The Douces visited Haiti.

It was acceptable, and considered a compliment, to borrow ideas from each other. One idea Dr. Douce "borrowed" was a sign that Dr. Wesche hung at Tenwek Hospital that read, "A doctor treats; Jesus heals." The Douces hung a sign on their Saraguro clinic that read, "A doctor treats; God heals."

SWMC doctors practiced a maverick concept in which physicians from various specialties could share ideas, expertise, and experience with each other and even shadow one another to learn. For whatever reason, especially several decades ago but to some extent even now, physicians of different specialties generally felt competitive or mistrustful of each other, and fail to appreciate each other's various points of view. Discussions, quick telephone calls for on-the-job advice, and especially joining a medical practice together were unheard of in the 1970s. Yet SWMC strongly encouraged the camaraderie. Dr. Douce said this invaluable habit spread from SWMC doctors to South America, and he believes this is now common in mission settings around the world, at least in part due to SWMC's influence.

Another invaluable philosophy at SWMC, according to Dr. Douce, was that even permanent SWMC doctors were encouraged to work on the mission field short-term. He said it gives U.S. physicians a global concept of medicine and helps them appreciate and understand the philosophy that sustains the clinic. Physicians naturally grow more supportive of missions after spending even short-term time out in the field.

Another bonding tradition at SWMC was the get-togethers, including annual Christmas dinners. One year someone asked if Dr. Douce would sing a hymn in Spanish. He agreed if Dr. Bill Wilkinson would sing along. Then, providing further musical entertainment, Dr. Douce played his flute. Dr. Schindler's bushy eyebrows shot up and his wide smile came out. He said he'd known Dr. Douce for years and never knew he played the flute.

The get-togethers were invaluable in building personal rapport among physicians. This rapport led to them helping each other beyond the professional setting in many personal ways, as they each jockeyed mission field work and returned to SWMC for furlough.

When the Douces would learn they were coming home on furlough, they'd contact Don Gast, and he would plug them in somewhere.

Don provided leadership and helped even with seemingly mundane things far beyond what the administrator of a typical clinic would provide in such a situation. Don opened the basement under the pediatric clinic in Berrien Springs to store the Douce's belongings. Don also encouraged the Douces to buy a home in 1979, while they were still full time missionaries in Ecuador. Whenever the Douces left the states to return to Ecuador, Ilene said, "Don arranged renters for the house…The mortgage was paid for by renters Don helped us get. Some renters were other SWMC doctors" coming home on furlough for a year while the Douces were away in Ecuador, including the Joneses, Ringenbergs, and Bakers. By 1993, when the Douces came home to "retire," their mortgage was completely paid.

This first "retirement" was not by choice. Over the years, OMS's enthusiasm about the tiny clinic in Saraguro waned. Like the prophet Isaiah experienced, troubles seemed to shadow the Douces in Ecuador. While their SWMC colleagues in Africa and Haiti reported exponential spiritual growth, with thriving clinics sometimes growing into hospitals and little churches popping up all over the wilderness, for decades the Douces saw little result from all of their evangelism efforts.

The Saraguro community did grow to appreciate Dr. Douce. On March 10, 1993, as part of the town's Independence Day ceremonies, Dr. Douce was presented with a special award acknowledging his 36 years of service to their community. Dignitaries, including the governor of the province, congratulated him on his work. Around that same time, Dr. Douce and Ilene were interviewed on videotape in their apartment above the shop for a "Men For Missions" documentary.

Just two months later, in May 1993, their sponsoring organization sent them home, and they came to SWMC with their heads spinning. Discouraged and feeling he had no option, Dr. Douce prepared to retire from Ecuador.

Don Gast found Dr. Douce a job with the health department, working at the Benton Harbor High School health clinic for about 10 years. The Douces did leave one or two summer months open in order to hold portable clinics in Ecuador. All that time, Saraguro did not forget the Douces.

In 2003 OMS reconsidered, and Dr. Douce was asked to go back to Ecuador full time. He returned to the same clinic and eventually began to see growth. The clinic moved into a larger building and trained nationals to assist in the clinic. A church formed and erected a building in town. Dr. Luis Vacacela became president of an indigenous church association — the Christian Association of Saraguro Indians.

In 2009, Dr. Douce again retired from SWMC. He and Ilene still fly to Ecuador for about one month each year to conduct mobile health clinics, staffed by short-term medical missionaries deep in the mountains. Often scores of people come to the Lord in addition to hundreds getting treated medically. At age 85, he led a medical caravan two hours upriver into the tropical wilderness with his son, Phil Douce, who runs a ministry to Ecuadorian street kids.

The clinic in Saraguro is now run by an Ecuadorian national pastor, Miguel Guaman, who started a local foundation and purchased the clinic from OMS. Miguel has been instrumental in organizing local doctors, both Protestant and Catholic, and has started an alcohol rehabilitation center.

Dr. Bill and Ilene Douce's home base is their little house that Don Gast helped them get. They live in SWMC country, and they continue to pray for SWMC and their missionary physician friends around the world. Looking to SWMC's future, Dr. Douce predicts that if the clinic "keeps the Lord first, it will keep on growing."

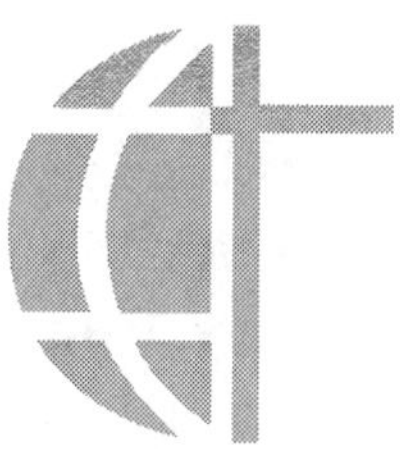

Chapter 8

Haiti

Chapter 8

Haiti

In 1957 when Dr. Bill and Ilene Douce saw their future in Saraguro, tucked under the shadow of the Andes, for the first time, Dr. Norbert "Andy" Anderson took a week in Haiti. He attended the inauguration of Haiti's new president Francois Duvalier (later nicknamed "Papa Doc"). The officials thought Dr. Anderson was a reporter, so they showed him to a seat up in the inaugural chambers. A University of Michigan graduate, Dr. Anderson had heard President Duvalier had attended U of M for a year.

When Dr. Anderson shook the hand of the new President, he commented about the university, and President Duvalier enthusiastically responded: "Ah, University of Michigan, Artes, Scientia, Veritas!" (the school motto, which means Arts, Knowledge, Truth).

Three years later, President Duvalier gave Dr. Anderson a presidential citation for his work in Haitian medical health. Because of the infamy surrounding "Papa Doc," Dr. Anderson didn't dare display the citation for 20 years.

Dr. Anderson was not the first young pre-SWMC American missionary doctor in the poor island nation. Dr. John Edling and his wife, Priscilla, a nurse, and their young family had been in Haiti since 1952. Dr. Edling's grandmother was a missionary to the Armenians in Turkey, and he was born in the African country of Angola. His parents were missionaries: his mother a nurse, and his father a minister. He grew up a missionary kid. Therefore, as an adult, he moved to Haiti with his eyes wide open, experienced beyond his years. Dr. Edling devoted each day of the week tending to medical and spiritual needs and alternating between three medical clinics operated by the American Wesleyan Mission.

One of those clinics was on the remote island of La Gonave, accessible only by outboard motor across a deadly channel. Home to some 50,000 people and one of the poorest regions in Haiti, La Gonave had just the one clinic staffed part-time by Dr. Edling. The coral island did not have a beach or dock, and there were no roads, no vehicles, nothing but foot trails and donkey paths wandering through the brush.

In 1955, the need for motorized transport for the clinic became evident. The first vehicle, a one-ton flatbed truck with sides, slipped into the ocean while they were trying to get it onto land. Forever burned into Dr. Edling's memory is the image of that truck, "onshore afterward, totally unsalvageable, sitting there like a skeleton, a monstrosity on the shore."

Finally, a Jeep was successfully delivered to the clinic. However, that did not immediately quicken transportation. To get around the island "you had to build your own roadway… foot by foot you built whatever you wanted," Dr. Edling recalled.

In the spring of 1958, Dr. Anderson returned to Haiti as La Gonave's first full time doctor. Almost immediately, he formulated plans for a hospital. One sunny day Dr. Edling sat on a concrete block with Dr. Anderson and said, "What do you want the hospital to look like?"

Dr. Anderson got some paper and began sketching. A design developed, loosely based on the beloved old University of Michigan hospital. He drew two Ys, with the operating room between the butts of the Ys. The legs of the Ys were long, wide hallways, letting tropical winds circle through. Though never formally trained in contracting or roofing, Dr. Anderson built Wesleyan Hospital with the help of Mr. Ed Harrington of Holland, Michigan, who stayed on La Gonave short-term with his young family. After Ed Harrington built the structure, he returned to Michigan.

Never having done a bit of plumbing before, Dr. Anderson took the task into his own hands with a length of pipe and a big wrench. Today, the plumbing still works, although some might complain it's a bit crooked. Dr. Anderson also laid all the electrical wiring, hooked up a diesel generator, and found and installed a used x-ray machine, building darkroom tanks for it.

In 1960 or 1961, an AT-6 airplane crashed in front of the hospital. The U.S. had provided about 50 of these old basic trainers for Port au Prince's military airport, and the pilots there were trained to fly in them. A couple of hotshot lieutenants dared each other to land on a tide flat just below the hospital. One pilot came in too low, nicked his tail wheel on some trees and landed upside-down. Dr. Anderson put a Band-Aid above his eye. The military chopped what was left of the airplane up in little pieces to haul it off.

Another time, while the government was working on a geographic survey, a helicopter had a failure just above the hospital on the mountain. During engine failure, a servo helicopter rotates upside-down. Four men in military uniforms walked to the hospital, no injuries, casual as can be, and said, "Hello, we just crashed up there."

Dr. Anderson considered those just two of many miracles he witnessed on La Gonave. He and his family – and the Edlings, too – experienced miracles in the treacherous 15-mile crossing to the mainland, where fine weather can switch to horrible seas within minutes.

As far as medicine was concerned, God was planning more big work in Haiti. Dr. E. Dewain Silvernale graduated in the class of 1960 from the University of Michigan. He worked with Dr. Anderson at Wesleyan Hospital on La Gonave as a senior medical student, went back and finished the year at the U of M, and returned to Haiti, where he personally delivered both Anderson boys. This time, Dr. Silvernale stayed in Haiti, where he felt God calling him into politics. He became head of the Haitian health department. Responsible for health needs all across Haiti, he spent less and less time on La Gonave.

Dr. Anderson received the monthly newsletter of the Christian Medical Society, although it arrived at a snail's pace at La Gonave. In the early 1960s, he read Dr. Cooke's small advertisement. In corresponding with Dr. Cooke, he was assured he could learn a lot about surgeries, an exciting prospect. Dr. Roland Stephens was an exception at Berrien County Hospital, having done a full surgery residency in Chattanooga before he went to Africa. Most other physicians who responded to Dr. Cooke's ad were looking for experience in surgery and were glad to receive it.

Dr. Anderson arrived at Berrien County Hospital on July 1, 1962, as a preceptor for one year under Dr. Cooke. Dr. Cooke became a personal friend and was helpful professionally throughout the years in other ways, but during that year at Berrien County Hospital, he kept Dr. Anderson busy outside the operating room. A baby boom hit central Berrien County. Dr. Anderson delivered more than 250 babies, many to migrants. Though he didn't mind too much, it was a far cry from what he came for.

While Dr. Anderson spent his year with Dr. Cooke, he attended an American Medical Association meeting in Chicago. He met Dr. Marilyn Hunter. "You're going to be a missionary," Dr. Anderson said.

"No, that's the one thing I refuse to be," she shot back. He bought her a cup of coffee. She spent at least 15 years at Wesleyan Hospital, La Gonave, and also worked at SWMC.

Dr. Anderson planned to return to Haiti after his year with Dr. Cooke was up, but a violent revolution locked the country tight. He went north instead, to Michigan's Upper Peninsula, still planning to return to La Gonave. In 1964, when his year in the UP was finished, some medical problems were developing in the Anderson family. Dr. Anderson decided to start a psychiatry residency.

Dr. Anderson kept track of various University of Michigan medical school graduates. One was Dr. Roland Stephens. The Stephens family had lived next door to the Andersons while they were interning in Lansing. One cold winter day, when little Dan Stephens was about six or seven years old, he bundled up a little too industriously. He zipped part of his chin into his coat. Kathy Stephens ran next door to Dr. Anderson. While Dan howled with pain, Dr. Anderson was able to unzip the skin.

Dr. Anderson was never able to return to La Gonave full time. He did serve on short-term trips, and in 2008 was honored as a dignitary at Wesleyan Hospital's 50th anniversary. The little town of grass-roofed huts had grown into a city of 30,000 people. Expanding with it, the hospital continued to do well.

In Dr. Anderson's absence, Dr. Edling carried on. He kept the Jeep in running order, repaired the water system, tinkered with the electrical wiring, and, naturally, doctored the 50,000 people on the island.

Meanwhile, at the University of Michigan, Dr. Chuck Pierson was interested in international medicine. However, being still in medical school, he had no money. In January 1968, a round-trip ticket to Port au Prince from the U.S. was $99. He wrote to Dr. Silvernale and Dr. Edling, and they invited him to visit them in Haiti and see international medicine first-hand.

On the second Sunday of January 1968, Dr. Pierson found himself at a Haitian revival service. That night Reverend Robert Lytle, assistant director of Wesleyan World Missions, spoke in English. The message was translated into Creole, so there was a pause between sentences for Dr. Pierson to think. Dr. Pierson had warmed a pew for 25 years in a liberal church without ever understanding the way to salvation. He had heard Billy Graham on television. Finally that night in Haiti, he gave his life to the Lord Jesus Christ.

Thus, Dr. Pierson's spiritual birthplace was Haiti. He felt at home there. His short-term trip to Haiti had changed his life. The Lord would bring him back later to change the lives of Haitians.

When Dr. Edling was in California on furlough in 1969, Dr. Anderson wrote him a letter. He suggested Dr. Edling get in touch with Dr. Cooke. Dr. Edling's furlough stretched into a nearly 10-year hiatus from Haiti while his children, Gary and Nancy, went through school. In the autumn of 1969, they stopped in Berrien Center to meet and possibly link up with SWMC. Dr. Cooke had written letters describing several possible open positions at the clinic. Dr. Edling planned to take one of those positions. The Edling family stayed several nights in Berrien Center.

Subsequently, they lived in their camper one month that fall while Gary and Nancy attended Berrien Springs Public Schools, but the house they wanted was pulled out from under them. After continuing to look around and feeling oddly out of place, they moved on to New York state, to a tuberculosis sanatorium in Mt. Morris.

During his 1955-1956 furlough, Dr. Edling had worked at a different sanatorium in Syracuse. He had profited from learning there and profited again at Mt. Morris. Not much was being done for TB patients when Dr. Edling first went to Haiti. These patients were dying in the countryside, and he felt called to do something for them.

In addition to principles of diagnosing and treating TB, at Mt. Morris Dr. Edling learned an important technique that was not used widely throughout the states because x-ray methods replaced it. It was a form of auscultatory percussion, which proved very successful in Haiti.

In 1971, the Edlings did come back to Berrien Center. This time it was the Lord's will that they stay. They remained seven years. Dr. Edling learned more about TB treatment from Dr. Wesche, who had worked on TB cases in Kenya. Dr. Wesche took care of the TB patients when he was home at Berrien General Hospital, and Dr. Edling worked in geriatrics and other long-term cases at the extended care facility connected to the hospital. Dr. Wesche turned over his TB cases to Dr. Edling when he had to be absent for a while.

Under these two men, the TB treatment program at Berrien General received statewide attention. The TB treatment program was heralded in a 1973 issue of Health, a publication produced by the Michigan Tuberculosis and Respiratory Disease Association.

Dr. Edling became director of the extended care facility, which included the long-term TB patients. He has been compared to Dr. Roy Ringenberg, taking forever to do rounds because he sat and talked with people at their bedside. His attentiveness to his patients became legendary, and the extended care facility grew to have a waiting list. Dr. Cooke wrote glowing words about Dr. Edling in his Christmas letter 1977:

John continues his full time work with the hospital's Extended Care Facility, as well as medical director of several nursing homes. Recently, it was reported to the hospital board that the percentage of ECF [extended care facility] patients who have been able to return home and care for some of their own needs has increased to 50 percent, up from 25 percent when John first came, which makes us doubly aware of the tremendous job he is doing. John provides coverage for furloughing missionaries in Haiti whenever possible; this year he spent December and January (1978) on La Gonave.

Dr. Cooke visited La Gonave five times, taking one son each trip, to help with surgery. Dr. Edling's daughter Nancy traveled along as Dr. Cooke's interpreter. Dr. Cooke pulled her into the OR to assist in surgery, taking pulse and blood pressure. She said he was so gifted as a teacher that she fell right into step and felt part of the surgical team.

By this time Dr. Silvernale had become legendary in Haiti. Largely because of Dr. Silvernale, Haiti, the poorest Caribbean nation, completed a TB vaccination project and treated TB and other illnesses ahead of wealthier nearby countries.

Dr. Silvernale started with SWMC in 1969, served as chief of staff for a while, and did his flight training at the Andrews College airport in Berrien Springs. He bought a little airplane during the Haitian TB vaccination project of the early 1970s. He was flying to these remote, little, rutted, grassy airstrips, and Dr. Anderson flew with him sometimes. One day Dr. Silvernale spotted what looked like a soccer field and attempted a landing. They bounced at least 10 feet in the air when they touched down. The plane survived, completely intact. They never told their wives.

Dr. Cooke included an update about the Silvernales in his 1977 Christmas letter:

Beryle and Dewain sent word that they are enjoying another Haitian Christmas, with sunshine and flowers 'while some of you are shoveling snow'! They have been busy with the massive TB immunization program, and have vaccinated 520,000 people with BCG. They are active in the rapidly-growing English church in Port-au-Prince. Dewain is still a medical officer for Berrien County, so he comes back quarterly and we are able to see him occasionally." [Handwritten notation: "He was at our last corporation meeting.]

Dr. Silvernale worked part-time with SWMC and part-time as director of the Berrien County public health department in the 1970s, when not in Haiti. In December 1978, Dr. Edling returned full time to La Gonave for 10 more years. Dr. Silvernale took Dr. Edling's former position as director of the extended care facility at Berrien General Hospital.

After nearly 50 years in Haiti, Dr. Silvernale retired. He died April 20, 2007. Dr. Edling and Priscilla retired to Florida. They cashed in their own life insurance policy and generously gave it to the people of Haiti. Then they decided to move into a modest trailer park populated by Haitian immigrants. They ministered to their neighbors until they were physically no longer able to do so. Unknowingly, they had moved only a few miles down the road from one of Dr. Cooke's sons, Dr. John Cooke, who had been a senior in Berrien Springs High School when Nancy was a junior.

Looking back, talking in his quiet, gravelly voice, Dr. Edling considers the lives of the SWMC doctors themselves, such as Dr. Schindler, Dr. Atkinson, Dr. Wesche and Dr. Roland Stephens, as the greatest evidence of God's miraculous work at SWMC. He is amazed at their Christian influence in their hospitals and communities abroad. Naturally, in his humility, he does not include himself in that list, but, without a doubt, his name belongs there, too.

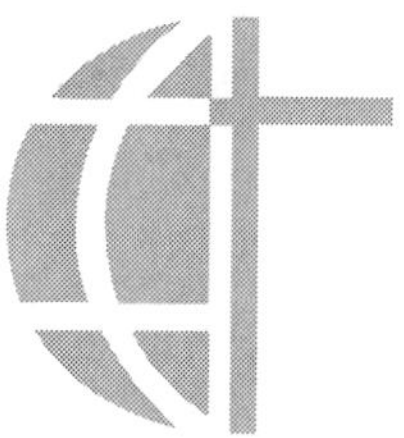

Chapter 9

The Early Seventies: Finances and Growth

Chapter 9

The Early Seventies: Finances and Growth

Though God blessed SWMC in many ways, He did not deliver abundant riches. Instead, He provided many faith-growing opportunities. In several white-knuckled financial situations, Dr. Bob Wesche displayed unwavering faith, and his memorable example encouraged his peers. Dr. Herb Atkinson talked about one meeting ca. 1973-1974 when Dr. Wesche was home from Tenwek Hospital in Kenya:

> *"One time we all got up for a night meeting, everybody tired and irritable, trying to find a penny...We just couldn't make the payroll. We didn't have the money; we were quite a bit short. Dear old Dr. Wesche, he just said, 'We're going to stop sweating it. We're just going to pray.' So we got down on our knees and prayed. Ever since then, we've made payroll."*

Like Dr. Bob Patton and others, Dr. Chuck Rhodes recalled another legendary meeting when – faced with yet another shortfall – the clinic's financial adviser strongly suggested reducing the 10 percent tithe to missions. After letting the adviser fully explain his reasoning, Dr. Wesche piped up and said, "Well, sir, if we can't stay afloat tithing 10 percent, why don't we up it to 15?"

Clearly floored, the financial adviser looked around the boardroom table at a crowd of steady faces. They didn't actually raise the tithe, but they certainly did not lower it. "The way the Lord met our financial need is an outstanding demonstration of his provision over us," Dr. Rhodes reflected. "At that time I wasn't on the finance board. All I know is, the monies came in. I suppose we got more surgery... orthopedic things, and were able to get the income from the surgeries...We never did stop our missions giving...ever."

Meetings featuring near-crisis financial discussions were normal. As the clinic grew, its finances did not improve, despite diligent efforts by highly qualified financial officers. Dr. Schindler often referred to the genius and stupidity of combining missions work and a for-profit business. Those who joined the clinic came with their eyes open. They knew they would face the struggles and blessings of the dueling duality: missions and business.

One of the first tests of each physician's commitment to SWMC's duality was the very real sacrifice of income. Dr. Robert Patton put it this way:

> *"I heard some people around the table say, 'I'm happy to come here and take a financial sacrifice of a thousand dollars a year to be able to do that' (referring to their missions giving). I kind of laughed to myself. A thousand dollars a year? It was more like 20 or 30 thousand dollars a year loss to come here (due to much smaller salaries than elsewhere). Nobody...came for financial success. In each case, it was the opposite. Interestingly, in the long run, (as missionaries) financially we ended up probably coming out ahead in the sense that we've received quarterly support now for almost 25 years. Add four thousand a year times almost 25 and you see I've received about 95 thousand dollars just from SWMC's quarterly gift alone. Plus, there was all the support from former SWMC colleagues, who give above and beyond SWMC's tithe. Think about it that way and God's blessings really add up."*

Another test of commitment to SWMC, at least for Dr. Wesche, was postponing overseas work to fill a dire need in the states. Dr. Wesche, a key surgeon and leader, was getting ready to go back overseas at a time when SWMC and the hospital were already short-staffed and struggling. Dr. Wesche believed God was calling him back to Africa, but his SWMC colleagues argued that God told them he would remain at Berrien General. "I think we shamed him into staying," Dr. Helene Johnson joked. "God is on everyone's side!"

Despite sacrificial salaries, potential career detours, and the clinic's financial woes, Dr. Cooke set up an unprecedented bonus system for all clinic staff and employees, according to financial secretary Virginia Stover. Quarterly, he spread around productivity bonuses to the doctors, giving the assistant as much money as the surgeon. At the end of the year, bonus gifts were divided among everyone, physicians and employees. Also, early on, Dr. Cooke set up pension profit-sharing and a 401(k) plan.

Dr. Cooke was very considerate of physicians returning from the field. Beyond just updating them on the latest surgical techniques and medical advances, he always made a place for missionary doctors to come back to work while home, and made sure they got their continuing education. He also thought of their families' welfare. While doctors were overseas and obviously not bringing revenue into the clinic, the clinic sent them $500 every quarter. Additionally, while doctors served overseas for typically a four-year cycle, Dr. Cooke instructed Virginia Stover to put $500 per quarter into a fund. When the doctors came back to Southwestern, they would have $8,000 in escrow to purchase a vehicle or make a down payment on a home, or however else they wanted to use it.

Generosity, trust, and equality spread beyond finances to the sharing of power. At corporate meetings, before SWMC grew into the need for a formal board of directors, every doctor had an equal vote. Also, during voluntary weekly prayer meetings, as noted earlier, doctors took turns leading devotions and prayer times for each other, patients, and the clinic. Everyone was important.

The voluntary Monday morning prayer meetings reflected their very real faith. Dr. John H. Edling said that while Pastor Schoen of Berrien Center Bible Church and other local pastors visited the hospital, mostly it was SWMC doctors who took care of the spiritual needs in the hospital. Dr. Roland Stephens, Dr. Wesche, and Dr. Atkinson were especially effective, according to Dr. Edling. These men spiritually inspired the staff and all the patients at Berrien General. Making rounds in their bow ties and soft-soled shoes, they visited patients in long-term wards and all through the hospital. They won many souls to the Lord.

Other doctors who joined SWMC and made rounds at Berrien General in these years included: Dr. James L. Wierman (1965, 1968-1969, 1973-78); Dr. Almarose Cooke Worden who returned 1969-1970; Dr. Robert A. Chapman (1966-1967); Dr. Cesar B. Cabascango (1969); Dr. Joseph H. Schoonmaker (1969-1970); Dr. E. Dewain Silvernale who joined in1969 and returned from Haiti many times over the decades; Dr. Eunice Wilson (dates not available); Dr. David Drake (1970-1972); Dr. Roland G. "Ron" Snearly (1971-1972); Dr. Richard A. "Hirsch" Hirschler (1970-1971, 1975-1977, and 2008); and Dr. John H. Edling (1971-1978).

Dr. Helene Olson (later Johnson), Dr. Janet Frey, and Don Gast all came in 1972. The end of 1972 saw Drs. Drake and Snearly leave. Dr. Kenley F.

Burkhart came around that time (ca. 1972-1978), as well as Dr. John Hanson (1972-1973) who became a career missionary in Asia. Dr. Wierman returned in 1973 for several more years. Dr. William F. "Bill" Douce (1973-2009) came, as well as Dr. Connie L. Landrum (1973), who didn't stay long before relocating to an Air Force base in Oklahoma, where she became the head of the ER. More doctors discovered SWMC. They crowded into BGH's narrow halls, stuffing more little secondhand desks into overcrowded offices and closets, hiring extra support staff to handle the increasing paperwork. Working out of the ER was busy and hectic. They talked of having their own space.

On Valentine's Day 1973, an article ran in the Journal Era regarding SWMC's request to lease land at Berrien General for an office. In part, the article read:

> *Richard Goodman, BGH administrator, said Thursday the Southwestern Medical Clinic – a private corporation – has asked the board to lease land beside the hospital...The corporation, headed by Dr. Weldon J. Cooke, presently leases space at the hospital for examining rooms and offices, and runs the ER during the daytime, Goodman said. 'They've always wanted a building here on the grounds...and if they can tie it right on the end of the hospital, they'll do it,' Goodman said. 'They've requested this plan for several years now, but nothing has seemed to transpire on it.' The proposition raises legal questions about leasing county-owned land and private ownership of property on county-owned land...*

Dr. Cooke ordered architectural plans drawn up and enthusiastically shared them during a special SWMC staff dinner at a riverfront restaurant in Benton Harbor. Much celebration followed. However, the drawings were never used.

Instead, Don Gast learned of a physician in downtown Berrien Springs who was leaving the area. Don went over and talked with Dr. Lutz, and they reached an agreement. It was a superlative deal. Instead of paying through the nose for new construction somewhere, and having all that hubbub to contend with for several months, they got an established practice in a finished building, and they could move right in.

By July 20, Drs. Silvernale, Atkinson, Wesche, Burkhart, Edling, and Cooke shared the office at 200 North Cass Street in Berrien Springs as an "extension" of their offices at the hospital and in addition to their duties in covering the ER. The Journal Era reported:

> *"The SWMC will provide regular office and emergency coverage from 9-5 Mon-Fri. After-hour emergencies will be rendered by the same physicians in the ER at BGH. This multispecialty group provides services in general surgery, OB, internal medicine, and pediatrics, combined with the family concept of medical practice."*

In addition to acquiring Dr. Lutz' office and his patients, SWMC also kept Dr. Lutz' assistants – medical assistant Bonnie Howe and receptionist Lou Bergey. Lou later recalled that part of the agreement between Dr. Lutz and Don Gast was that SWMC would retain the two. Lou said, "Before the clinic took us over, Dr. Lutz gave us 50-cent raises and told the clinic I was making $2.75 an hour rather than $2.25."

Initially uncertain about joining the clinic, Lou and Bonnie quickly grew to love Don and the physicians. Don even once loaned Lou $75 out of his own pocket for a washing machine.

They worked hard to ease the transition for the patients and for the doctors. Eventually Drs. Atkinson, Burkhart, Olson, and Wierman hung out their shingles and fell into regular hours at the Cass Street office. Lou was given the opportunity to learn Medicaid billing alongside Lela Harper, who did the coding. Lou also took a terminology course to learn coding. She soon learned that if she had a question on surgical procedure, she could ask the doctors anything.

"Did you do a biopsy also?" she could ask, and they'd be more than happy to take the time to explain.

This kind of teamwork, adding up the nickels, kept SWMC solvent during extra-tight months after its big purchase. The first satellite office proved successful. The clinic adapted the philosophy of locating near the patients, not vice versa.

Meanwhile, Berrien General Hospital needed to renovate and expand. At the end of the February 14, 1973 article, Goodman reported that architects had proposed a $3.5 million building program for the hospital, but the board members scrapped the plans because they "only had $300,000 to correct deficiencies cited by the state health department."

Working out of a new satellite office, in addition to facing health department deficiencies requiring immediate renovation, SWMC doctors and staff had never felt more stress. It took its toll in different ways. For Dr. Helene Olson (later Johnson), working obstetrics in less-than-optimal facilities as well as "regular doctoring" out of the ER and the Cass Street office contributed to serious personal health issues. Dr. Cooke was credited for saving her life at least once.

Dr. Olson practiced timeliness. "If patients were 15 minutes late, she wouldn't see them. She'd have the receptionist reschedule," Lou recalled. "Dr. Cooke, on the other hand, enjoyed feeling admired and needed. He was amused by having a roomful of patients waiting until 8 p.m."

Harried, some doctors didn't take time to speak to staff when they came rushing through. "They didn't last as long as the others," Bonnie Howe pointed out. She remembered Dr. Burt Sutherland as tall, dark, handsome, and very personable. He always spoke when he went through. Dr. C. Albert "Al" Snyder (1975-1998) had dry humor. He'd tell a joke and 10 minutes later, you'd figure it out and laugh. If Dr. Cooke didn't speak, it was because he had half a sandwich crammed in his mouth while running down the hall.

Dr. Cooke faced physical and mental exhaustion. He juggled managing the new satellite as well as his duties as acting hospital administrator. But he was also hospital medical director, chief of staff, president of SWMC, and even a third-term board member for the Berrien Springs Public Schools. In December 1973, Dr. Wesche succeeded Dr. Cooke as chief of staff. It wasn't as if Dr. Wesche had extra time to kill to devote to his new role. Dr. Wesche also served as director of the hospital's TB treatment program, as well as its poison control center (the first and only such facility in Berrien County).

At the BGH staff Christmas party that year, Dr. Wesche and his wife, Dora, were honored. Among others, Dr. Cooke received a 15-year pin and Mrs. Sandra Bruce, business office manager, received a five-year award pin. The event took place in the gymnasium of the county juvenile home across the parking lot from the hospital. As acting administrator, Dr. Weldon Cooke stated that Berrien General had the highest occupancy of any hospital in the county.

In late fall of 1974, Berrien General promoted business office manager Sandra Bruce to administrator, relieving a huge workload from Dr. Cooke. Sandra Bruce's mantra, "Progress," revealed itself in new equipment, remodeling, and construction of a direly needed new OB/surgical wing.

When this was completed in spring of 1975, the 1936 building was relegated to administrative and laboratory uses. An April 23, 1975 article in The Journal Era describes the 11,390-square-foot, $1.1 million addition as coming "in the wake of state mandates for upgrading the former facility." Berrien County Commission building and grounds committee chairman Otto Grau emphasized, "Through the use of revenue-sharing moneys, this fine and necessary addition…is paid for and no additional taxes are needed."

On April 24, the first child was born there, delivered by Drs. Atkinson and Olson. Of the addition, 7,169 square feet comprised the OB facility, with 10 patient beds, two labor rooms, two delivery rooms, three nurseries, and a fathers' lounge. When Bonnie Howe had her son there, Dr. Cooke helped with delivery after having been up three days straight. Dr. Olson also assisted in the delivery, though she had a 102-degree fever.

While the expansion cleared more room in the 1936 building for the clinic, it still didn't feel like home. Vocal resentment still railed against the clinic for having "unfair" access to patients through the ER and much-reduced overhead.

Finally, in 1975, a solution was found. The county had outgrown its juvenile center and planned to build a new one. It sold the old building to the hospital. Now the hospital offered to lease the building to SWMC for 10 years, with the agreement that the clinic would remodel the facility to meet its needs at its own expense.

Don Gast put his experience working in his father's Baroda hardware store to use. Acting as general contractor, he oversaw the renovation of the former juvenile center into Southwestern Medical Clinic's first independent facility. September 8 was moving day. They shuttled their clinic practice out of the hospital ER and most of their support staff out of the 1936 building.

Dubbed "Location One," and later "Location 10," their new office was within easy running distance across the parking lot from Berrien General Hospital. The front interior of the building was rearranged to create an east wing and a west wing, with enough rooms to allow four physicians to work simultaneously – two on the east wing and two on the west. The back halls contained support staff offices. Yet, they still did not stop dreaming. In his Christmas letter, Dr. Cooke wrote:

> *"So for all you skeptics who thought that SWMC would never build, at least we have gone this far. We are not strictly hospital-based*

any longer, but we are still close to the hospital…Several of us have speculated that we may own a building within five years. Perhaps we'll construct a building adjacent to the hospital and move back to a hospital-based type of practice; however, that is still a dream for the future."

Due to the move, Don Gast gained a beautiful office suite featuring a high wall of square windows facing north into the woods. Ginny Stover also acquired an office as well as a promotion to the clinic's first financial secretary. And, as Dr. Cooke wrote, "she continues to perform mathematical feats to keep us solvent."

Pat Caporale learned to use a switchboard for the clinic's new private telephone line. Lela Harper, the clinic's coding clerk, "changed medical procedures into dollar amounts for billing." Bev Stover "transmitted the voluminous clinic transactions from the office to the even more voluminous computer," which, though cutting-edge for its time, took up its own room in the back hall of "Location One".

The clinic's billing department included Ernestine "Sarge" Wilkes, in charge of insurance billing; Arlene Perry in Medicare billing; and co-op and college students handling Medicaid. Rose Hand, Pam Furman, Ruth Ann Stover, Theresa Porter, Donna Woods, and Lou Bergey also helped in the offices. The skeleton in the closet moved to "Location One" as well, and he showed up in various places. One day he sat behind the desk of SWMC credit manager Russell Bruce (Sandra's husband).

The physicians' secretary, Ruthie Leer, who replaced Karen Allred after she moved away, and "Captain" Jean Kistler, R.N., who ran the eye clinic, remained in the hospital as SWMC staff.

By the first snowfall of 1975, SWMC patients could choose from three office locations: the Ferry Street Office, "Location One" across from the hospital, or a tiny new Bridgman office above Dr. Smith's dental office. SWMC was the first clinic in Berrien County that expanded from one site to multisites, with satellites.

The clinic was finally physically independent of the hospital. The team had much to celebrate. Their habits of organizing picnics, birthday parties, luncheon meetings, and other special occasions increased. These events strengthened ties among staff of various locations. One time, they decided they wanted SWMC T-shirts. Ever adept at cost-cutting and creating opportunities for big laughs and great memories, they screened the shirts themselves in someone's basement. A few of those shirts might yet survive, but more importantly, the memories and the tight relationships continue to thrive. These memories and relationships compelled Southwestern to persevere through the tough times ahead.

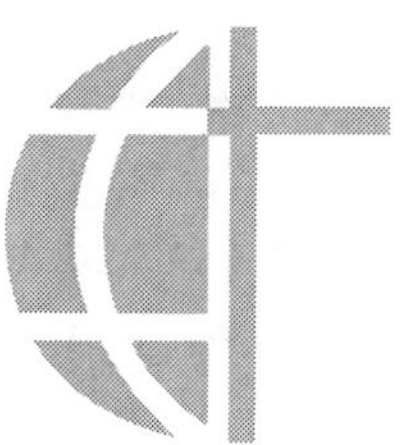

Chapter 10

The Birth Place

Chapter 10

The Birth Place

The story of Dr. Helene Olson Johnson's conversion is almost apocryphal. Everyone who was there wants to take a small part of the credit for it. The funny thing is, Dr. Johnson credits The Apostle John's epistle for her conversion, and God Himself, and says most everyone else just bugged her about it.

Well, of course they would. How a clinic staffed by Protestant, missions-minded physicians even took her on board is a mystery to begin with. She claims she heard long afterward that the only person who voted to take her into the group was Dr. Cooke, who had aggressively recruited her in an hour of dire need.

She didn't know what a Christian was. She didn't understand the group's vision. She answered an ad in a throwaway journal that said the group did some mission work, which from her liberal background sounded like a good thing, though she had no idea what it actually meant. SWMC ended up being her only interview anywhere.

Dr. Cooke rarely traveled to recruit, and he didn't call it recruiting. It seems he was in California anyway, having eye surgery, and it just worked out for him and his wife, Fran, to look up this young, unmarried doctor interning in the Army. They rode the trolley and ate supper at the wharf. When the bill came, Dr. Cooke tried to pay for their dinner with an out-of-state check, which the restaurant refused. He never carried much cash. So, the broke little intern had to pay the bill.

Regardless, Dr. Helene Olson agreed to spend three summer months in Berrien County, helping with seasonal migrant clinics before backpacking around Europe. It was something to do.

The Jewish lady from Berkeley and San Francisco stuck out garishly among the Christian conservatives in the sticks. She brought her one suitcase to Berrien Springs, worked with the migrants, and kept a wary eye on these weird Christians working alongside her. At the end of the summer, she went to Europe, but within a few months she grew cold and ran out of money.

Despite reservations, the clinic invited her to return and formally join. Despite her own reservations, she accepted, and she toted her one suitcase back to Berrien Springs. She spent two weeks in the labor room in the OB, and that's where Dr. Olson's legendary obstetrics career started.

She also worked the ER from Friday evenings to Monday mornings. Whatever case came in, she took. She didn't have a lot of practical experience, having just gotten out of school. She installed her first pace-maker using the directions on the package insert. Southwestern Medical Clinic, at that time, was heavily populated by surgeons, so by default she became the internist. She started their ICU and received some equipment she'd used in San Francisco.

Meanwhile, these mission doctors and their wives all had a burning desire to introduce this Jewess to the Messiah. They might have been a little clumsy at it. Dr. Atkinson pressed literature about Jews converting to Christianity into her hands. Later, he'd ask if she'd read it. "Yep," she'd say. Conversation closed.

For two or three years, Dr. Atkinson gave her literature, pursued conversations with her about Christ, prayed. Seeing absolutely no progress, and perhaps reading her growing annoyance, he told the Lord she had a hard head. He gave it a rest for a while.

Dr. Olson scrutinized the doctors with whom she worked. She considered Dr. Schindler special, the greatest influence on her as an example of what you'd want to be as a Christian. She even married a lab tech at Berrien General Hospital, a solid, quiet Christian man who did not badger her or confront her about the Lord.

When she was ill in bed, which happened a number of times, Frieda Atkinson visited her faithfully and talked about nothing but the Lord. Such persistence became almost offensive. Dr. Bob and Liz Patton also took on the task of winning her soul. They witnessed to her tenaciously and invited her to evangelistic meetings, and she went to them unfazed.

One time Liz asked her, "Helene, if I could show you from the Bible unquestionably that Jesus Christ was the Messiah of the Jews, would you declare your faith in Him?"

Dr. Johnson hesitated, saying she was not sure. Then Liz said, "Helene, your hesitation, then, is not intellectual, but a decision of the will."

While well-meaning, these tactics did not succeed to in converting Dr. Johnson. The actual event had to do with a nurse who worked with

Dr. Johnson. The nurse became pregnant with her first child, and Dr. Johnson took care of her. According to Dr. Johnson, a lot of things happened during labor and delivery. She did everything technically correct, but the baby came out severely brain damaged. She felt it had been preventable and couldn't fathom how it had happened. The situation weighed very heavily on her.

Within a few months, the burden was too much to bear. Dr. Johnson considered that someone larger than the doctors has to be in charge of life, death, and everything in between. Someone else has to be in control because she wasn't. She no longer wanted to believe that humans alone were responsible for everything.

She pulled out a Bible and opened to The Gospel of John. Alone with The Word, she read and became convinced that Jesus was, indeed, the Messiah.

Afterward, she spoke to both Dr. Atkinson and Dr. Bob Patton on the phone. The lesson Dr. Atkinson learned: Just trust the Lord for things that look to be impossible. This was 1979, nearly six years since she had begun working with the clinic. The Pattons invited the Johnsons to a weekly Bible study in their home, and according to Dr. Atkinson, "She just ate it up. Next thing we knew, she put a wing on a Bible plane."

Dr. Olson had no local family, so she spent a great deal of time in the hospital. She struck up a working friendship with one of the on-call lab techs, a man named Mark Johnson. When there were tests that required repeating in an hour or so, they played cards and spent time in conversation. Also, in those early years, from 1972 to 1975, she had a number of illnesses, and he was the best blood drawer around.

In addition, while he was a committed believer, he never bothered her about religion, just accepted her as she was. For him, it seemed a nonissue.

On a Friday afternoon, September 8, 1975, Dr. Olson and Mark took their next-door neighbors and 20 dollars to the courthouse and got married. They did not tell anyone of their plans, but the neighbor who stood up with them worked in the clinic and later surprised them by organizing a party. When the foursome went out to dinner afterward, half the clinic was there. It just so happened that the judge who married them went out to dinner with her husband at the same place. Dr. Olson and Mark Johnson were the first from the group to marry. Their son Eric was born in 1976 and Corey in 1978, both in Berrien General attended by Dr. Johnson's nurse practitioner, Betsy Zech, and Dr. Weldon Cooke.

Southwestern already had five surgeons when Dr. Helene Johnson née Olson arrived, so they put her in charge of internal medicine. She didn't really like internal medicine. She looked around and saw another need, and an idea began formulating.

As the county hospital, Berrien General delivered the children of folks who didn't have insurance or were on Medicaid. They saw a healthy number of deliveries but had no OB practitioner. She attended a conference, came back, and set up a prenatal clinic. But SWMC still saw her as its internist.

Then Dr. James Wierman, an actual internist, arrived. Another internist came after Dr. Wierman. SWMC moved Dr. Olson into pediatrics, but then as the clinic swelled, more pediatricians came. Finally, she got to work in OB.

During her training, she'd seen an epidural, so she began offering them. For at least five years, she was the only doctor in Berrien County doing epidurals, and even after that she was the only one who would give an epidural to a Medicaid patient. Berrien General experienced a booming baby business.

She introduced Lamaze as well, and Berrien General became known around the area as the place to come to have natural childbirth. Additionally, Berrien General was the first in the state to allow fathers into the OR during a birth. The University of Michigan took credit as the first in the state, but that was several years after Dr. Johnson and her staff had been allowing such a practice. When asked why she allowed it, she explained that it was mainly because she hadn't had formal OB training, and she "didn't know fathers weren't supposed to be in the room." The local newspapers wrote articles about fathers, siblings, and other family and friends allowed in the room during childbirth. Due to this, young married couples flocked to Berrien General Hospital.

"Back in the '70s, we just did what worked," Dr. Johnson says.

In addition, the hospital became a local legend for its kind treatment of every mother including the poor, nonresident migrants, or women of any variety of assorted backgrounds. It has been said that some migrant families planned their pregnancies so they could deliver at Berrien General during whatever fruit crop they came to Michigan to harvest.

Eventually, Berrien General was doing more deliveries than much larger hospitals in the area. Between 1970 and 1980, births at Berrien General increased 147%, far surpassing Berrien County's birthrate statistics.

In 1974 the clinic acquired an ultra-modern fetal heart monitor, used at that time only in special situations. In 1975 the hospital built a new OB unit to try to keep up with the demand. Two delivery rooms, three nurseries, 10 patient beds, and a family lounge comprised the happy, busy space.

Another difference came when Besty Zech, Dr. Johnson's right-hand-woman, started full time (in 1973) at Berrien General under the mentorship of head nurse Donna Borst. Betsy had come and gone as a nursing student working summers. As a nurse practitioner, she helped Dr. Johnson implement numerous programs. They worked well as a team. Eventually, Betsy became head nurse in the OB department.

Dr. Johnson and Betsy Zech developed Berrien County's first Family Birthing Program. The new program encouraged siblings and other family members to visit the new infant and made additional provisions for the father to participate in labor and delivery. In a Journal Era article on May 1, 1979, Dr. Johnson reassured the community that there would be no increased risk of infection due to a family member's presence. The South Bend Tribune followed up with a circa April 1980 article describing, at the program's infancy, fathers' attire in the delivery room: gown, mask, shoe covers.

Far ahead of the progress curve, the OB department installed infant intensive care equipment including one instrument that had the ability to do an ultrasound. These investments were worth the expense. In 1979 alone, Dr. Johnson and her team delivered 836 babies at Berrien General Hospital. Dr. Johnson and Betsy also did about 150 home births. They became too busy in the hospital to go to people's homes. This struggle prompted the "Birthing Room" concept. Lamaze classes had been offered in the community for several years. On March 29, 1984, the first Lamaze class was held at the hospital. In June 1984, the hospital unveiled its new BirthPlace, an addition to the OB wing, featuring a birthing suite named The Apartment, a birthing room, and an exam room. Dr. Johnson even handcrafted a cradle for the facility.

The BirthPlace generated a lot of excitement in Berrien County. All the newspapers within a 30-mile radius lavishly covered the opening of the facility, the first of its kind in southwestern Michigan. Much larger hospitals, such as St. Joseph Hospital in Mishawaka, Indiana and Borgess Medical Center in Kalamazoo — as much as an hour drive away for many southwestern Michigan residents — could not even boast of such modernized birthing options. Berrien General Hospital president Sandra

Bruce and Dr. Johnson, named Chief of Obstetrics Services at the hospital, had a lot to talk about. BirthPlace cost just under $150,000 to construct and covered only 1,417 square feet, but it changed the outlook of the hospital for several more decades.

Around that same time, Betsy Zech unveiled a "Get Acquainted" program, which opened the doors even wider for hospital-gown-wearing brothers, sisters and grandparents to touch and hold their new baby. In that era, it was not uncommon in other hospitals for mothers to have exclusive, but still surprisingly limited, hands-on rights aside from the hospital doctors and nurses. Infants spent a lot of time in the nursery, and families could view them only from behind glass.

Not so for Dr. Johnson. By 1989, families were removing their sterile gowns. Visitors only needed to wash their hands. When asked about the new practice, Dr. Johnson said she merely listened to her patients. "The families were so happy with it, that it was all worthwhile, and they proved to us that they weren't going to spread infection," Betsy Zech said.

By the spring of 1985, SWMC announced plans for a new women's clinic, "fulfilling the women's concept." Located in a renovated brick farmhouse on Niles Road near St. Joseph, the women's clinic featured an "attractive homelike setting with specialized services devised for women," according to a March 13, 1985 Herald-Palladium article. When the office opened on January 21, 1986, it was touted as the first health center for women in southwest Michigan. A twin opened in Buchanan two years later — a satellite to a satellite.

In 1986, Dr. Johnson was presented with a community woman of the year award. At that time, she'd delivered more than 10,000 babies — some 500-600 a year. She estimates conservatively that even with changes in medical practice and reimbursement, the closing of Berrien General Hospital, and her 30-minute commute now to Niles to work, she has delivered far more than 13,000 babies in her career.

Because God led her to SWMC and the SWMC doctors took a chance on a Jewish nonbeliever, and because she listened to her calling and pursued obstetrics, Dr. Johnson has delivered more babies than all the other doctors combined in Berrien County.

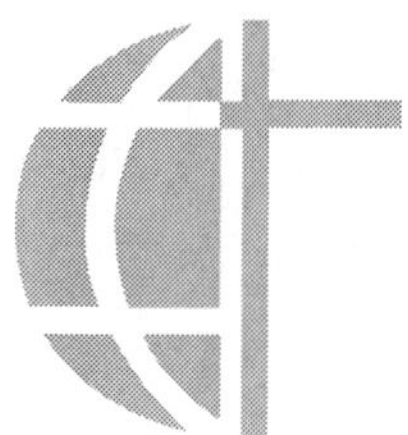

Chapter 11

Christmas and Other Good Times

Chapter 11

Christmas and Other Good Times

Dr. Cooke's annual Christmas letters have become the stuff of legends. He especially wanted these letters to go out to all the doctors on the field, no matter how far away they happened to be, so that they could hear news about their colleagues around the world at Christmastime.

There was one problem, however: Dr. Cooke didn't usually start these letters until December 23. As Christmas Day loomed, he'd feverishly begin scribbling that year's letter, then race off mid-sentence to take care of sudden emergencies. Then the next day, with a sandwich in one hand, he'd find another few minutes and rummage around, searching for his draft. He'd call out, "Ginny, where's that Christmas letter I was working on?"

They'd look everywhere together, eventually find it, and then he'd have to rush off again. Some years, this process stretched out way into the New Year. People began joking that it wasn't a Christmas letter, it was an Easter letter. Dr. Al Snyder, working in Africa where mail could be delayed for months, once said that he wasn't sure if it was a very late Christmas letter, or a very early one.

These beloved letters contained news about current and past SWMC physicians and their families, were often peppered with humor. Dr. Cooke finished the letters by writing about his own family. Before email and Facebook and cell phones, these mimeographed pages kept far-flung missionaries abreast of each other's "latest" news.

In March of 1976, not long after Dr. Cooke's Christmas letter was mailed, one of Olympic champion boxer Muhammad Ali's daughters, Hana, was born at Berrien General Hospital. After Dr. Cooke delivered the baby, the proud father cruised in his little sports car up the long, tree-shaded hospital driveway the wrong way, beaming at the staff.

That same year, Bev Stover's husband, Dick, suddenly became acutely ill. His hemoglobin dropped out of sight, and no one could discover the cause. Dr. Cooke called everyone over to get matched blood for transfusions. One Tuesday night, Bev returned to the hospital from a sporting event and found her husband's hospital bed empty. Frantic, she raced to the nurse's station and learned he had been transferred to the critical care unit.

Learning that Bev was there, Dr. Cooke came out of a meeting where the doctors had been praying for Dick.

When they got Dick's hemoglobin up to five, Dr. Cooke removed the man's spleen. Slowly, he began to return to good health. One day Dr. Cooke gave Dick some freedom and allowed him to go home for lunch. The man returned to the hospital for several more days.

Dr. Cooke and the other founders instilled flexibility. This creative approach to solving problems allowed for trial and error as SWMC grew. "We made a lot of changes in the 70s and early 80s," Don Gast recalled. "A lot of experimentation. We were the first clinic in Berrien County to expand from one clinic site to multiple sites."

Especially at the outset, SWMC considered its satellites experiments. At one time or another, SWMC ran sites in: Dowagiac; Bridgman; Sawyer; Benton Harbor on Pipestone across the street from the health department; Benton Harbor High School; Mercy Hospital's rural clinic, which eventually morphed into InterCare; two different buildings near the Berrien General Hospital; two locations in downtown Berrien Springs; a woman's clinic on Niles Road south of St. Joseph; Stevensville's Cleveland Avenue location; and locations in Niles across from Pawating Hospital and on U.S. 31.

"[In] first setting up the clinics, we'd put a family practice, an OB, surgical, and internal medicine doctor in each site. That way we had the range of doctors in each clinic instead of all OBs in one clinic. The doctors rotated from clinic to clinic so people in each community could see all doctors in their area," Don Gast said.

Lou Ellis said, "The clinic's philosophy was that we go to the patient, not vice versa."

Don further explained, "I always thought the doctors rotating was a good deal for the patient, to see a medical person right in your town. But it made it too inefficient for the clinic, too expensive, and impractical."

Several factors dictated the major paradigm shift to stop the doctors' multisite practices: time on the roads and increasing gasoline costs.

Other issues popped up as doctors rocketed to multiple locations daily. Dr. Schindler got stacks of speeding tickets, Dr. Janet Frey topped out the odometers of a dozen beaters, and there's no telling how many deer Dr. Atkinson hit on Dean's Hill Road while trying to get back to the hospital to deliver babies.

In addition to running numerous satellites, they also staffed mobile migrant clinics and worked with Mercy Clinic Rural Health. They opened a counseling office on Ferry Street and an eye clinic within Berrien General Hospital run by Jean Kistler and Dr. Julia L. Wixted.

Several doctors from the Twin Cities who had their own practices helped out when SWMC needed a specialist. Dr. William Bock — a general, thoracic and vascular surgeon who throughout the years served as Chief of Surgery at both Mercy and Memorial Hospitals and later co-founded the Cedarwood Medical Clinic — came to help on special cases as needed. Also, Dr. John H. Carter, a cardiologist who served as Chief of Staff at Mercy Hospital and implemented the first intensive care units at Mercy and Memorial Hospitals, helped SWMC when a specialist was needed.

Additionally, SWMC experimented by employing on call and short-term specialists. For several summers starting about 1977, a semi-retired physician from California, Dr. Fisher, helped in the migrant clinic, and Dr. Hinn, another doctor from California, came other times.

Doctors who came to SWMC during these years included: Dr. Thomas D. Burns, ca. 1976; Dr. Robert D. Patton, 1976-1986; Dr. Frederick"Rick" Johansen, 1977-present; Dr. Barton Comstock, 1977-present; Dr. Wallace "Wally" A. Donaldson, 1977-1978; Dr. Andrew A. White, 1981-ca. 1983; Dr. John R. Slater, 1981-1998; Dr. Daryl R. and Gina Erickson, ca. 1979-1981; Dr. Richard R. Roach, 1978-1992, and Dr. Gregory Adams, pre-1983-ca.1985.

Where did all these doctors come from? Word of mouth played a large role. When SWMC doctors went to the mission field, they networked with other missionary doctors, such as Dr. Hal Kime's referral of Dr. Bill Douce. SWMC doctors informally recruited while attending professional conferences — which is the way Dr. Janet Frey came.

Drs. Schindler and Atkinson avidly recruited at conferences and everywhere they went, as well as Dr. Wesche. All three traveled widely and "met missionaries all over the country and encouraged them to come to Southwestern," Don said. "Physicians wanted to come back to Southwestern to work alongside Dr. Wesche. His commitment to missions was unusual."

The doctors set up a sort of mission-recruit weekend. Medical school students, through their school's CMDA chapters, learned about these retreats and came to find out more about medical missions. While there to learn about medical missions in general, some remembered SWMC and later joined the clinic.

Don Gast came up with the idea of offering foundation grants to physicians looking to go abroad for residencies. He saw these grants as a natural result of the vision of the clinic. The grants turned out to be another avenue to bring in young, like-minded doctors. Returning from their missions residencies, which were partially paid for through the grant, they'd look up SWMC and "come home."

Don never wanted to let go of a physician who was called to overseas missions. He persuaded many to "come back on furloughs, to automatically come back after their long-term mission. A number of them did come back," he said.

The clinic thrived on the revolving door: new doctors recruited at conferences and numerous far-flung locations, returning missionaries, and specialists and others who came at their convenience. It was unusual in the business world to plug doctors in regardless of their strengths and the clinic's need. Outsiders considered it opposite thinking, rather than searching for a specific specialist to fill an open position. "That's how we grew and added sites," Don explained. "Whenever a doctor came home or arrived for the first time, we'd get a building or add a room or something. We made a place for him or her."

Don also made connections in local high schools to acquire co-op students. Many students were later hired full time and moved up the ranks for the rest of their careers. Judy Koebel Kubsch was one example. She worked as a co-op student in July 1977 in Medical Records in Berrien Center and then became the receptionist at North Cass Street. When the new Family Clinic opened on Ferry Street in Berrien Springs in December 1979, she just moved locations. Promoted throughout the years, she is now Practice Manager Specialist in Niles. Another later example was Sheila Lavallee Kipp.

Bonnie Howe, a medical assistant hired into SWMC when the clinic bought out Dr. Lutz' Berrien Springs practice, served as secretary and president of the Berrien County chapter of the American Association of Medical Assistants. Like all the staff, Bonnie provided comic relief for those straining under heavy loads. Once Bonnie accidentally blew chewing gum into CPR Annie's mouth during a staff training class. After a coding insurance meeting in Grand Rapids one summer day, Bev Stover and Millie Hoadley saw a billboard advertising dune buggy rides. Millie begged Don to stop. Don gave in and pulled off the highway, and all three of them rode the dune buggies.

Some SWMC staff might argue that the dune buggy rides weren't that far removed from a normal day's commute to work. Dr. Wally Donaldson, who worked at SWMC for about a year, had reckless transportation that was actually coveted by some. Dr. Helene Johnson recalls that Dr. Donaldson had bought an old beater to get through the year at SWMC. Not long after he joined around 1977, he had to make a trip into Chicago. He parked downtown, and someone stole his car. Getting himself to a nearby used car lot, he purchased a geriatric taxi for $150. "Ace Taxi Company" was still clearly emblazoned one side. On the other side, covering most of the door was "#6." An early 60s model, the thing had clearly given some wild rides in nearly two decades of service. People could hear it coming for miles. SWMC staff all knew to whom it belonged. As long as Dr. Donaldson was with SWMC, Dr. Cooke tried to deal him out of Ace #6.

In between trips to Madagascar, Dr. Richard Roach was a great storyteller. Dr. Roy Winslow and Dr. Rick Johansen are often called upon to share humorous stories. These are among the avid storytellers who have regaled Christmas partygoers with amusing adaptations of stories and fairy tales.

The doctors and staff planned unforgettable Christmas parties at various locations throughout the years. Everyone got dressed up and brought spouses along. Gast children and other young recruits served Bev Stover's raspberry punch. Entertainment completed a jolly time. One year in the 1990s, the pediatrics group sponsored the Christmas party entertainment. On a stage in the cafeteria at Woodland Shores Baptist Church, they performed a rendition of "'Twas the Night before Christmas." Dr. Bart Comstock narrated. "Every good storyteller needs a throne," he intoned, and he took a seat on a toilet.

"Not a creature was stirring, not even a mouse," he said. A medical student walked across the stage wearing an old, scruffy beaver costume. "Not even a beaver," Dr. Comstock corrected.

"Ma in her kerchief and I in my cap," he continued. Dr. Johansen and Dr. Schultz capered onstage in nightgowns. Marilyn Comstock was one of the kids and Dr. Dick Hines was the other child, dressed in red-and-white-striped nightgowns.

At the appropriate moment, they pulled a plastic Santa Claus and sleigh along a wire strung across the stage. Santa tipped and tottered and nearly brought down the stage.

A handful of years later, Marilyn Hurrle organized "The Little Boys' Choir." She recruited Dr. Chuck Pierson, Dr. Ken O'Neill, Dr. John Spriegel, Dr. Troy Thompson, Dr. Ron Baker, and Dr. Daniel Mitchell. They practiced and clowned around, but Marilyn did not tell the doctors everything she had up her sleeve.

She told them to wear Bermuda shorts and a white, short-sleeved shirt. The night of the party, she passed around knee socks, suspenders, and bow ties. She gave them blackjack gum to black out one of their front teeth. They greased their hair and parted it down the middle. Dr. Pierson had to wear a toupee. When he marched onstage, his shocked wife, Ruth, in the fourth row squealed, "Oh, Chuck looks so young!"

When the laughter quieted, Dr. Schindler paraded onstage. "Every good director needs a coat with tails," Marilyn said. She presented Conductor Schindler a corduroy jacket from which dangled fox and raccoon tails. For a baton, he waved a cheerleader's glittery baton decorated with streamers. Again, everyone laughed. Marilyn had pulled it off. She felt smug.

But then Dr. Schindler announced, "Every good director needs to have the right hair." He ducked down behind the rostrum and fiddled around, and Marilyn knew she was about to be outdone. He popped up wearing a wild white wig with blue and pink stripes. "Just call me Herr Rodman," he chortled, a la basketball celebrity Dennis Rodman.

"I laughed so hard I was crying," Marilyn recalled. Under Herr Rodman's direction — and flying hair — the talented and colorful boys' choir did sing several Christmas songs. It's uncertain how many words the audience heard. Herr Rodman and his boys brought down the house.

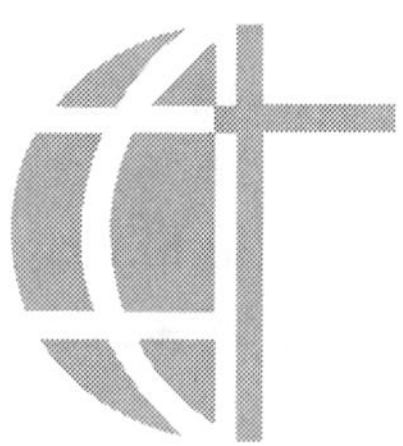

Chapter 12

To and from Ferkessédougou

Chapter 12

To and from Ferkessédougou

Apart from — or including — the good Herr Rodman and the Little Boys' Choir, from the clinic's birth, doctors had practiced in ways similar to mission field work. In the early 1980s, Berrien County and SWMC began seeing the need for specialized medicine. Dr. Kenneth O'Neill was one of the first specialists at SWMC, and Don Gast saw that his focus was to upgrade internal medical care in the local setting. The era of specialization brought many new and exciting changes for SWMC. But these changes did not alter the clinic's primary vision to help missionary physicians succeed on the field and at home.

One great example of an old-school general practice missionary doctor who sensed the needs for greater specialization in Africa, as well as in the states, and who successfully met those needs with the help of SWMC, was Dr. John Slater.

Dr. Slater joined SWMC in 1981 during a furlough. Having been in Africa on and off since 1959, he'd been in the Belgian Congo in 1959 when "everything just blew up" amid the revolutionary war that created the country of Zaire. In fact, Dr. Slater's rescue by the United Nations' Nigerian "blue hats" created a sensation on national television and in Newsweek and Time. God was in charge of that rescue. He prepared another half-century of amazing work for Dr. Slater to complete.

In 1961, less than a year after the Cote D'Ivoire (the Ivory Coast) declared independence from France, Dr. Slater and his brother moved to this western African country, to the "tongue-twisting town of Ferkessédougou." By the next year they re-opened a Baptist mission hospital. With three nurses and approximately 50 trained Africans, Dr. Slater and his brother treated 45,000 patients a year.

In 1965, Dr. Slater pursued a general surgery residency in Detroit's Grace Hospital. Then, armed with practical surgical training and experience, he returned to Ferkessédougou, nicknamed "Ferké." In 1972, he felt the need for further intensive training. He went back to Grace Hospital for an OB/GYN residency. From 1976-1981, he worked again at the Baptist Mission Hospital in Ferke.

Dr. Slater joined SWMC in the late summer of 1981, and worked as an OB/GYN in both the Berrien Center office adjacent to Berrien General Hospital and in the Dowagiac office at 417 West High Street. SWMC's short-lived Dowagiac office was opened on September 17, 1979, by Dr. Daryl Erickson during an early furlough as pioneer surgeon at Oasis Hospital in Abu Dhabi, United Arab Emirates from 1976-1985. Dr. Cooke filled in at the Dowagiac office. When Dr. Slater prepared to return to Ferké in June 1982, he closed the Dowagiac office.

Though he was a quiet-looking man who squinted behind large glasses, Dr. Slater made quite an impression on Dowagiac that year. An avid story-teller, he certainly entertained many with his real-life African adventures. At the time of Dr. Slater's departure for the Cote D'Ivoire, Dowagiac Daily News editor John Eby wrote a lengthy and glowing article.

In the early 1980s, the Cote D'Ivoire progressed comfortably under a stable government led by Felix Houphouet-Boigny, himself a doctor. The former capital city of Abidjan was, John Eby wrote, "a success-story locale that has been favorably compared with Miami Beach and Beverly Hills. Balconies overlook bays, glass towers gleam, and tapering skyscrapers change colors as their tiled facings climb toward the clouds."

"At rush hour in Abidjan, you'd think you were in Paris," Dr. Slater said, adding, "They have ultra-modern skyscrapers. Americans would not believe it."

Many rural areas, while predominantly dotted with shacks, saw the arrival of electricity, good roads, schools, and "every week or so a ceremony to open a new health center or rural clinic," Dr. Slater said.

In the second-largest city in the Cote D'Ivoire, Dr. Slater and his wife, Marion, a nurse, lived in a concrete house near the hospital, equipped not with glass windows but with rain shutters. "We come back to America and have claustrophobia," he said. "We're used to living outdoors."

Included is Dr. Slater's first known letter back to SWMC. As a typical letter sent by a SWMC colleague on foreign mission, it was big news. It was read aloud during weekly prayer meeting and also printed in the clinic's News Briefs, which were distributed to everyone at all the satellites.

Dear Don, Virginia, and all –

Enclosed is a check for $200 to cover the hepatitis vaccine we got from the clinic just before we left. I asked our mission treasurer to pay it, but he preferred that I do it. Sorry for the delay!

Our trip was long and tiring, but the reception by our African staff was marvelous. How we praise the Lord for a greatly improved attitude toward … [illegible].

A T.V. crew from M.A.P. International arrived soon after we did to film a documentary on the hospital. They filmed in Kenya, India, and Ecuador for a M.A.P. T.V. special. I asked Guy Condon to send a program schedule to you. We filmed a C-section the night the crew arrived at Ferkessédougou. I felt all thumbs; the instruments were different from when I left and even more so from the set at Berrien General. I was given a #15 blade for the incision — the size used for fine surgery like plastic surgery. I thought I'd never get through the skin. At least they can make it look decent (I hope!) by editing.

I look back with real pleasure to my time in Berrien Springs at the clinic. Lord willing, I'll be back. Greetings to all!

John Slater's next known letter to SWMC was dated December 19, 1982:

…Our baggage has arrived in generally good shape. I was concerned when the ultrasound case was lying on its side in the shipping container instead of upright as marked. When I readjusted the main voltage switch and plugged it in, my fears were confirmed! We got a grid image and caliper markers, but no picture.

A Wycliffe missionary, Jim Cooper — Wheaton '55 (a master fix-it), offered to look at it. The main fuses (where I checked) were fine, but the fuses on the freeze unit were blown. The Toshiba salesman only showed me one switch to adjust to 220 volts. Apparently he did not know there was another soldered adjustment to be made inside. Fortunately, the machine now works beautifully. Thanks again to those of you who helped make its purchase possible.

I look back with pleasure on my time with you all and a twinge of nostalgia hits me. Lord willing, I hope to return to SWMC in a few years. May the Lord bless you all.

Several years later, in 1987, Dr. Slater wrote a humorous call for help that surely spurred his SWMC colleagues to his aid. John titled this letter, "Lazarus II… The Saga of an X-ray Machine."

1962 – When we reopened the hospital after it had been closed for four years, our x-ray was a leftover Picker military field hospital portable unit used in World War II. It took mediocre x-rays of extremities and if we were fortunate, a weak chest film. But it was better than nothing!

1967—We were ecstatic! From special gifts, a new big Picker x-ray was purchased. Our joy was short-lived. The unit arrived rusty and many of the automatic features never worked. After much correspondence we learned we had to "live" with the machine. It functioned sporadically for a while and was worked on by various technicians over the years. Eventually it died. We resurrected the old portable World War II x-ray unit and called it Lazarus II. It was better than nothing!

1984 – The big Picker x-ray was rebuilt with used components by a French technician. It felt good to have a better means of diagnosing. But the big machine died again. Out came Lazarus II… it was better than nothing!

1986 – March: we missed two fractures and a dislocation in Marion's foot because of a poor x-ray. August: the big Picker machine was again rebuilt, this time with new parts by a talented Liberian technician. December: the big Picker machine died again. We wheeled out our good friend Lazarus II. It was better than nothing!

1987 – Lazarus II is still taking poor x-rays…but it is better than nothing! It is now over 45 years old and ready for retirement. Can you understand our frustration in trying to give good medical care with

Lazarus II as a means of diagnosis?

But here is some exciting news. We have decided to purchase a new x-ray machine through REAP, a Christian organization in California that services medical equipment for mission hospitals. The cost is $16,000. Our field has now approved a special project for the hospital: 'Ferké Hospital X-ray Machine.' We are excited to see how God will provide the funds for this tremendous need. Won't you join us in praying for it to become a reality soon? In need of your prayers, John and Marion Slater.

In February 1989, Dr. Slater returned on another furlough. From 1993-1998 he worked at SWMC until he retired to Florida, where he died on February 3, 2010. His nephew, Dr. Dwight E. Slater, also served for 17 years at the Baptist Mission Hospital in Ferké. The hospital in Ferkessédougou continues its life-saving work, owing much to the tireless efforts of Dr. John Slater. SWMC is blessed to have called him one of their own.

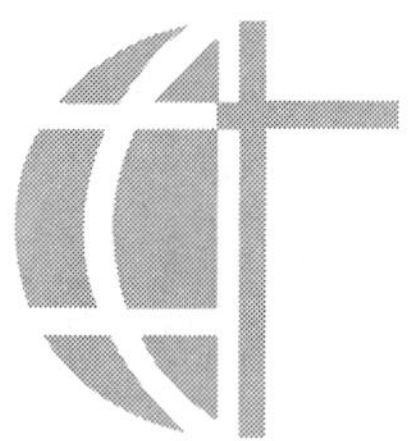

Chapter 13

Stories of Faith's Significance

Chapter 13

Stories of Faith's Significance

Many doctors come and go at SWMC. They spend a number of years abroad and then return stateside to work at SWMC for a year or so before returning to their mission. This has been an ongoing circuit for years.

Unlike most missionary physicians associated with Southwestern, Dr. Robert E. Patton worked at SWMC for a solid 10 years (1976-1986) and then cut ties and turned to the mission field full time in Suriname, South America, never to return to work at Southwestern.

Dr. Bob Patton (no relation to Dr. Charlie Patton) first went overseas in 1971 as a self-described "liberal do-gooder" to set up a department of internal medicine in a new medical school in Liberia. Two doctors witnessed to Dr. Patton and his wife, Liz — Dr. Bob Schindler, while he was in Liberia, and a replacement for him, Dr. Bud Hurst. Dr. Patton didn't listen too hard. He read his Bible "like a good boy" and went to church every week. He says, "Everybody thought we were model Christians, but I had never received the Lord."

In 1974, he was saved in Liberia while reading the Gospel of John. As a fledging servant of Christ, Dr. Patton faced dark, desperate days in Liberia as well as major life decisions.

Liberia's political scene was descending into the chaos of what would erupt into a 30-year war. Meanwhile, Dr. Patton began to realize that the students he had come to help train weren't very interested in his training. He and Liz discussed leaving Liberia. Looking back now, he can ironically say he considers it fortunate that the government had set up a financial deterrent to leaving before the end of the term. He gritted his teeth and made it through the five years, and along the way, he made a lifelong friend whose advice altered the course of his career.

Dr. Schindler and Dr. Patton became friends first on a professional level. Dr. Schindler appreciated Dr. Patton's efforts to bring internal medicine practice to a new level in Liberia at the JFK Medicine Center. The two started a training program. Dr. Schindler also asked Dr. Patton to consult on a number of his patients. Soon the two couples befriended each other and kept in touch even while Dr. Schindler returned to the states for about a year and a half, finishing his training to become board-certified as a surgeon.

Along the way, Dr. Schindler told Dr. Patton about Southwestern. Dr. Patton had planned to stay in academic medicine, which he loved. He recalls, "I had a couple of other solid opportunities...but felt the Lord wanted me to come to Southwestern. It truly was a personal struggle for me to give up my academics...I came to Southwestern because I felt the Lord wanted it, no other reason."

As it turned out, Dr. Patton thinks back that "it was the time at Southwestern there that our spiritual lives got on a firm foundation."

The way Dr. Patton tells the story, God had SWMC in mind for him, not the other way around. But he definitely made his mark at the clinic, both as a founding physician at the Stevensville office in 1980 and as Chief of Medicine at Berrien General Hospital by 1985.

When Dr. Patton arrived at Southwestern, Dr. Wierman was "basically the internist until I came along. A few years later, he went into private practice for himself in Dowagiac." Dr. Patton also opened a satellite office in Sawyer and was one of four who founded the Stevensville office, along with Drs. Rhodes, Schindler, and Atkinson.

As the years progressed Dr. Patton and Liz led a Bible study together, and Liz led a women's Bible study. Liz also took on the task of keeping various Southwestern offices supplied with evangelistic tracts. The couple earned reputations around Southwestern as being ardent soul-winners. Probably because of their own long journeys to faith in Christ, the two witnessed boldly to everyone they encountered...even the new Jewish physician on staff at Southwestern.

Once Dr. Wierman left, Dr. Helene Johnson "basically covered for me in internal medicine while I was gone," Dr. Patton recalls.

Dr. Patton couldn't have been gone too much. In his 1977 Christmas letter, Dr. Cooke wrote:

> *Bob's practice as internist and cardiologist has grown by leaps and bounds. He has taken charge of our ICU, including the setting up of a cardiac monitoring system whereby patients on Ward A can be continuously monitored in IC. Then Bob talked Don Gast into trying it out for us. I guess Don was unimpressed with it, however; he made Bob release him after a week or so. We have enjoyed welcoming the Pattons*

into our Berrien Center Bible Church family as well.

Handwritten note: "The Pattons run a bus service for the Sunday school."

Miraculous Resuscitation Survivor

If Dr. Patton wasn't busy enough working nonstop at Southwestern and leading a Bible study, he and his wife had a bus route for eight years for their church, mainly to pick up and minister to children. One woman, a patient of his at the clinic, agreed to come to church on Easter morning, and the Pattons arranged to pick her up along their bus route. Dr. Patton normally preached on the bus, and the woman came to salvation on the bus.

Dr. Patton recalled: "She was on Medicaid, food stamps, and really was in very difficult financial situation. We began to see her every week on the bus route. We'd visit the kids and adults every week on Saturday and encourage them to come and make a schedule to pick them up the next day. This lady invited us to stop by her house, and she'd make us soup afterward. So my wife and I and our four kids stopped every week for several years and she'd make soup for us. She'd run one 25-watt bulb every night to save electricity. She piled on extra sweaters in the winters to keep costs down.

"One day in church this lady started feeling bad. She normally sat with us or right behind us. I took her down the hall. She would've been in her early to mid-60s. She fell to the floor and had a cardiac arrest. I could not detect a pulse. At this point I was alone in the hall. I did resuscitation.

"...Later in the hospital, there was no evidence of a heart attack or stroke or anything of that sort. We couldn't give a reason, but she had no ill effects from that episode. She's now a 30-year resuscitation survivor."

One day she asked Dr. Patton, "What is this tithing business?"

Sympathetic to her financial situation, Dr. Patton wanted to say, "Tithing's for other people. I think you're exempt." But he explained tithing to her. After that, a check showed up in the plate every week for eight dollars. "Oh, my goodness," he said, "she's tithing."

Some time passed, and one Sunday he saw she had a new microwave. She got excited and told the Pattons, "The government said I paid too much in taxes and they gave me money back!"

A little later she got her house painted. She'd been chosen for a gift.

One week, as the Pattons began raising support to go overseas, a check came in for $1,038 — a personal check from this lady. "From the day we'd talked about going overseas, she'd started putting a little money aside," Dr. Patton recalls, still marveling.

"She then committed to saving $25 a month for our missions funds. Later on, she also took on my daughter for $25 a month. After a while, she also took on my son, who's a missionary in Hungary. When the Rasmussens started, she took them on. Here this lady was putting out $100 per month as an offering. She's on several hundred dollars a month for Medicaid, her only income. This continued to go on for a number of years.

"Finally, she broke her shoulder age 89 and had to go into a nursing home. She apologized, she couldn't give us support anymore.

"Now, this lady has a private room in one of the nicer nursing homes in the area. She has a big-screen TV, a lift chair, a nice hospital bed. I asked her once, 'How'd you get all these things?'

"She said, 'The government changed its mind after I had to sell my house, and they told my family, as long as the money from the sale of the house is used for me, it's not a problem.' She's been there about five years. The Lord continues to take care of her."

Another Story

"We were covering the ER in rotation at that time. We were required to take a resuscitation course. My turn came, and I learned something new: mouth to nose resuscitation.

"The following day we were riding the bus. I led a program to the kids along the route, so my back was to the front. Suddenly, the bus stopped. There had been an accident in front of us just a minute before. As a physician, I jumped off the bus. I went to the first car with several people in it. One guy was complaining of chest pain, a cardiac patient, so I instructed the passengers to give him a nitro.

"The second car seemed to be empty until I got there. A lady in a little VW had been thrown diagonally across, so her head was actually where the feet of the passenger would be. She was totally unresponsive; her face was black or purple. I was at first afraid to move her, but decided I must take a chance of back injury because she had no pulse.

"I faced her up with her back straightened out, but I found I could not give her mouth to mouth. Her teeth were clenched tight like she was biting on something. So I started blowing in her nose and pressing on her chest like I had learned just the day before. A few seconds later, her pulse came back and she began responding.

"Paramedics arrived shortly afterward and carried her off to the hospital. Well, to follow up, my wife had the opportunity to lead her to the Lord in the hospital a few days later. That woman had absolutely no residual [effects from the accident]!"

Dr. Patton later also went to the woman's husband, who was not at all interested in the Lord, but very grateful his wife was alive.

Suriname

Meanwhile, Dr. and Liz Patton began getting restless. They wanted to return to full time overseas missions — and not necessarily as medical missionaries.

"My wife, Liz, and I knew that we would eventually go full time on the mission field, but it wasn't a come and go," Dr. Patton says.

The situation in Liberia was basically closed because of a horrendous civil war that lasted almost 30 years, so to go back would've been extremely difficult. The country was in total chaos.

"We looked at going to another place and talked to our pastor about it. He said, 'Your kids are all in high school doing very well. Wait a little while,' and I totally agreed with him."

The Pattons delayed going one year, so they were in the states for their youngest son's senior year. Then they packed up and headed out of the country, not back to Africa, but to South America to the country of Suriname.

Dr. Patton says, "Originally, we asked the Lord to give us at least 20 years [on one mission field]. I thought it would require that time to get a church properly built and be self-sustaining, so if I left things would keep on going — basically a generation to train nationals."

He had a heart attack around 2005, a small one, and wondered if God was cutting things short. But the Pattons remained in Suriname and have been church planting there now for 25 years.

When Dr. and Liz Patton left for Suriname, they did not follow the same path that many of their colleagues at Southwestern chose. Dr. Patton explains, "The clinic would plan on having [its missionary doctors] come back every four years, and they put a thousand dollars away for you per quarter while you were gone. That added up when you came back to rent a car, rent a house. The idea was that during that year you would work at the clinic, help the clinic, and improve your knowledge."

"When I left, I told them, 'I won't be back, don't put a thousand dollars away a quarter. When I leave, I leave.' And I wrote a [farewell] note and put in an evangelical tract for all of my patients. I wanted to burn my bridges. Sometimes it's too easy to turn around if it gets tough and doesn't go well, so we sold our house, gave money away, closed down shop, and basically burned the bridge."

It did get tough in Suriname. But by then, after a decade of spiritual growth, the Pattons were solid in their commitment to missions. They never seriously considered heading back to the states.

This second time overseas, in addition to their spiritual maturity, they had another support: all their mission-minded friends from Southwestern. They didn't burn any relational bridges. Through a quarter of a century of work in Suriname, they kept in contact with Don Gast, Dr. Herb Atkinson, Dr. Helene Johnson, Dr. Bart Comstock, Dr. Bob Wesche, and others.

As Dr. Patton sees it, "Christianity is all about relationships. Those are things you don't toss away. They're also examples of faithfulness, and they're prayer support and financial support even now."

"We were building our first church in 1991 and we were assured we had accumulated the kind of money to finish it, very erroneous. All of a sudden, we could see in the next month I would be $3,000 short. We started to pray about it. I wrote three or four of my doctor friends about it. I was really concerned. My wife wondered, 'Where is your faith?' At the end of the month, $3,000 came in, but not from any of my three or four doctor friends, not from anyone who knew about it.

"Next month, we were also $3,000 short. That time I did not ask anyone to send emergency money, and Helene, unknowing, sent me $3,000 just in the nick of time.

"God's done the same sort of thing in our second and third church builds. Property owners refused to give it to us and then changed their mind a month later, and in both cases the fluctuating exchange rate over that long month saved us about $15,000.

"At one of those times, we got the money together and made arrangements. Another missionary and I had gone down to sign the papers. Somehow we misunderstood the time and got there an hour late, and the seller had been there already and left. That day one of our nationals came up to us. He'd had a dream and said, 'Something is not right about this deal.'

"The next day we did a more thorough investigation and found the seller did not actually own the property. He thought he owned it, but actually owned a different property that had three or four squatters sitting on it. It's virtually impossible to get them off. After a bit of hunting we located the real property owner of that land we were hoping for. He was out of the country, and it turns out, he sold the property to us for much less than we had arranged to pay the first seller."

Dr. Patton still sends a weekly prayer letter to SWMC and many of the friends he made while he was here. He credits faithful prayers of so many stateside, at least in part, for the miraculous provision of God in Suriname. The Pattons are now raising money to finish the construction of their fourth church in Suriname. Currently, the church meets in a "tenti," a lean-to structure with a concrete floor and a roof "and some lath to keep the beasties out and the people in," he says. The building is now semi-built to the level of the windows. They're hoping to return to Suriname with enough money to finish the building.

SWMC taught the Pattons valuable lessons in faith's significance in tallying finances. Dr. Patton credits SWMC for a great time of spiritual growth in the decade he was rearing his family and considering a future in missions. He faithfully sat in on the prayer meetings and witnessed faith in SWMC's finances. These experiences played a significant role in how he handled financial crises later in Suriname.

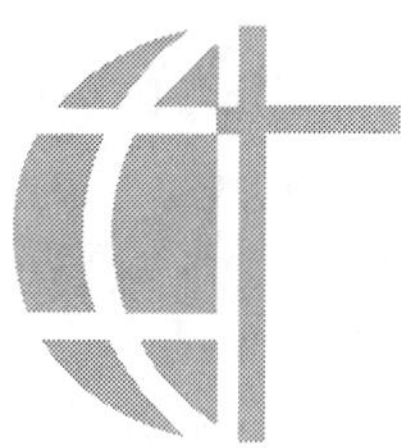

Chapter 14

Crisscross Cultures at SWMC and Beyond

Chapter 14

Crisscross Cultures at SWMC and Beyond

Dr. Frey

Another person who did not participate in the revolving-door habit, but ran up her odometer traveling from satellite to satellite was Dr. Janet Louise Frey. She started working at SWMC a few days after Don Gast came.

Back in June 1971, Dr. Frey completed her radiology residency and began job hunting. She had hoped for work in Columbus, Ohio, her hometown. Her husband, John, was working on a research project there. She contacted every radiology practice within 50 miles of Columbus. No one had an opening. The Freys prayed, "Lord, what do you want us to do?"

About that time the federal grant paying for John's research project was terminated. After a few weeks he got a job plating metals for computer chips, using dangerous materials for not much money. They had an infant daughter to support.

Summer came and went. Their prayers continued: "Well, Lord, we can't pay the bills, but you've taken care of us thus far. What do you want us to do?"

The leaves colored and fell, and a cold wind sprang up, and still Dr. Frey had not even a hint of a job. Being a fourth generation Free Methodist, she wanted to go to the Free Methodist Medical Fellowship in Cadillac, Michigan. She had nothing better to do. So she borrowed her in-laws' car for the long weekend in October.

At one conference meal, she happened to sit with Dr. Robert Wesche. Claiming they needed a radiologist, he invited her to visit the Southwestern Medical Clinic. The Freys scraped together the money to visit during Thanksgiving weekend. They looked around and said, "Well, Lord, is this what you want? You've sort of been priming us to move."

The Lord said, "Come to Michigan."

God even directed the weather to accommodate their move. The Freys moved to Berrien County between Christmas and the New Year in shirtsleeve weather. By the following weekend, Janet's first weekend on call, the thermometer fell to 13 below zero.

While Dr. Frey stayed, many doctors came to the SWMC and left a year later, or a few years later, for foreign mission assignments or to further their careers elsewhere. After working at the SWMC for two or three years, Dr. Andrew White, a general practitioner, felt called to go back to school to get a degree in malpractice law. Praying about it, he felt God wanted him to have a dual view as a physician and a lawyer.

Shortly after Dr. Frey's daughter Jeanette was born, a doctor in the Holy Land contacted the SWMC with a pressing need. The doctor's mother had contracted a rare form of cancer, and he being the only son, had to go home and take care of her and her affairs. This doctor, a radiologist, wondered if Dr. Cooke knew of any radiologist in the states who could fill in for him for several months while he was gone. For years, Dr. Frey's husband had longed to visit the Holy Land. The Lord said, "Here's your chance." The Freys lived on a hospital compound between Bethlehem and Hebron for six weeks. Jeanette learned to crawl on the flat stone roof of their house.

It was Dr. Frey's first-ever mission trip. The adventure was one of the highlights of her career and her life, made possible because not only did the SWMC support missions, but the clinic learned of this opportunity and arranged it.

Providentially, in her internship and residency, Dr. Frey had learned to do old-fashioned radiology with red goggles and without image intensification. In Israel they hand-developed each slide in the dark room with tanks. They hung it on a rack and took it outside to dry in the sun. One of the local boys had to watch that the dogs on the hospital compound didn't come up and urinate on the slides.

The hospital was in the West Bank. Most of their patients were Arabs, who were not seen in hospitals in Israel proper. There were only a few hospitals in the West Bank. The Arabs traveled by taxi or bus, some from 90 miles away north of Jerusalem, with a physician's scrawled order for an x-ray. The patient sat quietly while Dr. Frey made and looked at the x-ray. Through an interpreter, she told the patient what the x-ray showed and wrote her findings. Then she gave the patient the x-ray and her notes in a big zip-close bag to take back to his or her doctor. These were experiences she could share with her colleagues back home, her own mission stories, after soaking up everyone else's.

In 1980, a doctor came to the clinic for a year from the United Arab Emirates. Dr. Daryl Erickson, a surgeon, worked mostly in Dowagiac. Once when he was at Berrien, he talked with Dr. Frey about the need for an ultrasound machine at the hospital in Al Ain, in the United Arab Emitates.

Seeing Dr. Frey's love of adventure, Dr. Erickson filled her imagination. "Al Ain is an oasis in the middle of a vast desert," he told her. "Do not go wandering across the road from the hospital. You'll be in wilderness, in the empty quarter. There's not another road that side of Saudi Arabia. You don't want to lose sight of the highway."

The SWMC arranged for a U.S. ultrasound company to donate a machine to the hospital. Dr. Frey and her family — with four children by this time — traveled to Al Ain for six weeks. Dr. Frey taught the hospital staff how to use the machine, including Dr. Andy Rutherford, who would later come to SWMC. Dr. Frey did not get lost in the empty quarter.

In 1984, Dr. Frey transported another ultrasound machine, and she trained staff at Kibogora Hospital, the Free Methodist Hospital in Rwanda. This time her son James was a newborn, and her next son was born nine months later.

As Dr. Frey's family increased, SWMC grew. Change was expected and exciting. When the Freys first moved from Ohio, they rented a farmhouse in the country between Berrien General Hospital and the little town of Eau Claire. The large farmhouse presented opportunities for storage for missionary doctors going overseas. At least one SWMC doctor, Dr. Helene Olson, lived upstairs in the farmhouse before settling into a place of her own. Dr. Olson worked at SWMC in the summer of 1972.

Dr. Frey saw the hand of the Lord in the frequent house swapping and sharing. Many times one doctor and his family were moving out en route to Africa or South America at the same time as another doctor was arriving at the SWMC. It just made sense to welcome the new family with open arms and an available place to live. If the other family could move in and use the same furniture, no one had to crate up anything and put it into storage. No one had to sell or buy a house in a rush.

They shopped each other's garage sales. In preparing to return to Africa, Dr. Richard A. Hirschler and his family held a giant yard sale. Dr. Frey bought their set of china, which had been to Africa and back. Except for a slight difference in some serving dishes, the Hirschlers' set matched the Freys'. The Freys also bought their little yellow foreign car.

Another garage sale provided a windfall of props for Dr. Frey's children's church missionary lessons. Dr. Bob Patton had been in Liberia, and then worked at SWMC until he felt the call to go to Suriname. The Freys bought liberally at the sale, knowing the proceeds would help finance the Pattons' trip. Spying African artifacts, Dr. Frey bought a carved ivory tusk and a chieftain's robe given as gifts to the Pattons. She took home a Liberian drum intricately decorated and carved from a single hollowed log. The drum came with stories of the hands that played the drum, both African and American. Now the friends of the Freys' seven children play on the drum.

Dr. Bruerd

Imagine working at Gorgas Hospital in the Canal Zone — a beautiful and historic edifice looking down upon Panama City from breezy Ancon Hill. In the mid-seventies, white-coated Dr. Charles E. Bruerd interned at this legendary U.S. Army hospital, described as the finest and most modern in the tropics. He considered a career on the mission field.

He talked with Dr. Hal Kime, on furlough from Ecuador, and applied to the same mission Dr. Kime was with. Dr. Kime described SWMC and urged Dr. Bruerd to join, but instead he took a family practice job in Delta, Ohio. About a year later, in 1976, that job fell through. Dr. Bruerd contacted Dr. Kime again. It just so happened that SWMC needed another family practice doctor. This time, Dr. Bruerd, a.k.a Dr. Bird, took the position at the rural clinic in the cornfield. According to Dr. Cooke's 1977 Christmas letter, Charles Bruerd built a successful pediatric practice at three SWMC locations, and when he left, two doctors filled the position.

In 1977, Dr. Bruerd and his wife, Yvonne, started the process of moving to Ecuador like the Kimes and the Douces. But it wasn't meant to be. Dr. Bruerd wasn't able to get his license. Somewhat disappointed, but still certain of his call to missions, he returned to SWMC in the spring of 1979.

About 1980, Southwestern held a round table to discuss the purpose of medical missions. Southwestern wanted to hone in on its focus. About 200 to 225 years of combined medical mission experience was sitting around that table. Dr. Doug Taylor had been a missionary in South Africa for 30 to 35 years. Dr. Atkinson, Dr. Schindler, Dr. Wesche, and others collectively formulated their primary purpose: "First, to disciple the nationals with whom they worked. Second was providing healthcare in the name of the Lord as an open, intentional witness. Third was to evangelize and plant churches. Fourth was to train nationals in healthcare. Those principles we all took to heart and tried to implement as best we could," said Dr. Bruerd.

Fascinated with foreign missions, Dr. Bruerd soaked up everything he could from his colleagues who served overseas. Wanting to prepare him the best they could, those medical missionaries did not sugarcoat anything.

"The guys at Southwestern, knowing I was going overseas, treated my time there as a mini-residency, said Dr. Bruerd. From their experience, knowledge, and training, they taught me internal medicine and unique aspects of surgery, and some obstetrics as well, as part of my preparation for service overseas."

Dr. Bruerd also took advantage of education outside the clinic. He and Dr. Cooke took an early Advanced Cardiac Life Support (ACLS) course in 1980, and then taught the course together in Kalamazoo.

Even with Southwestern's rigorous schedule, encouragement to pursue further education, and vast amount of shared collective mission experience, it's impossible to preconceive accurately the difficulties of life overseas. Some doctors left with romantic ideas — as evidenced by the flowery language in Dr. Bruerd's farewell note:

> *On July 14 [1982] my family [wife Yvonne and sons Barak and Joel] and I will be flying out of Chicago headed for Kamakwie, Sierra Leone, West Africa. We will be serving under the Wesleyan World Mission board in a hospital with only one other doctor. We would appreciate very much your prayers on our behalf. Even a letter or card would be most welcome. Thus, I bid you goodbye, expecting to see you again in a couple of years.*

Life got real in a hurry. Note the tone in the first known letter back to SWMC from Kamakwie, dated October 10, 1982. To his credit and for God's glory, Dr. Bruerd did stick it out…

> *Dear folks,*
>
> *We do have goats here in the country and in Kamakwie. They do not use them for milk, but for meat and ceremonial sacrifices only. There are also some mangy cows locally, but I fear that they may be contaminated with TB and other diseases.*
>
> *Saturday evening, I and two nationals "dug clay." Actually, it was a*

large termite mound made of clay. This I will use to make brick for my oven. I think I'll use mud block for the base.

Enclosed is a sketch of the stove I built and one of the proposed oven. Oil drums here are at a premium. We have to save them all for storage against weather, bugs and rodents. So that was out. What I did was use solid cement 4" blocks, which I had made. As you note it has two fire boxes: one long one on the left with heavy wire for a cook surface; the one on the right has two holes with ½" steel rods to set pots on. The fire boxes are shaped like cones so all the heat goes up to the cook surface. I formed the fire boxes with sand, as a mold, then poured cement over them with a form siding. After drying, I removed the sand and had a good fire box. For the top I inlaid pieces of terrazzo tile I had found which had been thrown out years ago after flooring had been put down in the hospital. It makes a nice hard, smooth, good-looking top. The oven will have a dirt block base with fire box. Above the box will be a heavy metal plate heat baffle to deflect and distribute heat. The oven box will be one cannibalized from an old non-working oven, surrounded by 2-3 inches of air space. Then there will be a 6-10" clay brick heat retainer/radiator which will then be covered with a cement plaster surface to make it weather proof. I would also like to make a solar oven, if just for heating/drying things. After the oven, my next projects are to install glass windows in the house, build a solar water heater and a solar dryer. …

To date, in addition to the hospital work and the garden, I've built the cook house, stove, blackboard, one window frame, two shutters, clothes line outside, clothes line inside, water drainage pit, rebuilt six shutters, supervised construction of our new veranda and desks for each of the boys, and supervised construction of our pantry. I've repaired the stove, the refrigerator, the toilet, the sewer drain, the shower, and a hand crank ice cream freezer I found.

I also rebuilt our bed and either replaced or fixed locks on all our outside doors. And I found or begged and appropriated five old drums and two trunks which I scraped, sanded, refurbished and painted…

In a letter later sent back with a mutual friend:

Pray for us, we are in a real pitch battle with Satan for these people, and even for the church. They know of salvation from sin, but do not have deliverance… Witchcraft, Satan and demon worship, devil dancing, human sacrifice and cannibalism are only scratching the surface. Sexual and other immorality in high places in the church by elders, deacons, lay leaders is common and the rule. Seldom seen: a hungering for the Word or righteousness.

Kamakwie Wesleyan Hospital averages about 390 patients an afternoon in the out-patient clinic, after doing the rounds and surgery in the hospital in the morning. There are two doctors and four nurses on staff.

To get an idea of the number of such letters being carefully opened and read during weekly prayer meetings, here is a list of other SWMC physicians also overseas while Dr. Bruerd was writing and sending his above letters. At the same time, Dr. Ron Baker was serving long-term at UBC Mission Hospital, Mattru Jong, Sierra Leone, West Africa. Other physicians overseas in November 1982: Dr. Hirschler at Kinshasa, Republic of Zaire; Dr. Charles Rhodes, Baptist Mid-Missions, Bangui, Central African Republic; Dr. Bill Douce, Hospital Vozandes, Quito, Ecuador; Dr. David Drake, Hatfield, Zimbabwe; Dr. John H. Edling, Hospital Wesleyan de LaGonave, Haiti, West Indies; Dr. Daryl Erickson, Oasis Hospital, Al Ain, Abu Dhabi, United Arab Emirates; Dr. John Slater, Baptist Mission Hospital, Ferkessédougou, Cote D'Ivoire; Dr. Clarence Snyder, Kigali Hospital, Rwanda; and Dr. Robert Wesche, Tenwek Hospital, Bomet, Kenya.

From 1982-1984, while Dr. Bruerd served in Sierra Leone with the Wesleyan Mission, he recruited Dr. Chuck Pierson, Dr. Chuck Paine, Dr. Tom Ritter, and Dr. Ron Baker. Like Dr. Kime had done for him, Dr. Bruerd told them all about SWMC and encouraged them to check it out.

Yvonne Bruerd credited Southwestern with greatly impacting her husband's skillset and career. "Charles got all this training from surgeons there. What a great concept it was. As government regulations get tighter and tighter and have more control, it's more difficult for a hospital to take under their wing a physician…I know they can't train a physician like those surgeons trained Charles."

Dr. Bruerd, formally trained as a general practice physician in the states, was able to perform surgery in Sierra Leone because of his significant experience under Southwestern surgeons. In Sierra Leone, there were no surgeons around. Yvonne talked about the dark, lonely nights at the hospital in Sierra Leone:

> *Charles knew this person was going to die, but he came back and opened up his books [thinking], "How am I going to do this?" He laid a textbook open on the table in the OR and asked the Lord to help him do the surgery. That patient left a week later from the hospital. It was because those surgeons like Dr. Wesche were able to train Charles, and the impact because of those surgery skills. He can't walk into any hospital in the U.S. and do surgery, but because of what he learned at Southwestern, he can do [it when necessary] overseas, and he has saved so many lives because of it. I just appreciate that so much.*

Dr. Charles Bruerd was also able to pass along his knowledge to others. While the Bruerds were in Sierra Leone from 1982-1984, it was common to have one or more medical students living in the guest house on the hospital compound. Yvonne shared that one young medical student who came for about a month got sick. Yvonne took him food. He recovered quickly and was able to work at the hospital that month before returning to the states.

"Years later," Yvonne said, "we visited Southwestern at an annual party or something. A physician came up and talked to Charles and me. He remembered our two little boys, and he thanked me profusely for the food I had brought him and the prayers. Dr. Mike Chupp. I didn't remember him. I had taken food to so many. But he certainly remembered us and was very thankful."

Dr. Chupp, with SWMC, is now working at Tenwek Hospital in Kenya. "It's amazing how your lives can crisscross with these Christian physicians in different places," Yvonne said. "We certainly had that happen to us."

Dr. Bruerd brought more than medical experience and encouragement from Southwestern to Sierra Leone. He took the first computer to Sierra

Leone, and he ran it off a solar panel with a deep-cycle battery and an inverter. Seeing more possibilities, he talked at length about solar light with the mission board. After the Bruerds were there a year, World Wildlife Fund set up a game preserve a few miles down the dirt road, and they set up their camp with solar. Dr. Bruerd convinced everyone coming to visit to bring parts and pieces. They soon had a solar hospital, laboratory, and solar refrigerator. Missionaries are still using solar lights and fans and other 12-volt equipment.

"You had to be a little visionary and innovative," Dr. Bruerd said. He also introduced diagnostic ultrasound to their hospital in Papua, New Guinea while they were there from 1988-1995. Because they had limited x-ray capabilities, they used their ultrasound in outpatient as a diagnostic tool from the beginning. Using it they could diagnose hepatomas, osteomyelitis, pericarditis, typical kidney and renal problems, as well as OB problems and tuberculosis pericarditis. Dr. Bruerd was able to share his hospital's experience with this at the national medical meeting in Papua New Guinea around 1993, and it revolutionized how other hospitals began using ultrasounds as a diagnostic tool.

Later in the 80's, the Bruerds returned to Southwestern. The corporation made Dr. Bruerd its representative for alternative healthcare financing, which allowed for emerging trends, including HMOs and PPOs. He became a board member of the HMO the clinic began participating with in Kalamazoo, called Health Circle. In this position, Dr. Bruerd learned more than he'd ever wanted to about healthcare finance and quality improvement. He remembers one day coming home and telling Yvonne, "I went into medicine to treat people and actually practice. What is the Lord preparing me for?"

A few years later, they found out. As Chief Medical Officer in Papua, New Guinea, Dr. Bruerd set up bylaws, appointed a chief administrator, and implemented many other changes. Not only do the national government and people recognize their private mission facility as the best in Papua, with the highest quality care even without the big budget and equipment of other facilities, but the prime minister formally approached the hospital and asked them to assume management of all government hospitals. Instead, they helped convert the other hospitals from being government-based to community-based hospital systems. Their little hospital was able to revolutionize the organization — and, indirectly, the care given by — most of the hospitals in the country.

Dr. Bruerd said, "This was a God thing God did, based on everything I learned while working at SWMC."

At SWMC, Dr. Bruerd sensed spiritual warfare which manifested itself mostly in terms of finance, because the clinic felt a need to take care of the poor. The clinic provided care to a large percentage of Berrien County's Medicare and Medicaid patients, the TB program, and more than half the manpower of the seasonal migrant health program. "You don't get paid much for all those kinds of things, taking care of the entire Medicare and a fair proportion of Medicaid patients as well," he said.

The clinic had opened offices in Berrien Springs and Bridgman, and more expansion seemed necessary. "There was a lot of discussion about whether we should go to St. Joseph and Stevensville, more affluent communities," Dr. Bruerd said. "People there had options. Other communities didn't. We cared about the poorer communities, but the Lord did lead us to St. Joseph and Stevensville."

Another topic of discussion was what to do with physicians coming on furlough. "We just added water to the soup. We put them into clinics, and in one year they couldn't be super productive, but some of us cut down our hours for them so they could practice and update their skills and knowledge, giving them time for adequate continuing education, and supplementing their incomes that year out of our pockets, and some didn't want to make that sacrifice," but that was central to the clinic's goal and philosophy, so at the end of the discussion, despite obvious financial sacrifice, furloughed physicians were welcomed.

SWMC had much to think through. For newer doctors, the ideals of supporting missionary doctors wavered under the hard reality of financial difficulty and professional stature in the community. "Some felt that returning doctors weren't up to par knowledge-wise to meet the standard of care that we were expected to give in the community," Dr. Bruerd recalled.

He found their concern unwarranted and quite ironic. Dr. Wesche, a SWMC surgeon who returned many times from Africa, was one of the best surgeons Dr. Bruerd knew. After a dozen years as an anesthesiologist in California and a career spanning decades in general practice and emergency room medicine, Dr. Bruerd still considers Dr. Wesche one of the best he's ever worked with. And other mission doctors at SWMC were stellar as well.

Mission doctors aren't leaving the United States to practice because they're second-rate. On the contrary, they're top of the line. They're God's cream of the crop, and they're sent out to do His special work.

Dr. Helene Johnson agrees. When she first came from California, she "was surprised at the quality of medicine, then I realized that the people came here because they were drawn here by their faith, overqualified. Other small rural hospitals…didn't have nearly the quality of medicine that we did. Dr. Patton [was the area's] first invasive cardiologist, and [without SWMC] we wouldn't have had anyone like his caliber here… [before] the age of specialization," she wrote in an email.

Some perceive that God used financial issues and other issues as spiritual tests to weed out candidates. Sometimes a physician would come, look things over at Berrien Center and realize what a monetary sacrifice was required to join the clinic, and would decline to join. Others would come, look at the structure of Southwestern with hopes of starting up other similar clinics, but leave discouraged because it was so difficult to begin.

Southwestern doctors and their families did not drive flashy new cars like their fellow medical school graduates. Their kids didn't always wear the most fashionable clothes. They didn't invest in luxurious real estate. But God was using that money to help people around the world. Knowing this was a great blessing to the Bruerds and to the other Southwestern families. Even now for the Bruerds, who are both still working rather than retired like their peers in New Mexico, short-term missions is still a focus in their lives.

Even after the Bruerds left SWMC and moved out west, they kept up with several couples they'd met at Berrien Center: the Wesches and the Kimes. Over the years, they've gone on numerous short-term missions trips with the Kimes. They also exchange prayer letters and letters of encouragement with the Piersons, who are back in Sierra Leone. Ruth Pierson has had two rounds of chemotherapy, and the Piersons and Bruerds have both been faced with other difficulties and victories, "so you get cards going out both directions," Yvonne said.

As the Bruerds have traveled around the world, if they mention SWMC, often people will recognize the clinic. Someone might say, "Oh, that's where Dr. Schindler worked. Didn't he publish a book I read?" Or they might be working with someone associated with SWMC in some remote place.

"Given today's climate, I don't know how what was done then could be duplicated," Dr. Bruerd said. "I thank God for Southwestern and the part that it played in our lives. The background there helped to set the tone."

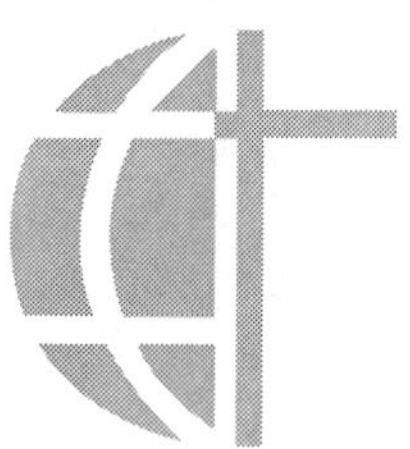

Chapter 15

Recruitment, the Lost Box Seats, Decision-Making Secrets, and Other Stories

Chapter 15

Recruitment, the Lost Box Seats, Decision-Making Secrets, and Other Stories

When Dr. Rick Johansen explains, "Most of us were not wooed to come here," it appears to be something of an understatement.

Bright-eyed, fresh-faced, optimistic, young Dr. Johansen arrived from New York State in a blizzard. The ever-overworked Don Gast picked him up and hurtled top-speed through the storm to Berrien General Hospital, not slacking pace even on Dean's Hill Road, an old Indian trail infamous for its serpentine curves down through the ravine.

After brushing off a foot or so of heavy snowfall just inside the hospital doors, Don introduced Dr. Johansen to the doctor on call, who was instructed to give Dr. Johansen a facility tour.

Dr. Hirschler, a very capable doctor and a respected Mennonite missionary to China and other places, had many great qualities. However, even on the best of days, he was not a vibrant conversationalist. It being a wintry Sunday evening, he was completing another busy weekend on call — perhaps one of many recent weekends. Dr. Johansen remembers the tour to be one of the quietest in his experience.

After a long, somewhat silent tour, Dr. Hirschler said, "We should probably eat now."

Dr. Johansen was hungry. It had been hours since he'd eaten somewhere back in New York. By this time, it was 8 or 9 p.m., so they went down to the hospital cafeteria just before it closed.

The cafeteria's menu at that hour was limited. They posted chicken tetrazzini or something like that, which Dr. Johansen had already learned you never get in a hospital cafeteria because it's always filled with miscellaneous leftovers from the week. The other item on the menu: Vega Hot Dogs.

Andrews University was not on Dr. Johansen's radar. Thinking Vega a regional brand name, he ordered two. He and Dr. Hirschler leaned across a table in the virtually empty cafeteria while the kitchen staff scraped the pans and cleaned up for the night. Dr. Johansen asked his tour guide a few questions, to which the answers were either yes or no.

He took a giant bite of the first hot dog, upon which, a "torrent" of four words suddenly flowed from quiet Dr. Hirschler: "So, you're a vegetarian?"

Dr. Johansen said, "What?"

It dawned on him that the hot dog was especially rubbery.

That was the first recruitment question Dr. Johansen remembers being asked. Conversation lulled after that. Dr. Hirschler drove him to the house where he was to spend the night, Dr. Bruerd's home. Dr. Bruerd was a family practitioner with SWMC at the time.

Dr. Johansen walked in and he met Dr. Bruerd and his lovely wife, Yvonne. Within four minutes of being in the house, at close to midnight, she said, "Would you mind doing us a favor? You're a pediatrician, right?"

Dr. Johansen said, "Yes."

She said, "Well, our son has one leg we're a little concerned about. Would you examine it?"

With that she ushered Dr. Johansen into a darkened bedroom. She woke her toddler from a deep sleep to inform him that a nice doctor was here to look at him. The boy began to scream because there was a strange man in the room messing around with his knee and ankle. That was Dr. Johansen's second SWMC experience.

Before dawn, he was taken to a devotional time. He got into a medical discussion with a surgeon, Dr. Cooke, who argued that all kids who were going to get a spinal tap should be sedated, which was contrary to popular medical opinion. Later, Dr. Johansen learned that despite Dr. Cooke always raising questions, he was actually a brilliant guy. That was Dr. Johansen's first clinical discussion at SWMC.

After that, he had lunch with a guy whose name won't be mentioned, who looked around, lowered his voice and told him, "You really don't want to come here."

So, that was the trip. That was not a recruitment trip that would've wooed anyone.

Dr. Johansen's joke is, no matter your theological persuasion, if you end up at SWMC, there's a good chance you have a Calvinistic perspective, believing you were sent, you didn't choose to come.

SWMC Family Housing

SWMC hospitality is legendary. During recruitment and often for a period of time afterward, rather than putting doctors and their families up in some hotel, SWMC families would offer their own homes. Many new families spent time in the Gast house.

When Dr. Johansen and his wife and their two little children first came, Dr. Silvernale allowed them to stay in his home while he was in Haiti until they found a place of their own. The Johansens shared this living arrangement with another family, a newly married couple. The wife was meticulous: one evening she spent 45 minutes cutting her husband's hair in the kitchen. The Johansens had two hungry preschool kids, and the other couple was in the middle of the kitchen cutting hair.

While generosity was much appreciated, staying in homes did have uncomfortable moments.

Don Gast: SWMC'S Godfather

Doctors sometimes arrived home without planned notice from mission assignments. Often, they flew in without much notice, on red-eye transcontinental flights in a state of culture shock and not exactly in tune with what was going on.

One such doctor arrived in South Bend Regional Airport with an amazing collection of bags. Two valets carefully piled the bags, one after another, onto the back of a truck. When the whole loading experience was done, the kind doctor reached into his wallet and gave them each a dollar. These guys were incredulous, and they thought it might be a joke. Don Gast quickly and quietly slipped them a more appropriate tip.

Don was always good about covering for inadvertent faux pas and cultural insensitivities. That's the way Don was. Don was also SWMC's Godfather. He was a licensed plumber and a licensed electrician. He always knew someone or would send someone to help fix anything, anytime. It was common for him to call the South Bend supply company and finagle expertly to get plumbing and electrical supplies at discounts.

Sometimes, however, his help was a little bit convoluted. You'd have to meet guy X at store Y to help you get a deal. When you got there, the deal wasn't exactly what you wanted. So there were some moments when Don's arrangements were "interesting," so to speak. But, overall, Don knew everything and would help to do anything.

People Who Actually Failed Recruitment

There were also people whom SWMC didn't hire. Throughout the years, some very interesting individuals found their way across Berrien County's back roads to the clinic in search of a job.

One was a promising-sounding guy, a brilliant internist who'd received his training in some of the best places. Dr. Johansen picked him up from the airport. He came walking through the gate wheeling this one-year-old kid in a little red wagon. He proceeded to roll his son on the wagon through the airport. Wagons aren't the safest modes of transportation for one-year-olds. Sometimes if turns are made too sharply, the whole thing will tip over.

Later, at Dr. Johansen's house, the brilliant internist took his son and wagon out onto the Johansen driveway. One of Dr. Johansen's kids wanted to take the kid for a pull around the drive, but Dr. Johansen said, "No way." A moment later, the family was looking out the picture window and the dad turned it around, and there went the little guy, head first on the concrete. Dr. Johansen heard the crack of his head through the picture window. This happened more than once. Needless to say, SWMC did not take this individual. He was a little out of touch.

Another time, a recruit and his family stayed in the Johansen home. The family and their visitors were watching television and having what Dr. Johansen thought was a reasonable conversation. Suddenly, in the middle of everything, the recruit stood up and announced, "Well, we're going to go and have our family devotions now."

He walked over and turned off the Johansen's TV in the Johansen's family room and took his wife and kids down to the guest bedroom. Dr. Johansen and his wife sat for a minute in the dark and looked at each other, trying to figure out what had just happened. SWMC did not hire this individual either.

Corporation Benefits

SWMC had tickets to the White Sox. They were spectacular seats, second row, and right behind the plate. SWMC physicians had virtually no perks or benefits, but this was one thing that Dr. Cooke had actually gotten a long time before and just let the doctors and staff use the seats. Everyone got to pick a game.

During one monthly meeting in the board room at Berrien General Hospital, probably in the middle of another discussion about the tight finances or some pressing mission need, an unfortunate digression occurred.

One of SWMC's returning missionaries, a rather devout man, Dr. Bob Patton, brought up the fact that he did not feel it was appropriate to use SWMC finances to buy baseball tickets. All extra money should be going overseas. A long debate ensued. Dr. Johansen actually sided with those who said it was nice for employees to have the benefit for families and even for returning missionaries. The discussion swelled. People became teary-eyed over the issue. They took a vote. Majority ruled. They went around the room, and Dr. Johansen's was the last vote.

Dr. Patton sat directly on Dr. Johansen's left at the table. There Dr. Johansen was, having to make the deciding vote with Dr. Patton sitting beside him, emotional, trembling. The whole issue had become a spiritual test for the group. Dr. Johansen regrets this vote to this day, but he did say, "Okay, we'll get rid of the tickets."

That was the sad end of SWMC's White Sox tickets, and Dr. Johansen is still sorry.

There was another legendary set of tickets. Dr. Bob Wesche lived in South Bend and commuted each day. He had two beautiful Notre Dame football tickets. Fifteenth, twentieth row, right behind the goal posts, just gorgeous seats. He didn't want to go to all the games, so there were always a few games for his SWMC family.

One year he was going to be in Africa around the time he expected the ticket renewal notice to come in the mail. A fast response is essential because other contributors are waiting for available tickets.

While in Africa, Dr. Wesche was letting someone else live in his house in South Bend, and he told them exactly what the envelope was going to look like. He described the envelope to a T — it always came packaged just so. He stressed that this was of utmost importance: The other mail, the bills, everything else could sit here on the counter, but as soon as this envelope came, they were to get it to Don Gast immediately, and Don would know what to do.

No envelope like that ever came. Notre Dame switched to a different mailer that year, and the envelope came looking like a bill with no Notre Dame logo. It was just a standard kind of envelope with a window saying, "Remittance to." The house guest put it in the pile and kept waiting for the described envelope.

Dr. Wesche came back a day or two after the thing had to be in, opened his mail, and experienced temporary heart failure. He called the Notre Dame ticket office with his sob story, "I was in Kenya serving the Lord, can you give me a couple of days grace?"

They said, "Nope, our deadline is our deadline and that's it. Those tickets have already been spoken for, for another donor."

The tickets were gone forever. Poor Dr. Wesche. Poor SWMC.

The 401K Stipulation

SWMC had a 401(k), an investment program. A nice gentleman oversaw the investments for the group, a great fellow who always wanted to please.

Some people would stress, "It's not as important to us the percentage of return we're getting. We want to make sure that none of our investments go to alcohol, tobacco, or gambling." For them, this was the all-consuming issue.

This guy kept trying to explain that with all the conglomerate companies now, it was almost impossible to know that indirectly, a company might have ties somewhere. After a while, it got to be a little joke, to help relieve some of the pressure for him. Although he was going to try, there was no way that some of SWMC's money wasn't going to some of this stuff.

Buildings

The main office in Berrien Center had been a juvenile center. While renovated for clinic use, its layout retained a few quirks. To get to the best bathroom in the place, you had to go through Don Gast's Chief Executive office. If he was talking to someone else in his office, which he often was doing, it was a trip.

The only other bathrooms in the building were patient bathrooms up front in the clinic area, which sometimes weren't so good. The better bathroom did have a drawback. The toilet had an industrial-strength flush. It was right on the other side of the wall from Don's office. If you happened to be sitting in his office when someone was using the bathroom, it sounded like an explosion going off at the hospital next door.

Another drawback in the construction of the Berrien Center office: a flat roof. Michigan is known for its torrential rains, which quickly overpower the unfortunate horizontal surface of such a roof. In the spring and the fall, and partway through the summer, and on sunny winter afternoons, choreography became routine for office staff, maneuvering around buckets. Sometimes patients had to step around buckets to be seen.

The first Stevensville pediatric office, located in a small office building on Fairview, also had some layout quirks. The pediatrics office was down below where counseling is now — a very small place. There were three exam rooms, only one of which had a window. There was only one entrance to the pediatric office — a basement stuck in the side of the hill.

So, as a physician, if you came late, every patient sitting in the waiting room knew exactly when you arrived. There were probably more doctors on time there than any other SWMC facility.

If a doctor really had a good excuse, such as he or she was late because of doing an emergency C-section in the hospital or something like that, the doctor was quick to mention this to the receptionist in a very loud voice. Whether the patients believed it or not was entirely up to them.

Actually, that was not the worst structural feature at Fairview. The pocket-door "office" measured, at most, six by eight feet. It also served as storage. Stuffed in there, in addition to a very small desk and a child-sized chair, were all the medical samples and cleaning supplies. If anyone sat slightly wrong or leaned wrong while standing, that person might get a sigmoidoscopy from the vacuum cleaner handle. Inadvertent medical procedures performed — it probably happened to most of the staff at least once.

The new Berrien Springs pediatric office more than made up for the lack of storage at Fairview. With a full basement for storage, it didn't take long for Don Gast and the missionary doctors' families to take full advantage. Having such accessible storage turned out to provide for some interesting scenarios.

This scene opens on a sick boy reclining stiffly on a cold medical table. Not too keen on the doctor's office anyway, he's trying to be brave and praying he wouldn't need a shot or some sort of surgery. As he waits there, he hears voices coming from some vague place nearby.

"Shine the light over here. I think I've found it."

"No, it wasn't way in there."

"Yes! Look! This is it!"

"Oh, no, that's way too big."

"It has to be right. Let's just take it out and get a good look at it."

"I'm telling you, don't mess with it. It's not the right size."

"Here, lift up that corner. I'll shine the light on it. Then we'll know for sure."

"Ow! You dropped it on my foot!"

"Sorry."

"See, I told you, that's not it. The color is all wrong. And it's too..."

"It sure is heavy. You'd better go get the doctor. We're going to need some help."

The nurse enters the examining room. She has heard the conversation as well. Seeing the boy's growing horror, she gives a funny little laugh. "Don't be alarmed. It's just a missionary and his wife in the basement. They've come home from Kenya and they're trying to move their couch and furniture out of storage down there."

Patient Care

This is the saga of the doctor who fell asleep.

In Bridgman, SWMC rented the bottom half of Dr. Dale Smith's old dental office. It contained one patient room that consisted of an examining table and a counter with a sink. Leaning on the counter over a chart, Dr. Bob Patton was taking the medical history of a gowned, middle-aged woman.

Dr. Patton was an incredible workaholic. He translated many books of the Bible into Surinamantango, one language they speak in Suriname. When in the states, Dr. Patton went to church in South Bend and drove the bus around picking up kids for ministry. This day was probably a day after one of those Sundays, following a full work week and a weekend on call. While the woman was talking, and Dr. Patton was in the middle of taking down her history, he dozed off. He was out, pen still in hand, but totally asleep.

Very politely, the woman walked out of the room and down the hallway, still in her gown, and very calmly told the nurse, Cheryl Baggett, "My physician fell asleep. I tried to wake him up a couple of times." The woman was probably a mother, who understood sleep deficit firsthand.

Cheryl and the patient walked back to the room. Cheryl woke Dr. Patton. He said, "I'm sorry," and the interview continued as if nothing had ever happened.

Some of the More Unusual Pediatric Cases

Understandably, SWMC doctors were especially good with exotic cases. In various corners of the world, SWMC doctors have seen anthrax, TB, malaria, and a quite a few other unusual cases, so they are not surprised by anything. But a few cases are memorable:

One nice little girl from Benton Harbor went on a trip to Guatemala. When she returned, she grew a sore on her cheek. The girl's mother called and said, "There's something that sticks up out of her face and then goes back in again."

Sure enough, a pediatrician took a look and quite easily diagnosed it — a parasite, a bot fly. These things are like little maggots that live under your skin with a burrow almost like a ground hog.

Dr. Johansen once had a call from a mother who thought her son had stuck an eraser in his nose. She said, "There's something pink way back up his nose." Dr. Johansen took a light and did see what could have been the end of a pencil eraser. In retrospect he thought maybe he saw it move, but it could've just been the kid moving. Dr. Johansen reached in with long forceps specially made for the nose, while the mother restrained the kid. He grabbed ahold of what he thought was an eraser. While the mom and nurse watched and the kid howled, out came about a 10-inch-long worm, an ascaris. Most tend to go south. This one had decided to head north. Ascaris is a native species, and the kid had probably picked it up while playing in the sand box.

SWMC offices have always featured great diversity, financially and ethnically and everything else. It is really special. In four rooms in a row, you could see a Whirlpool executive's kid, a farmer's kid, a foreign national child of an Andrews University seminary student, and an inner-city homeless kid. Dr. Johansen, coming from cosmopolitan New York out to the boondocks, never expected waiting rooms looking like the United Nations.

Historically, SWMC doctors have also been very good with grand entrances. Dr. Bill Douce came from a little clinic in the Andes Mountains and needed work. SWMC found him a place to work at the school-based clinic in Benton Harbor. Dr. Douce is a quiet older guy, very unassuming, and he walked in and got right to work with hardly anyone noticing him. On his first or second day on the job, they called him to an emergency in the high school cafeteria: a kid was choking on something he ate. Dr. Douce gave him abdominal thrusts and dislodged the food at once, and the kid's coloring and breathing returned to normal. Dr. Douce earned instant credibility and became a hero in the school.

Patient Care

In the beginning, SWMC doctors had to cover the whole hospital on weekends and nights, even pediatricians such as Dr. Johansen. So there were some interesting moments where Dr. Johansen found himself doing things he'd never done before, like pulling a tube out of a patient's gallbladder.

He's bent over this tube with an ear plastered to a telephone receiver, being coached over the phone by the surgeon telling him, "You can do it, Rick, it's no big deal. Just hold it like so, cut that suture there, pull the thing out."

Doctors like Dr. Johansen were thankful for good nurses when they covered the ICU (intensive care unit) full of cardiac cases. In situations where they walked in on things they hadn't seen or couldn't quite recall doing, they'd go humbly to the nurses and say, "Could you tell me about this?" Although the SWMC doctors enjoyed exposures and experiences beyond their formal training, at the end of the day they'd thank God the nurses were sharp.

SWMC's patient care was often on the cutting edge. They had fairly avant-garde doctors who wanted to do the latest and greatest things.

In the OB world, when Dr. Johansen first came, SWMC was already allowing a lot of fathers in the room during C-sections. That was unheard of at the time. Even the most liberal, suburban hospitals in New York weren't doing that yet. And fathers could cut the umbilical cord. No one other than a doctor was doing that in those days, but Dr. Helene Johnson read about some hospital in California doing something new, so she decided it would be good to do it at Berrien General. Another "cutting-edge" trend was allowing wives to watch their husbands' vasectomies on Friday afternoons.

These innovative practices were encouraged by Dr. Cooke, the founder, who was always a step ahead. Back in the old days, he checked the urine of every hospitalized patient to see a precise history of the patient's blood sugar levels during the previous 4-5 hours. He said, "While they're in the hospital draw their blood four or five times." Some people objected to all the finger pokes, but he wanted to know the complete picture, and it was sometimes amazing to detect unexpected, non-symptomatic problems. Now, 35-40 years later, that is the national medical standard procedure.

More recently, pediatrician Dr. Georg Schultz has been one of the first pediatricians nationally to go digital. He was a leader. Despite being keyboard challenged, he has been on the forefront doing electronic records.

On the topic of pediatrics, throughout the years there have been a few turf battles regarding circumcisions. SWMC physicians have weathered the successful transition from OBs to pediatricians doing circumcisions in the hospital. The pediatricians wanted to do circumcisions rather than the obstetrician. If the pediatrician was going to be following the child out of the hospital, he or she wanted to do the surgery.

Here's the story of Dr. Schindler's highly successful pre-Viagra medication. In a lot of places, if a doctor saw a 50-something male at the clinic who appeared healthy, there was a good chance he was worried about possible impotence. Dr. Schindler became tired of seeing so many of these guys because in those days there was no treatment for impotence. Finally, an idea for a remedy came to him. He gave his male patients a little packet of vitamins, but he didn't tell them what the pills were. He had instructions attached and also gave them verbal instructions to take one pill, wait seven days, and then your problem should go away. It worked. For the average male, if they had to wait seven days before being intimate, their impotence problem was solved. People would show up with little babies, thanking him and lauding his pills. They probably thought his wide smile was for the baby. Dr. Schindler told them, "Don't forget the instructions."

Maverick Missionaries

Missionaries generally lived a frugal and austere life; they did not spend a lot of extra money on themselves. SWMC did have a physician who was on the cutting edge of that, too.

Dr. Schindler had a condo in Spain. Back in those days, no missionary coming back from Africa stopped off for R and R to decompress on the way back. But Dr. Schindler did, and it was no secret. He readily shared his condo with anyone else who was traveling. Even today, missionaries are aware of austere expectations put upon them, and they talk about how it's not a good idea to drive up to a sponsoring church in a high-end rental car. Dr. Schindler apparently didn't care what others thought.

Dr. Richard Hirschler was a one-time missionary to China and other places, and he was also a pilot. He convinced a couple of public health officials in Berrien County that instead of driving up to a conference in Traverse City, he would fly them there. On the way home, somewhere near Muskegon, Dr. Hirschler said, "We're getting pretty low on fuel, but I think we're going to make it."

The two looked at him wide-eyed and said, "Shouldn't we stop at another airport?" He squinted at the gauges again and said, "Nah, I think we'll make it." They weren't exactly excited about this flight anymore.

Sure enough, as they approached Andrews Airport, the plane did run out of fuel, and Dr. Hirschler gracefully and safely glided the plane in under no engine power.

A number of missionary physicians served in the DMZ (demilitarized zone) in the middle of war. Dr. Roland Stephens served in a Zimbabwe bush hospital that ended up in the middle of battle lines of a brutal civil war. No one touched his hospital, however. As the legend is told around SWMC, both sides put a white flag up and carried their injured into Dr. Stephens' hospital. In the wards, people on opposite sides of the battle lay in beds side by side actually talking to each other, but when they were healed, they'd raise up a white flag and walk back to their side and resume fighting.

One of SWMC's most saintly men is another quiet, unassuming gentleman, Dr. John Edling. He was the Dr. Van Oosterhout of his time, heading the extended care facility. Dr. Edling had a practice of prescribing innumerable medications. He had medications he was using to treat side effects of the medications he was using to treat the side effects of the other medications...A typical patient might take nine or ten different medications. When other physicians took over his cases when he was in Haiti, they'd have to whittle down the list.

What made Dr. Edling and his wife, Priscilla, a nurse, saints was their lifelong dedication to the people of Haiti. Dr. Edling devoted almost his entire life to the people of Haiti on the island of La Gonave at a mission hospital. He did everything for these people. When he finally retired, well into his seventies, where did he retire? He retired to Florida, not at the beach or in Orlando, but in hot, rural Florida, to a trailer park out in desolate nowhere. Guess who all of his neighbors were in that trailer park? Yes, Haitian refugees. And for the rest of their lives, as long as they were able, Dr. Edling and his wife ministered to the migrant workers living in that community.

Romance

Working with Berrien County Health Department, Dr. Johansen is fascinated with statistics — everything from to numbers of specific types of cases. An incredible statistic of SWMC, as best as Dr. Johansen has been able to determine, is that only two SWMC physicians have ever been divorced. The divorce rate of doctors nationally is something like 70%, and of more than 200 physicians who have worked with SWMC, the divorce tally is two. Not even 2% but two. It's not that SWMC doctors are better husbands or wives than others; it's just a remarkable statistic. Throughout the years, SWMC doctors have dealt with incredible stress: crazy working hours, time overseas, not being wealthy by any means.

SWMC has occasionally fostered romance. People at SWMC who met and fell in love and then got married include: Drs. Susan and Paul Lim, and Dr. Helene and Mark Johnson.

Honor and Influence Overseas

Dr. Schindler was honored by the Royal College of Surgeons and knighted in England. This was big news in the papers because very few Americans are ever inducted there. Another time Dr. Schindler was working at SWMC for a while when an inauguration took place in Liberia. This was during the mid-'70s, when Liberia was actually a democracy once before the revolution. The Liberian government paid Dr. Schindler's way and sat him up as a distinguished guest on the podium. The headline across the Monrovian Times: "Miracle Doctor Returns."

Dr. Silvernale, a SWMC public health doctor and pediatrician, was the director of the national immunization and anti-tuberculosis campaign of the government of Haiti in the mid-'70s and early '80s. He worked with the infamous despot Baby Doc. Baby Doc commissioned Dr. Silvernale to administer thousands of BCG vaccines across the country and later also initiate the HIV program. One thing they did right in Haiti was that they immunized virtually everybody. Dr. Silvernale was a recognizable name in medical circles worldwide because of that successful program.

Dr. Silvernale once planted a fruit tree on a plot in Haiti where nothing grew. He instructed the neighbors to water it carefully. People thought he was crazy. Someone took him aside and said, "Dr. Silvernale, why would you do this? You'll never enjoy the fruit from this tree."

He said, "But your children and grandchildren will enjoy the fruit from this tree."

Stories like Dr. Silvernale's fruit tree resonate in Berrien County, one of the fruit capitals of the world. SWMC doctors and their children remember such tales as though they were parables, illustrating the importance of laying the groundwork for the future, even if the planter won't personally benefit.

Miracle

Dr. Johansen worked his first weekend at Berrien General during the Fourth of July holiday in 1977. He wasn't supposed to be on. He and his family weren't even unpacked in the house they were sharing with another family. He'd been in the hospital solo about three hours when a guy crashed his motorcycle on the St. Joseph River Bridge. Both his femurs were sticking out. A pediatrician, Dr. Johansen phoned the surgeon on call, Dr. Cooke, and asked, "Where do I send this guy?"

At first, Dr. Cooke said, "Give him pain medication and stabilize him." Then, taking a minute to think, Dr. Cooke said, "Well, I've done some orthopedics. Let me come take a look at it."

Dr. Johansen figured he'd come in and say, "Sorry, get him out of here."

Dr. Cooke came in, looked and said, "Oh, yes, we can do this."

We?

Dr. Cooke thought it was a straightforward case. He got another doctor to come cover the ER for an hour or two. Dr. Johansen found himself scrubbed up and standing awkwardly across the operating table from the doctor who'd argued about kids getting spinal taps. "You're going to help me," Dr. Cooke said. "You hold this here, do this, and watch me screw this long rod in."

Dr. Cooke implanted the rod perfectly. The guy's circulation was fine. Then, as Dr. Johansen remembers it, Dr. Cooke looked over at Dr. Johansen and said, "You're in a better position on that side. You can screw the other rod in."

Dr. Johansen said, "I've never driven any screw into anyone's bones."

"Don't worry," Dr. Cooke said. "The real work you've already done, lining it up in the right position."

Dr. Cooke held the patient's leg in position and talked Dr. Johansen through the procedure. When the screw was in place, Dr. Cooke sewed him up partway before the doctor covering the ER called Dr. Cooke to look at something else. He left Dr. Johansen in the OR alone to finish the last couple of stitches. The guy left the hospital a few days later, and Dr. Johansen has since met that person walking around as though nothing ever happened to him, which to him is a miracle.

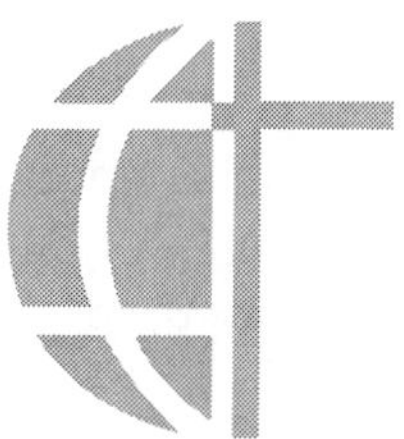

Chapter 16

The Founder's Story

Chapter 16

The Founder's Story

If Southwestern Medical Clinic was born on that summer day in 1968, it was inseminated a decade and a half earlier.

While young Weldon Cooke attended Wheaton College where his father taught, he got "the missionary bug." He listened intently to professors and visiting speakers about the need for doctors in third-world countries, and he felt called to go. Several of his classmates felt the same way, and they all encouraged each other.

After graduating from Wheaton, and medical school at Northwestern in Illinois, in between residencies at Cook County Hospital and Hines General Hospital (which later merged with Loyola), Dr. Cooke spent two years at Berrien County Hospital.

In the mid-1950s, Berrien County Hospital was run by a hospital board made up of supervisors and other county politicians. Dr. Cooke's supervisor was Dr. Charles W. Bush. Dr. Bush was a brash fellow sporting a goatee with a handlebar, "a very self-centered guy, and fairly good surgeon."

Drs. Bush and Cooke were the two surgeons at Berrien County Hospital in those years. Dr. Bush, acting as medical director, oversaw surgery. Dr. Cooke "did everything else: ran ER, deliveries...Dr. Bush was hard to get along with. I attended board meetings right along with him and got him out of a lot of jams — he was such an arrogant, impossible guy to work with. Soon as I left he got fired, and I had predicted as much," Dr. Cooke recalls.

While Dr. Cooke completed his residency at Hines, another surgeon took Dr. Bush's and Dr. Cooke's places at Berrien County Hospital. Dr. Andrews was a decent surgeon, but couldn't get along with the board either, so he expressed his desire to resign about four years later. Dr. Cooke's residency at Hines ended in 1959. He had no idea where he was going to go, though he had done some looking around.

On a Thursday in March 1959, Dr. Cooke was sweating through another feverish day in Hines' ER, seeing a patient, when he got an overhead page, which rarely happened. Dr. Cooke was just a number, just another physician completing his residency. He had a telephone call. When he got to a phone he immediately recognized the deep voice of the Berrien County supervisor and head of Berrien County Hospital board: Ted Katzbach.

"We lost Dr. Andrews and we're looking for a medical director," Mr. Katzbach said.

Dr. Cooke explained he would be finished with his residency in July. "I'll come if I can pick my staff," he said, his mind turning. He was hired while still on the phone.

Wasting no time, Dr. Cooke first called his sister Almarose, just back from four years in Honduras. She agreed to spend a year with him at Berrien County Hospital before returning to the mission field, the next time to Rhodesia.

Then he called one of his Wheaton classmates, tall, thin, bespectacled Dr. Charles "Charlie" Patton. Though they had gone on to different medical schools (Dr. Patton at University of Illinois), they kept track of each other. Charlie had placed an ad in the Christian Medical Society Journal, looking for a job for a year to spend with a surgeon. He wanted to learn surgery before going with his wife to the mission field in Brazil. He took the job right away.

In an hour Dr. Cooke had his staff. He knew it had to be the hand of the Lord.

On July 17 the threesome made rounds at the hospital with the outgoing Dr. Andrews. They went to work immediately. They inherited all the patients.

Dr. Cooke's desire was still to be a missionary doctor, but the way he tells the story, three of his kids were still in diapers and the timing just didn't seem right. He began realizing the possibilities of his position at Berrien County Hospital as medical director and head surgeon. In this quiet, rural hospital, he could train surgeons to go out on the mission field. He could teach them all he knew, while they had the freedom to stay at Berrien County Hospital as long as they needed.

As the story goes, everything was mountaintop and sunny in these early glory days. The three young, adventurous doctors had their lives ahead of them and built their skills and their dreams at Berrien County Hospital. In reality, work was hard and politics with Ted Katzbach grisly and grim.

Dr. Cooke considered quitting. Mr. Katzbach was trying to run everything and getting in the way. Mr. Katzbach told the newcomers he was in his 80s, and he thought he was entitled to expect them to listen to him about days gone by.

Sometime before the end of the year, however, about four months after Dr. Cooke came, Mr. Katzbach retired. Wryly, Dr. Cooke gives Mr. Katzbach some credit for SWMC's existence: "If he hadn't called that afternoon in March with his deep voice, it wouldn't have been." But they sighed with relief when his deep voice no longer droned on over their shoulders.

When Dr. Almarose Cooke and Dr. Charles Patton left for their respective mission fields a year later, neither ever to return on staff, Dr. Cooke found himself in desperate need. He advertised in the Christian Medical Society magazine, and the Lord supplied him with two of the finest people he had ever met.

Dr. Roland Stephens had completed three years of surgical residency and needed an externship for two more years. Dr. Wayne Meyers, by Dr. Cooke's definition a genius, a very academic type, planned to return to Africa but needed a place to work until then.

Dr. Cooke credits those two more than any others in helping him get the fledgling, disorganized medical clinic off the ground. "The whole medical society in Berrien County hated Berrien County Hospital," Dr. Cooke recalls. "It was used so the local politicians could get taken care of for free. They never considered that the doctors were any good. I did my best with those two to improve that image a little."

Dr. David Drake (ca. 1970-1972)

In another desperate need sometime around 1970, Dr. Cooke located Dr. David Drake. Dr. Drake had served with Dr. Roland Stephens in Africa and had a Canadian license, not an American license. Back then there was no quick way for Dr. Drake to get an American license, but Dr. Cooke needed a doctor, and Dr. Drake needed a place to work. Dr. Cooke determined to make it happen.

He had to concoct a program to be approved by the state medical society — nothing was in existence at the time. He had to drive to Lansing and win over the state medical society during a committee meeting among the big shots. The meeting was scheduled for 11 a.m.

Foul winter weather was predicted. Well, Dr. Cooke thought, at least I have my brand new Oldsmobile.

The car didn't have more than 30 miles on it before starting the trip. Dr. Cooke gave himself plenty of time. Even as he started out, snow was falling fast. All of a sudden the car conked out. The engine would not revive. Dr. Cooke didn't know what to do. There were no car phones then. No cell phones either. He sat at the wheel, fingers growing cold, and all he could do was pray.

After praying a while, he thought he'd try to restart the car. It started and ran fine. At the next town, he had someone at a gas station look under the hood. They couldn't find anything wrong with the car.

Dr. Cooke had never driven in such a storm — no wind, just sheets of snow. Maybe 30 miles down the road, his new Olds conked out again. Staring at his stack of papers, determined to make it to Lansing, he waited and prayed and got the engine going again after a time. It went this way all the way to the state capital.

When it became evident he would not arrive on time (not to mention dubious that his car would get him there at all), he stopped along the way and called the medical society on a pay phone. Explaining his car trouble and the weather, he got them all sympathetic. They agreed to listen to him when he got there.

He arrived just as capital clocks tolled noon. The committee was breaking for lunch. The head of the committee graciously invited Dr. Cooke to dine with him. So it turned out that Dr. Cooke had a whole hour to bend the man's ear about the program.

When they reconvened, they wasted no time; they just passed his proposal. Meanwhile, snow buried Lansing. Though he'd planned to return that night, Dr. Cooke left three days later when roads were cleared of the blizzard. He had no further trouble with the car.

It turned out Dr. Cooke used the program only for Dr. Drake, but that program got Dr. Drake approved for a U.S. license to practice medicine, and he spent two years with the clinic. Dr. Cooke never questioned that the efforts were worthwhile. He probably had no time to contemplate.

Dr. Cooke became desperate again in 1972. This time, he and his wife traveled to San Francisco to woo a Jewess to work at a male-dominated clinic for Christian missionary doctors.

Dr. Helene Johnson — Olson at the time — was interning at a military hospital in San Francisco. Dr. Cooke and his wife picked her up at the hospital, and they took the trolley up and down the hills to the wharf, where they ate at a restaurant. Dr. Cooke recalls Dr. Olson telling him later that she never liked him and didn't want the job. But he was desperate. He needed her. Somehow he wheedled her into coming.

As others attest, Dr. Cooke was a hands-on physician and medical director, taking care to make rounds daily and know the charts of every patient. By the early 70s, administrative paperwork was ramping up, and to get it all done and his rounds and surgeries, too, Dr. Cooke ran serious sleep deficits.

Medicare started in 1968. Other area physicians who already detested Southwestern Medical Clinic, jealous of the fact that these physicians had salaries from the county and free overhead at the hospital and built-in patients to inherit after their ER trips, now had many new reasons to be disgruntled. So under pressure, Berrien General began breaking direct monetary ties to Southwestern. The whole process took a year or two. At the end of it all, Southwestern had its own clinic and paid rent; worked as independent contractors for Berrien General Hospital; and Dr. Cooke's workload expanded exponentially. Still he thought not of himself, but of the vitality of the clinic for so many of his missionary colleagues.

Keeping The Clinic Viable

Dr. Cooke insisted that everyone have a vote. To keep a clinic viable, in his opinion, from day one, every physician had to have an equal vote. "I depended on everyone," he said. It was a struggle every year to fill doctors' shoes when they left. Every year was a repeat of that first crazy 24-hour hiring jag. "Who can I call? How can I convince him or her to come? What will I do if he or she says no?"

And then after a blur of an interview and tour, he hired his doctors on a handshake. Nobody signed anything; they just started working and worked until they needed to go on their mission.

La Gonave

Though Dr. Cooke never had the chance to work as a full time missionary, he was able to travel to Haiti on five different occasions. These trips were some of the highlights of his life, and they were also life-changing for three of his four children.

Dr. James L. Wierman arranged for Dr. Cooke to go to the Haitian island of La Gonave. Dr. Edling followed Dr. Wierman, who followed Dr. E. Dewain Silvernale, who followed Dr. Norbert O. Anderson.

Dr. Wierman spent several years in Haiti before coming to Southwestern for a year to learn surgery. After the year, he returned to Haiti. One day he contacted Dr. Cooke and said, "I'm up to my ears in surgery here. I sure could use some help."

La Gonave was the only hospital in Haiti doing surgery at the time. A government hospital in Port au Prince still had dirt floors and did no surgery. Later, Duke University put up Albert Schweitzer Hospital, but only allowed patients from one Haitian district to go there. People desperate for medical care boated to La Gonave, braving north winds with horrendous waves. Some boats sank in the effort.

From about 1971-1976, Dr. Cooke visited Dr. Wierman at La Gonave five times for two weeks each time. He brought his own anesthetics and his own first assistants: his children.

Due to a number of factors, women did not come for hysterectomies until absolutely necessary. Tumors the size of footballs were common. Dr. Cooke faced patients lined up with advanced gonorrhea infections, adhesions everywhere. "You sort of have to chisel them out," he said. "Right next to the cervix are two ureters. If you nick one of those, you have a destroyed patient." In Haiti, leaking urine constantly, a woman would be an outcast. By the grace of God, Dr. Cooke was able to avoid any of these devastating complications.

High spinal anesthetic was all he could get, and his young son would hold the retractor. He had to teach his sons not to say "Oops" if the retractor slipped. If the patient heard that, she'd stiffen up. "Oops" is apparently a universal term.

Wanting to be able to perform as many surgeries as possible for these needy people, Dr. Cooke worked as quickly as he safely could. Among many other types of surgeries, he performed about a dozen hysterectomies per trip. One time, when he got back to the states, he scheduled a hysterectomy for a Monday. It was a routine hysterectomy, and having a much lighter schedule than the long lines in Haiti, he took his time. After completing the procedure he looked at the clock. He'd been in surgery only 20 minutes.

Working on the mission field, even short-term, changes a person. It changes more than physician's speed or ability to perform under less-than-ideal conditions. It changes his entire outlook on medical practice and on life.

Dr. Cooke kept a photograph of a small girl sitting on his knee. The little seven-year-old girl, a daughter of one of the local Haitian preachers, came to La Gonave, suffering severe abdominal pain. The pain was too intense for an appendix, but Dr. Cooke had already learned nationals do not get appendicitis. He determined it had to be a ruptured something-or-other.

With no time to waste, he opened her up, not even knowing exactly where to cut. If she hadn't lived right next to the hospital, she wouldn't have made it through anything. He could see right away he was facing a perforation. They set up the spinal anesthetic and kept IVs going so she wouldn't collapse.

It turned out to be a big hole in the ilium, the small bowel, due to typhoid, not uncommon, he was told. They put it together and she made it. When Dr. Cooke returned to Haiti the following year, he met her again, and she sat on his knee, and someone took their picture.

Highs like these have remained with Dr. Cooke the rest of his life.

Dr. Cooke's Namesake

Dr. Cooke was named after Weldon Baxter Cooke, his father's older brother. Weldon Baxter Cooke was a stunt pilot, among other things. He flew the first airmail in the east around Baltimore. He had built about nine commercial planes before Douglas and others had built any. His two-cycle engine was lighter than any other, and Dr. Cooke has a photo of Weldon Baxter carrying one in his hand. He held the altitude record at the time he died. He did most of his air shows in and around Oakland, California. He went to Denver in September 1914, for an altitude record attempt. He may not have realized he was already a mile up before he left the ground. At any rate, he passed out and crashed, which ended his life.

Dr. Cooke's parents could not have been certain their son would inherit the fearless, creative innovativeness of Weldon Baxter Cooke. But they surely passed on a great heritage — and a great challenge — to their little boy to live up to this family legend.

The Crisis Regarding Berrien General's OB Department

Berrien General Hospital's facility was outdated, and Dr. Cooke had talked to the county supervisors for years about the necessity of a quality obstetrics department. Money was tight every year for decades. Year after year, the doctors continued to operate in the old section, until daily operations came into jeopardy. They faced closing the OB department and possibly surgery.

Dr. Cooke tried to convince the county supervisors and commissioners that Berrien General Hospital depended on a viable OB department. As soon as the OB goes, a hospital goes defunct. The whole county was against the outlay of money required to update the OR and OB departments. Everything was falling apart.

Under intense emotional pressure, Dr. Cooke developed a cutting-edge presentation. He turned to the two commissioners who seemed supportive and practiced his speech on them. They more than listened; they even gave him some tips. Going into the meeting, Dr. Cooke knew he had two positive votes out of 13. It was a closed meeting, but the public was in a furor. It wanted its little community hospital to stay open.

Dr. Cooke felt confident he had the support of the two commissioners, and as they introduced him to the rest of the board, he steadied himself and looked around the room. He can't remember his arguments, but he does remember those two supportive commissioners like angels, jumping in and saying "Yes, yes," voicing their strong support of the renovations.

Chart after chart he uncovered on his easel, graph after graph, showing his careful studies and tabulations, arguing for the renovations, no matter how costly they were. He appealed to those other 11 faces, knowing that if the majority became convinced of the hospital's worth to the community, they would swing his way.

After Dr. Cooke finished his presentation, he was asked to leave while they voted. He didn't find out until the next morning how it turned out. It passed 11 to two. Two were hospital administrators at Memorial Hospital and at Mercy Hospital. To this day, he is certain they remained against it.

Had the commissioners voted against the renovations, it would've been the end of Berrien General Hospital. Southwestern Medical Clinic would've had to move to one of the other hospitals — a huge hurdle at that time. No one from SWMC was on those hospital staffs yet. The whole clinic did all their hospitalization at Berrien General.

But 11 of the commissioners had voted for the renovations. The OB department was saved. The hospital and the community soon reaped the benefits of those renovations. Berrien General's OB department earned widespread praise.

Teaching Surgery

Dr. Cooke hired Dr. Rick Johansen in another tight spot. When Dr. Johansen came, Dr. Cooke had taken calls in the ER probably 20 nights straight.

Dr. Johansen, a pediatrician, was assigned in the ER his very first day at Southwestern. He called Dr. Cooke and said, "I have this 16-year-old boy, hit by a car. Both of his femurs are cleanly fractured. What orthopod should I call?"

"Let me look at the x-rays," Dr. Cooke said.

Dr. Cooke saw both femurs, both split cleanly in the middle. It was a good case for rods. The operation was straightforward, but tricky; if you put the rod in wrong, the foot sticks out. This kid had two clean, identical fractures bilaterally.

The way Dr. Cooke tells it, he told Dr. Johansen, "Let's set up the OR."

A little wide-eyed, young Dr. Johansen said, "You're going to do it?"

They put the boy on his side, cleaned him up and did the first side, Dr. Johansen assisting Dr. Cooke. Dr. Cooke sewed the first leg up, turned him over, gave Dr. Johansen the scalpel, and said, "Now it's your turn."

Openmouthed, Dr. Johansen just stared at Dr. Cooke.

Dr. Cooke told him, "You just saw one! You can do it!"

Dr. Cooke insists that he masterminded, but he let Dr. Johansen do the cutting on the second femur. Dr. Johansen had never done surgery before; he was a pediatrician. The next day, the patient walked out of the hospital. The rods, tight and placed correctly, enabled the patient to put complete weight on them.

That's the way Dr. Cooke broke in the new doctors at Southwestern. And they never forgot it.

Another thing he did with missionaries and those preparing to go on the field was to share his surgical cases to give those guys good, solid surgical experience. "Here," he'd say, handing over a chart. "Here's an interesting case for you to do."

He learned, however, that experienced missionary doctors weren't interested in appendectomies. They said, "We never see appendix issues in the mission field."

Later, Dr. Cooke found out why. The only appendectomies abroad were cases of missionaries who ate canned food brought from home. Nothing's processed in the third world. Dr. Cooke discovered research that proved that high fiber and low additives nearly eliminate appendicitis.

The Collection

Decades later, SWMC staff can describe in exaggerated detail a very individual collection that Dr. Cooke amassed on one wall of the OR. He had forgotten about this strange display. Remembering it brought out another great yarn.

For years coho salmon fishing was very popular just below the dam at Berrien Springs. What made the crowds so large was that "snagging the fish" was legal back then. The inventions they used bordered on the unbelievable: three-prong hooks as big as a man's hand with a chunk of lead at the center was common. Fishermen would line up on both sides of the St. Joseph River below the dam — elbow to elbow — and besides the coho they would occasionally snag one of their fishing buddies.

At first, Dr. Cooke used plenty of lidocaine, cut the hook with a wire cutter — sometimes there were two of the three hooks imbedded beneath the skin — and then with a needle holder push the barb out through a new puncture wound.

One day he was reading The New England Journal of Medicine — the prestigious, up-to-date periodical — and came across an article written by an avid fisherman doctor who had been reading Field and Stream. There had been a piece written by a commercial fisherman. He described the lives of these men who went for days way out in the ocean east of New England before returning with their catch. When one of them encountered a fish hook, it was impossible to return in the middle of their run, so these guys had devised a method of flipping the hook out backward without tearing the flesh and with little or no pain. The doctor was so impressed, he tried it out on patients who came into his ER with the problem. He used the method on a significant number of patients, and then submitted the description of the method and it became an accepted surgical procedure. Of course Dr. Cooke had to try it out.

One day a father brought in a six-year-old kid with one of those monstrosities in the top of his head. He had two hooks imbedded under the scalp. Fortunately, his hair was cut short. Dr. Cooke asked the father to check in at admitting, and while he was gone, Dr. Cooke examined the hook. The fishing line was still attached to the eye of the hook, so he didn't have to insert a heavy nylon suture material to replace it. All he needed was a couple of pieces of string. It looked so easy, he couldn't resist. He flipped it out on the spot. The lad sat straight up with his mouth wide open, but without a sound. Popeyed, he felt the top of his head, and a big smile crossed his eyes. When his father returned, the boy was ready to leave. The thought crossed Dr. Cooke's mind that the father might object to paying the bill.

It didn't take long for Dr. Cooke to collect a number of fish-hook specimens to make an impressive display. Since leaving SWMC, Dr. Cooke hasn't seen many fish hooks. He has discussed the technique with a number of ER doctors and others, but he's never met one who has ever used it or even heard of it. For all he knows, it may be a lost art.

Mountaintop and Dark Valley

Being hired as medical director of Berrien County Infirmary, and hiring his staff in a single day with the first hot flame of vision — in retrospect, Dr. Cooke considers this his mountaintop moment. The beginning was the peak for him. After that, it was a struggle all the way through. It was one hassle after another.

Dr. Cooke's innovation and creativity had always led him to be current regarding surgical practice. These characteristics that attracted young physicians to learn by his side before leaving, well-prepared for anything, for the mission field, proved to be nearly fatal. His same larger-than-life persona led him to the edges of propriety both professionally and personally and eventually to behaviors not compatible with SWMC's environment. He made some serious mistakes that would shape his own future and, inevitably, change the future of SWMC as well.

As a result, around 1980, he left. Walking away from the medical clinic where he had invested decades of his heart and soul felt surreal. This was a dark time for him — the worst of several. He started out one day with a note in his pocket. His son had recently bought an old clunker for $150. What may have stopped Dr. Cooke was that he couldn't get the jalopy going fast enough. He had read a study suggesting that 50% of doctors who lost their license or their job attempted or succeeded suicide. He felt very alone.

God did not leave Dr. Cooke at the bottom of the valley without providing a way out. Through an old connection made at SWMC from years before, Dr. Cooke found himself practicing medicine at Indiana State Prison. While there, as well as enduring trials of many kinds, he found good counsel and, eventually, rejuvenation. After nine years, Dr. Cooke left the prison system to open a new clinic in Michigan City, Indiana.

Dr. Cooke has not performed major surgery since his days in Berrien Center, but now as an octogenarian he has a part-time, solo, general practice. He considers his subspecialty addictionology medicine — addictions recovery. Rather than seeking this subspecialty, Dr. Cooke senses that God handpicked him for the job. Since he was seeing so many narcotic-addicted patients, the topic was at the forefront of his mind. In 2007, he attended a conference in Chicago to understand the legal restraints and pitfalls related to the contact with and care of addicted individuals. He went from knowing practically nothing about addictionology to accepting patients from a radius, including Berrien County. Not many physicians in the area take on large numbers of narcotic-addicted patients. Dr. Cooke estimates that he has treated about 500 — not all to recovery.

In the process he learned a few things and saw what needy and desperate people these individuals tend to be. Face to face with a mission field, he met it head on. He organized NA (Narcotics Anonymous) meetings in his office twice a month. Using a Recovery Bible as the basis, he stresses there's only one way out of addictions, and the Higher Power is the God of the Bible. Some of the biblical content of the meetings is not so different from the content of the prayer meetings back in Berrien General Hospital.

Dr. Cooke looks back to those years and says, "God has been good to me, I don't know why. No reason. I ended up destroying a lot of people's faith. While I've had a charmed life, I've had my share of struggles. But if I look back and count the blessings, I have way more blessings than I deserve."

Dr. Cooke had weaknesses, flaws, but that's not what to remember. His story mirrors the triumphs and despair of many great people. Men who follow after God are not flawless. Let us remember them for the ways they allowed their Maker to shine through them. We remember King David not for his faults, but for his amazing accomplishments; and his son Solomon we revere not as the king who built the synagogue before he erected temples to other gods, but as the wisest man who ever lived. As Dr. Atkinson and others would agree, even amid desperation and despair, God's provision must be acknowledged and, indeed, becomes more visible.

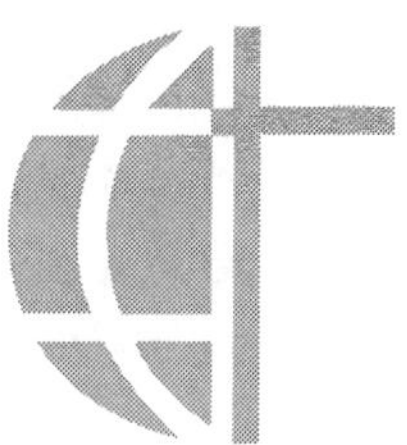

Chapter 17

Growth after Change

Chapter 17

Growth after Change

Dr. Bob Schindler was president of the clinic when Dr. Cooke left, but no one felt Dr. Cooke's absence more than Don Gast. "When Dr. Cooke left, I had more responsibility. Dr. Cooke had been doing so much, and now I had to do it. It took a lot of hours to keep things going. That was my responsibility," he said.

For 12 years, from the time he began with SWMC in 1972, Don never took a week off; he never took his family away; and he did this voluntarily to keep the momentum going. "The doctors also worked like that. Dr. Cooke was like that. Dr. Stephens is the same way," Don said. "It was my own commitment. They didn't drive me, they gave me the opportunity."

Not long after Dr. Cooke's departure, at one of Don's high school reunion banquets at Baroda, people kept saying, "Why are you still working for Southwestern?" The question began to eat away at him. In the middle of the night Don suffered from insomnia and doubt. He got out of bed and wrote down all the reasons why he was still working at the clinic. Once the list went down on paper, it renewed his resolve. Many times afterward he went back to that list.

Feeling God's provision in the midst of the difficult days, Don kept chugging away. "I brought my work home at night and over the weekend," he joked — quite literally, because often he and Jule hosted recruits in their basement.

"If I'd been smarter, I would've hired somebody else to help me. The clinic would've done that for me," he said, looking back. "But the ship was tight." He couldn't seriously consider adding another level of administration to the strained payroll.

Instead, he continued to grow the clinic. Don hired Dr. Daniel Metzger (1982-present), Dr. Ron Baker (1982-present); and Dr. Gregory L. Adams, a pediatrician. In 1983, God brought Dr. Kenneth J. O'Neill (1983-present), Dr. Thomas L. Ritter (1983-present), and Dr. Roy Ringenberg (1983-present). Tom Ritter said, "The summer Drs. O'Neill, Ringenberg and I came, the corporation had about a dozen doctors. The three of us that summer increased the corporation by about 25%."

In 1985, several more new faces came to SWMC: Dr. Charles B. Pierson and Dr. Richard Walton "Dick" Douce. And Dr. Lawrence "Larry" Cairns and Dr. Barb Boyd (1986-1991 and 2007-present) came in 1986. Dr. Georg Schultz and Dr. Andy Rutherford came in 1987, followed by Dr. Claire L. Scheele and Dr. Dan Stephens in 1989.

Dr. Cooke had been a one-man show, and after he had to leave, the clinic set up committees to keep the clinic going. Meetings were full of prayer and new ideas. Don called the committee chairs "the solid ones." They looked to each other as rocks, but ultimately looked to Christ the solid rock.

Dr. Ken O'Neill, who came in the summer of 1983, saw SWMC's transfer of leadership into a new model, from the visionary founder and a town-hall style of governance to a board of directors and committees. Whereas the event spurring this change was cataclysmic, the change itself was healthy for the organization to develop and grow. God used a difficult situation for His glory.

Another big simultaneous transition was the nationwide move in medicine from general practitioners to specialists. "In 1983, I was at the tail end of those transitions," Dr. O'Neill recalls. "General surgeons [at SWMC] were still seeing some people for physical exams. A lot of my patients were offloading from Dr. Schindler as he shifted" into administrative leadership and a solely surgical practice.

In 1983, Dr. Roland Stephens, as a general surgeon, was still taking care of patients in the hospital, such as pneumonia cases, but other doctors were beginning to push back. Internists started rounding. Dr. O'Neill did rounds at Berrien General, Memorial, and Mercy Hospital daily and was on call at all three hospitals. He didn't get to his office until 10:30 a.m.

Part of Dr. O'Neill's initial schedule involved emergency room work. Often he was on the telephone to other doctors for direction. But the shift to more specialty departments and segregation of duties started at Memorial and Mercy hospitals and percolated down to affect Southwestern Medical Clinic as well. Within a few years, by the mid-'80s, Dr. O'Neill no longer worked in the ER.

No longer running the hospital single-handedly on weekend and night shifts, Dr. O'Neill was able to focus on upgrading internal medical care in the area. Within a decade he followed Dr. Schindler's footsteps, splitting his time between administrative duties and his clinical practice.

From 1995-2005, he served as president of SWMC and also as medical director from 1998-present. In addition, he has sat on the executive committee and the board of directors of the local physician-hospital organization (PHO) Lakeland Care, Inc. since its formation in 1995. Dr. O'Neill also served as chairman of the ethics committee at Lakeland HealthCare, chairman of the department of medicine at Lakeland Medical Center, Berrien Center, and chairman of the department of medicine medical care evaluation committee at Lakeland Regional Medical Center, St. Joseph. On the board of directors of Lakeland Regional Health System, he serves on the board's strategic planning committee. Meanwhile he has fitted in short-term mission trips to Kenya, Haiti, Romania, and Pakistan.

Dr. O'Neill remembers that Dr. Schindler often talked about the genius and stupidity of combining missions and business. SWMC is a for-profit business that functions in many ways like a faith-based, not-for-profit organization. This dualism is both a strength and a source of internal conflict.

The way Dr. O'Neill sees it, the tabletop of SWMC's mission statement rests on two pillars: a financially successful business, and an organization whose focus is to support missions. Reading bestselling business writer Jim Collins' book "Built to Last" about long-term, successful business processes, Dr. O'Neill had several epiphanies regarding SWMC. Collins mentions two components of successful long-term businesses that SWMC clearly portrays: first, a clear sense of vision apart from making money that gives the organization its sense of identity. Second, the ability to bring together unique, compelling, and often seemingly mutually exclusive characteristics. These components resonated with Dr. O'Neill.

When the clinic directors wrote and later revised its mission statement, they clearly saw those components as the core of the clinic. They reduced the clinic's purpose into one easy-to-grasp sentence: "SWMC, by God's grace and following the example of Jesus Christ, strives to be a distinctive role model and leader in the integration of medical care, Christian witness, and missions."

When Dr. O'Neill first came, "the whole notion of governance was vague and muddled, with no clear mission statement. The leadership changed from visionary founder to town hall style, from family to board of directors to integrated health system. All of these changes were done with some fear and trepidation. Even when we were converting to the board of directors, there was a lot of discussion. Looking back, these changes were inevitable. We're living the next chapter now."

Sheila Lavallee Kipp lived through SWMC's transition from a small clinic to a corporation. When she started, SWMC had a staff of 70. When she left full time in 2007, the clinic had 350 on its payroll, and as director of human resources, she had interviewed most of them and knew them all.

Sheila started in mid-1986 as a Medicare billing clerk and rose through the ranks to director of human resources and head of risk management and a member of the senior leadership team.

She first worked in the Ferry Street office in Berrien Springs during a practicum in college. Don Gast told her, "When you get through school, give me a call."

She did. She started at "Location 10," the billing office on Dean's Hill Road, where administration worked too at that time. Doctors and nurses also worked in the front of that building. In that environment with so many people and departments, she observed the gears that made the corporation turn.

In 1986 when she started, about 17 doctors worked stateside. Dr. Ken O'Neill had joined two years prior. Drs. Bob Patton and Weldon Cooke had just left when she came.

The clinic worked out of Berrien Center, Berrien Springs, Stevensville, and Bridgman. At that time there was no Women's Center or St. Joseph. With four locations, it was not as difficult to maintain a clinic-wide family environment. As the clinic grew, each location began to develop its individual culture, its own family atmosphere. Each location began to celebrate its own birthdays and significant events the way the entire clinic had done when it was smaller.

Sheila remembers that as the clinic swelled and these mini-cultures began to develop, Dr. Herb Atkinson, who may still have been chief of staff at the time, set up weekly prayer groups at each location, and he attended them all. People were not offended, since the prayer groups were optional.

People also were not offended because Dr. A was Dr. A. He was a big lovable teddy bear, a Colonel Sanders. He even looked like Colonel Sanders, and he knew it. He loved people. People appreciated him because he was an old-time country doctor. He spent time listening to people. His waiting room could be an hour and a half behind, but his patients didn't mind, because after that long wait they got to spend time with him. More recently there has been an attempt to hold quarterly corporate worship. But it is difficult for all to come from so many locations to this corporate worship meeting.

When Sheila started, Don held monthly corporate business meetings as well. They got together to cover business, read missionary letters, and make major decisions together. Later, they also distributed information about what the board of directors was doing. In the meeting room by the cafeteria, Don sat near the head of the table along the side. Ruthie Leer, Carol Gonnerman, and Sheila all sat close to Don to help do whatever Don needed. Ruthie took the minutes. Doctors sat willy-nilly, wherever they could sit, and some never sat at all. They were on call, so they were coming and going during the meeting. A nasally voice would page overhead, and someone jumped to their feet and took off.

Devotions were upstairs in a small room in the old hospital. The education room, where they conducted staff orientation (a few times a year, with 12-15 people) and OSHA (Occupational Safety and Health Administration, government regulations) training, was above the laundry in the old hospital. The whole room would vibrate and all the materials jiggled when the old industrial driers came on.

While staff had been oriented for years, SWMC had no real formal doctor orientation until around 2005. Doctors were expected just to be able to jump in. As Sheila saw it, trial by fire is generally not good for physicians. In the clinics, the doctors did get some general orientation, usually a run-through of the physical layout the first weekend. The first weekend after they moved, new doctors were generally on call. SWMC was so short-staffed waiting for the new doctor that when he finally came everyone was like, "You're here! Yippee! You're on call!"

When they first came, a doctor and his family could be living at Don and Jule Gasts'. Don recruited, entertained, and helped them look for a car and house. Jule could be taking the doctor's wife out shopping and setting up bank accounts. Don worked around the clock. Don set the pace, with an unspoken statement, "This is how you're going to work."

In the old days surgeons did a lot of family practice, even staffed the ER. A couple of surgeons came out to this rural clinic, and it just wasn't for them. They liked missions but couldn't handle the pace. SWMC physicians did a lot for the team. When the hospital was short, they'd often have to cover two extra shifts a week. Sheila would be calling, begging people for coverage, joking, "I'm not a doctor. I can't cover it! You've got to help!"

At a clinic where missionaries came and went often without much warning, and where the whole staff lived with a sort of maverick mentality, as director of human resources Sheila compared her job to herding cats. When hiring, SWMC made a practice to hold two interviews. Sheila usually got the follow-up interview, she said, "because I could catch things." Sheila wanted to see that they loved healthcare, that they had a spirit of determination, and that they had compatibility in addition to skill. She didn't want to see a long history of job turnover. Do they have schedule flexibility? The walk-in clinics close at 8 p.m., so staff didn't leave until 9 or 9:30.

"Usually if I was unsure about a person and the clinic went ahead anyway, he or she didn't last six months," Sheila observed. "But it became evident throughout the course of time that God had place-holders sometimes, holding the position for the right person to come."

Ever since Carol Gonnerman Jewell started working at SWMC in August 1989, she always thought she would get to Tenwek Hospital. She'd even seriously contemplated retiring there. SWMC gave her many opportunities and memories, but she never got to Kenya at all.

She had a better job offer at the Point o' Woods Country Club, but she knew what kind of men Dr. Atkinson and Dr. Schindler were, and she was never sorry she took the medical clinic instead of the golf course. Virginia Stover was retiring. Ginny had come from a banking background; Carol Gonnerman's background was accounting, "and poor Don Gast had to try to figure things out," Carol recalled.

When Carol came, the accounts payable books were hand-tabulated. Accounts receivable had a computer, but across the hall all the checks were still written by hand. Carol felt transported into the Dark Ages. Only a few weeks after she started, she began talking to Don about getting a computer. His eyes glazed over. Carol knew the company needed to update, so instead of closing her mouth, she found other sets of ears. First she prayed: "Lord, if they can't get a computer by the beginning of the year, I've come to the wrong place." Then she talked to the administrative doctors. By October, they gave her permission to purchase a computer with the accounting software she thought would fit.

In January, they ran a parallel hand and computer system and everything balanced out perfectly.

When she applied for the job, she answered a blind ad in the Herald-Palladium. She sent her resume to a post office box. She had worked for another company for 37 years. The company had been sold, and employees who were over age 50 weren't needed by the new company. Carol was 54. Everyone said, "You'll never find a job." She was temping for the sheriff's department but needed a job with benefits.

The blind ad was for accounts receivable. Russ Bruce got Carol's application and took it to Don, knowing Ginny was retiring. Don never told Carol how much he was going to pay her. She had the offer from Point o' Woods Country Club. When Point o'Woods gave her an ultimatum, she told them she had another job, but Don hadn't called her back yet! She felt in her heart that SWMC was the place for her. In the end, SWMC gave her five thousand less than Point o'Woods had offered, but that's where she wanted to be. She wanted the great joy of working on Dean's Hill Road in the wintertime.

Carol remembered that Dr. Schindler had a "Rule of 72." If there was a disagreement, or a fight, wait at least 72 hours before doing anything. Write a letter maybe, to get emotion off your chest, he said, but don't send it until you wait 72 hours. Carol considers that some of the best advice she ever received.

After Dr. Schindler died, people often dealt with issues by asking, "What would Dr. Schindler do? What would Dr. Schindler say?"

Despite the endless financial tight spots at SWMC, Carol saw God's hand clearly in the midst of it.

Because the doctors felt called to see a lot of Medicaid patients, cash flow was always a problem. Almost every month, the clinic worried about having enough money to meet its obligations. One time the state and feds were very slow sending Medicaid/Medicare money. On her office door, Carol drew a couple of thermometers, one measuring Medicare and one Medicaid, showing how much was owed and how much was received. In administrative meetings, it was a matter of earnest prayer to get that money in. It always came in; maybe just in time, but it did come in. It was a community effort of prayer, and the doctors were keenly aware of it. They came face-to-face with those thermometers every time they went into Carol's office to pick up their paycheck. They walked by the thermometers when they stopped in to talk to Don Gast or Warren White.

Carol got to know many of the physicians that way. Dr. Keith Van Oosterhout, who can come across initially as quiet and aloof, "has a dry sense of humor and is a gem of a man," Carol said, and he always liked to come see her and the rest of the administrative staff when he picked up his paycheck.

Doctors sometimes get a bad rap for their impersonal bedside manner, but Carol saw the opposite in SWMC physicians. They deeply cared for their patients, just as they loved each other. During the Rwandan massacre, the physicians were concerned about Dr. Al Snyder's safety. They were glued to the news and craved updates from anyone. Don called Dr. Snyder's mission organization several times on the urgent request of the other doctors, and whenever Don heard anything, he immediately relayed it to the physicians and staff.

Even on days when no 7 a.m. prayer meeting was on the schedule, most of the staff was in the office before 7 a.m., updating each other on news needing prayer. When the Ivory Coast was bombarded, even if Dr. John Slater wasn't there, it was his mission field, so everyone felt compelled to pray earnestly. The Schindlers were in Africa when it was frequently ravaged by tribal violence.

Something was always going on somewhere in the world and needed to be taken to the Lord. Carol felt it was her privilege and honor to work for such a dedicated and professional group of people. She thought it was just a matter of time until integration with Cedarwood Medical Clinic or some other merger, or until the clinic would have to close. She figured Cedarwood with its flashy team of specialists and new building would succeed abundantly. When it failed, she found it interesting that SWMC survived.

Carol had always thought she would go to Tenwek Hospital in Kenya. She thought for sure when she retired she'd have time to go. Suddenly after retirement, she had knee replacement surgery, and then she got married and that changed everything. She never got to Africa. But she did get to work at SWMC with some of the "greatest people in the world," as a second career and a second chance. She receives prayer letters and updates from SWMC physicians on mission, so a decade after retirement, her globe-trotting prayers do the traveling, both short-term and long-term.

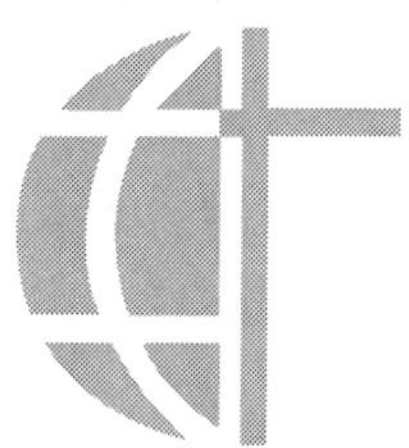

Chapter 18

Stories of Devotions and Devotion on Monday Morning and Always

Chapter 18

Stories of Devotions and Devotion on Monday Morning and Always

Dr. Richard R. Roach, an internist, worked at SWMC from 1978-1992. One time he referred a patient with carpal tunnel syndrome to Dr. Schindler. Later, Dr. Schindler told Dr. Roach about an unexpected complication during the procedure. The patient came into surgery and received only local anesthesia, so she was wide awake. Dr. Schindler eased into his chair to begin the surgery.

"Oh, no, you don't," the patient said.

Dr. Schindler rose from his chair. "What's wrong? Did you decide not to have surgery?"

"You have to sing before you do surgery," she said.

So Dr. Schindler took a deep breath and launched into a solo of "How Great Thou Art." When he was done the patient settled down, ready for surgery.

While at SWMC, Dr. Roach also befriended Dr. Doug Taylor, who had worked 25 to 30 years in Zululand. He still worked at SWMC into his 70s in order to set up his retirement. Dr. Roach invited Dr. Taylor to his house to watch "The Gods Must Be Crazy", a movie about Zululand. Dr. Taylor laughed so hard watching the movie that Dr. Roach was concerned he would have a heart attack. Still holding his chest, Dr. Taylor exclaimed, "Everything that happened in the movie has happened to me."

"Even cranking your jeep up a tree?" asked Dr. Roach.

"Yes, even that."

Dr. Taylor never tired of adventure. Dr. Roach had grown up in northern Minnesota and worked as a professional canoe guide in the Boundary Waters Canoe Area. When he offered to lead a Boundary Waters canoe trip with Five Pines Christian Camp, Dr. Taylor was eager to join the group. Against his better judgment, Dr. Roach agreed that he could come.

Several days into the trip, they were paddling upstream to reach a portage. They had two options: straight ahead was an easier paddle, but a longer portage trail. Around a bend, there was a shorter portage, but the current was strong and unpredictable. It was a difficult paddle against the swirling water around a rocky point.

Dr. Taylor wanted to try the shorter portage. Although Dr. Roach had serious concerns about it, Dr. Taylor was with two expert paddlers, so he allowed them to try. Dr. Roach, with his novice group from Five Pines, took the longer portage. He had hoisted the canoe on his shoulders when out of the corner of his eye he saw Dr. Taylor's overturned canoe drift by. As the empty canoe shot downstream, Dr. Roach spotted the two other paddlers, but not Dr. Taylor.

Dr. Roach ran to shore, threw his canoe into the water, grabbed one of his novice paddlers, and paddled furiously to Dr. Taylor's overturned canoe. They searched for Dr. Taylor, but there was no sign of him. Fearing the worst, Dr. Roach's mind reeled. Why had he let Dr. Taylor take the more difficult route? Why had he even let the 70-year-old, irreplaceable doctor and friend come along?

Early June in Minnesota, the river was ice cold. Minutes passed. Someone shouted. Halfway downstream, Dr. Taylor popped up, as purple as a grape. He hauled himself onto a grassy island, and Dr. Roach and his partner swept downstream to pick him up. Dr. Taylor was shivering and shaking, purple from head to toe.

"Are you pretty cold?" Dr. Roach asked.

Teeth chattering, Dr. Taylor grinned. "No, this always happens when I take my Inderol."

Perhaps at that moment it was Dr. Roach who needed blood pressure medication more than his elder friend.

Dr. Taylor really was irreplaceable as a colleague and friend. Once, Dr. Roach had a patient with a seizure disorder. He put her on Dilantin, which controlled her seizures, but she developed Stevens-Johnson syndrome. She sloughed skin from her whole body and she was critically ill. Stevens-Johnson syndrome has a 20% mortality rate, but she survived, treated with steroids and IV therapy, and got her skin back without scars. Obviously, she couldn't take Dilantin anymore. So Dr. Roach consulted a neurologist in Kalamazoo. "What other drug will control her seizures without developing Stevens-Johnson syndrome?"

The neurologist recommended Tegretol. About a month later she had had no seizures, but her skin started getting red. Dr. Roach took her off the medication. He met with her and her husband and told them, "I don't know of any seizure medication that's safe for her. I think it's better not to treat the seizure disorder with medication. Stay well rested and avoid alcohol and caffeine."

She accepted the advice, but her husband became quite upset. He said the seizures really scared her. About three weeks later, Dr. Taylor was staffing the emergency department. He paged Dr. Roach. Rather than answer the page, Dr. Roach saw it was the emergency department and to save time, he just ran down.

Entering the ER, Dr. Roach came into trouble. The husband saw Dr. Roach. His wife had suffered another seizure. He yanked the electrical conduit off the wall and came after Dr. Roach to spear him. "I'm going to kill you, Dr. Roach!"

Like a flash, Dr. Taylor disarmed him and pinned him on the floor. He asked Dr. Roach, "Why did you come down here? Why didn't you answer my page? I was paging you to tell you to stay away from the ER!"

Dr. Roach stood in awe. "How did you get him on the floor so fast?"

"Oh, I've dealt with lots of Zulu warriors," the silver-haired doctor said with a smile.

Physicians took turns leading Bible studies on Monday mornings. In Zululand, Dr. Taylor traveled the country to meet his patients. He slept in their huts and spent weeks at a time in the outlying villages. When it was Dr. Taylor's turn to lead devotions, he decided to talk about Psalm 23. It's not a very long psalm and well known already to the SWMC physicians. For some, it might not have been enough material for the entire hour. But Dr. Taylor had uncommon applicable knowledge. He started going through the psalm, telling stories about the Zulu shepherds to illustrate each verse. An hour later, Dr. Taylor was only halfway through the psalm, still telling stories. Everybody was fascinated, but they had surgery to attend to and patients to see. So, they asked him to continue the next Monday. The next week, he again took the whole hour sharing subtle nuances of the psalm. He could've continued another hour. Everyone agreed that it was the most magnificent dissertation they'd ever heard on the psalm. The 23rd Psalm would never be the same for those in attendance.

As Dr. Roach recalls, it was not Ken Taylor's brother but Dr. Wesche who was the first SWMC physician to present devotions from The Living Bible. Long before versions other than King James were widely read, Dr. Wesche habitually used The Living Bible. Dr. Wesche said the other versions were too hard for him to understand. It amazed his colleagues. Most thought of him as a spiritually profound person and were shocked that other versions taxed his understanding. An enriching exposure, it opened their hearts to take an interest in Bible translations and versions beyond the King James Version.

Even in a blizzard, Dr. Wesche came to work in a short-sleeved white shirt. As far as Dr. Roach can remember, Dr. Wesche never wore a coat in Berrien Springs. When asked, he said he was enjoying the cold weather, a refreshing contrast to Kenya.

Of all the miracles Dr. Roach witnessed, none was more vividly imprinted on his memory than Alma Fredrickson. Alma told Dr. Roach, "If you ever tell anyone my story, make sure you use my real name."

Alma came to Dr. Roach complaining of nausea. A CT scan illuminated a mass in her pancreas. Dr. Roach referred her to Dr. Wesche for a Whipple procedure. Dr. Wesche performed a laparotomy and found a pancreatic cancer with multiple metastases all over the liver and a sprinkling of metastases in the omentum. She was full of cancer.

Dr. Wesche saw it was futile to do any surgery, so he just sewed her back up. When she came out of anesthesia, he told her she had pancreatic cancer and didn't have long to live. Dr. Ray Lord, a Christian oncologist from Kalamazoo, came to do a consult. He told her honestly that he knew of nothing to cure her cancer, but if she wanted, he could give her some chemotherapy to see if it might give her a little bit of benefit. Alma agreed. She came every other week for her chemotherapy. She always ate a McDonald's hamburger before she came. She said the chemotherapy made her nauseated and she always threw up after the treatment, so eating the greasy hamburger wouldn't hurt her. This went on for months. The prognosis for metastatic pancreatic cancer is about three months.

After nearly six months, Alma was still walking into the office, symptom-free except nausea from the chemotherapy. She wasn't even taking pain medicine. She asked him once, "Dr. Roach, how long do I have to live?"

"Alma, you were supposed to have died three months ago," he told her honestly.

She found that hysterical. "God has work for me to do, so I won't die until I finish it."

From Benton Harbor, Alma owned her own home and was a solid Christian witness in her African-American community. He asked, "What work does God have you doing?"

"I plucked a prostitute off the street, brought her into my home, and I've been sharing the Gospel with her. She has accepted Christ as her Savior, and I'm teaching her to live as a Christian."

This gave Dr. Roach pause. One day several weeks later, the telephone rang for him. Alma invited him and Dorothy, the receptionist at the Benton Harbor clinic, over during their lunch break. Alma's house was immaculate, and she was feeling great. Dr. Roach and Dorothy met the young woman Alma was mentoring in the Christian faith. A sincere, most gracious young lady, she testified that Alma had changed her life. She told Dr. Roach, "Without Ms. Fredrickson, I would be dead today."

Eighteen months after Alma's cancer diagnosis, while she was receiving her chemotherapy, a nurse pulled Dr. Roach aside. "You need to go see Alma."

He interrupted his rounds and went down to her room. She was sobbing. "Alma, what's the matter?"

She huffed, "Dr. Roach, don't you think I can grieve my own death?"

Dr. Roach took a step back. "If you want to, go ahead!"

"Well, I'm done now," she retorted, and in an instant her grief was gone.

The next morning on hospital rounds she said, "Dr. Roach, I want to tell you I have finished teaching that girl everything I know. I have nothing more to teach her. Tomorrow I will die."

"Alma, are you having a lot of pain?"

"No, I feel fine," she said.

The next morning, Alma was comatose. Later that day she was gone.

If SWMC hadn't ministered to all in the name of Christ, if SWMC doctors hadn't taken time to get to know their patients' spiritual commitments, Dr. Roach wouldn't even have known Alma's story or so many others. Alma's was only one example.

Neighbors Dr. Roach and Dr. Ron Baker used to go running together down favorite trails and quiet roads before 6 a.m. and then have time to start reading EKGs by 7. Dr. Baker lived in Sierra Leone for many years and was fluent in Mende. They ran fast enough for exercise, but Dr. Baker could still talk because he loved to tell stories. One day he unconsciously slipped into Mende. It was a funny story, and when he finished he started laughing. He couldn't understand why Richard wasn't laughing with him. "Didn't you think that was funny?"

"Ron, I don't know Mende," Dr. Roach reminded him. Their laughter echoed down the ravine.

Many stories have been told so many times they've become legends. Dr. Atkinson was a great storyteller. One time when Dr. Roach and Dr. A were on call together, the former Belgian Congo came up. Dr. Atkinson had worked there during the 1967 Katamba revolution, seeking freedom from Belgium. Hundreds of Belgians were killed, and Dr. A had two Belgian friends he was helping to escape. In his Land Rover they drove through 16 roadblocks while trying to get those two guys out of harm's way.

The seventeenth roadblock wasn't just wooden; the rebels had stones piled up across the road. It was the last roadblock before getting out of the Congo, and Dr. A couldn't run it. The rebel army stopped the car. They grabbed Dr. A and hustled him to the sergeant. The sergeant started talking to him, found out he spoke English and French like a Belgian, and ordered his soldiers to execute him.

Within minutes, they shoved Dr. A in front of the firing squad. While the soldiers were loading their guns, Dr. A heard them talking the tribal language in the Congo. He said in their native language, "Why are you shooting a friend?"

Hearing him speak their language fluently, the soldiers refused to shoot. The sergeant got really angry. He went to the commanding officer, complaining about the soldiers refusing to shoot. "Bring the prisoner to me," the commanding officer ordered.

The sergeant yanked Dr. Atkinson into the room and dropped him at the commander's feet. When the commander looked at Dr. A, he broke into laughter. Dr. Atkinson had done hernia surgery on him and had given him a Bible. The commander had him untied and let him take his Belgian friends around the roadblock and exit the country.

Dr. Roach remembered SWMC as a wild place. One time at Berrien General Hospital, a man came running in breathless. "I need a chest x-ray," he said.

Dr. Roach said, "Let me check you over and then we'll see. Here, sit down."

"No, out in the parking lot!" the man gasped.

Dr. Roach said, "This is highly unusual. Slow down and tell me about it."

"It's not for me," the guy said emphatically. "It's for a horse!"

The man was a local veterinarian. He suspected the horse had pneumonia, but did not have equine x-ray equipment at the veterinarian hospital. He knew the hospital had a portable x-ray machine, so he had transported the horse to the hospital parking lot. Dr. Roach determined this was worth the trouble to don a lead vest, quiet the veterinarian, calm the horse, wheel the machine into the parking lot, hold the machine still in just the right position, and take the x-ray.

The horse did have pneumonia, which showed up on the film and allowed the veterinarian to give proper antibiotics. The horse recovered.

Not long afterward, Dr. Roach was appointed chief of staff and Dr. Atkinson was assistant chief of staff. Sometimes these places of leadership required tough skin. They had to lead the clinic through uncharted deep waters, and it required a lot of prayer. A brilliant, innovative surgeon, Dr. Cooke's innovation and creativity had always led him to be state of the art in surgical practice. But this time, as explained earlier, a critical mistake got Dr. Cooke in trouble.

Dr. Cooke lost his hospital privileges, and then lost his license, and the whole clinic felt their founder's pain. People were bewildered, aghast. It was hard to know what to do. But when Dr. Cooke lost his privileges, a bell tolled. According to the SWMC bylaws, one had to have privileges in Berrien General Hospital to be part of the corporation. By the bylaws of the corporation, Dr. Cooke could no longer be a SWMC member. Dr. Cooke had been one of four people who had written those bylaws!

Financially, the clinic struggled to stay afloat. It was a time of emotional and spiritual soul-searching. They refused to give up, grasping at every possible bit of assistance. An efficiency expert spent two weeks reviewing the clinic's function. He couldn't find anything to make the clinic more efficient and charged SWMC $4,000 for his time. He said SWMC was by far the most efficient clinic he'd ever evaluated in his career.

Regardless of efficiency, money got tighter at the clinic. Medicaid was paying SWMC $11 a visit. It cost more to get a haircut in Berrien Springs than SWMC was getting in patient reimbursement. When Dr. Richard Roach left, it was for two reasons: he was exhausted, and his salary had slowly been trimmed to half of his initial pay. The salary cut was not an efficiency problem, but because the government came up with all kinds of reasons not to reimburse for complex care.

Dr. Roach and his staff had wonderful times, but their Benton Harbor clinic literally went bankrupt. They just couldn't support that office anymore, and it really seemed Dr. Roach's time at SWMC had run out.

After Dr. Roach left, Don Gast went to Lansing. In Lansing they told him they would not reimburse any more until the clinic provided statistics on how many Medicare and Medicaid patients SWMC was seeing. Don collected the data to verify that SWMC was caring for 40% of those patients in three counties. Lansing's response: "We'll pay you $35 per visit, but you have to see all of those patients in one clinic."

It was inconceivable that needy patients across Berrien, Van Buren, and Cass counties had to travel to a single location to see a physician. Dr. Roach still believes this was the predicament that became the impetus for the formation of InterCare. SWMC physician's assistant John Kittredge had a yearning to help these patients, and Don saw that. So InterCare, which developed as a separate community health center not connected to SWMC, acquired SWMC's financially beleaguered Benton Harbor clinic (and eventually InterCare convinced the state to allow satellite offices in other parts of the tri-county area).

Dr. Roach believed that his leaving caused a crisis that, in the end, benefited the clinic and his patients. Now practicing internal medicine and directing the tropical medicine teaching program about an hour away at Michigan State University's Kalamazoo Center, Dr. Roach maintains good relationships with everyone at SWMC. Since moving out of the area, he no longer leads Five Pines canoe trips, but he still takes private groups every year. Dr. Baker and Dr. Ken O'Neill have gone on canoe trips with him.

An important part of being an SWMC physician has always been to go where their partners were working worldwide, to help staff their clinics for them whenever needed. Dr. Roach still takes short-term medical trips, mostly now to Madagascar. While at SWMC, he traveled short-term to see Dr. Baker in Sierra Leone, then to see Dr. Wesche in Kenya, and once even took his wife and kids along to help Dr. Al Snyder in Rwanda for four months.

Dr. Roach ran the tuberculosis and internal medicine program while Dr. Al Snyder did surgery for those four months, about five years before the Rwandan Holocaust. When the holocaust happened, the Roaches' beloved housekeeper Marceline, their cook and his nurse translator, were all killed in the first four days. Dr. Roach's daughter cried for two days straight when she heard that Marceline had been killed. Like tree roots, friendships run deep in rugged places.

One Christmas, it was Dr. Roach's turn to lead Monday morning devotions. He passed around slips of paper with references to 21 Old

Testament verses. Perplexed, the physicians looked up the verses and read them aloud. Finally, Dr. O'Neill piped up, "These verses don't have anything to do with each other, and furthermore, they have nothing to do with Christmas!"

"That's exactly what I wanted you to say," Dr. Roach said. "Does everyone agree with Ken? Turn to St. Luke."

They recited Mary's magnificat. Phrase after phrase, it became clear that Mary quoted the Old Testament in her famous song of praise, and Dr. Roach merely had them read the original passages first.

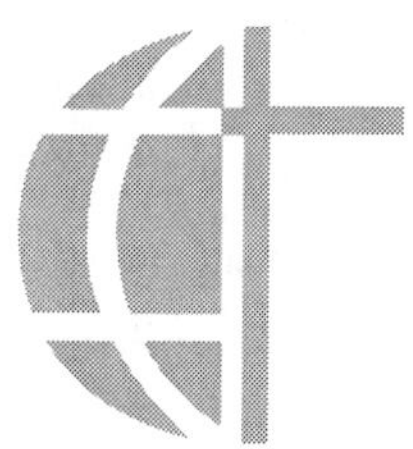

Chapter 19

Bridgman

Chapter 19

Bridgman

Southwestern Medical Clinic opened "The Cave" in late 1973. Located underneath dentists Drs. Dale and Neal Smith's office in the Colonial Professional Building on Toth Street in Bridgman, it was SWMC's third satellite (counting the office next door to Berrien General Hospital and downtown Berrien Springs).

Affectionately nicknamed "The Cave" because of its dank, windowless basement location, it was a part-time location for seven of SWMC's 12 stateside physicians. A Herald-Palladium article announcing the opening listed Dr. E. Dewain Silvernale, pediatrician; Dr. Herbert A. Atkinson, general practice; Dr. William F. Douce, general practice; Dr. Charles Rhodes, family practitioner with certification in general surgery; Dr. James L. Wierman, internal medicine; Dr. Roland R. Stephens, general surgery; and Dr. Kenley F. Burkhart, general surgery. These doctors traveled to all three locations and also helped staff Berrien General Hospital.

The staff at the Bridgman office included Cheryl Baggett, who has been a nurse with SWMC for more than three decades, probably the longest nursing tenure at SWMC. Others included Dr. Barb Boyd, specializing in pediatrics and internal medicine. She felt called to help the less fortunate and is continuing her local mission with InterCare. Another is Nancy Labis, long-time Bridgman clinic director.

Another of the Bridgman office's gems was radiology technologist Marilyn Willeman, RT. She came from Berrien General Hospital to the Bridgman office, where she worked until 2011 when mammography was discontinued at Bridgman. Patients loved Marilyn's gentle yet exacting personality. When she left, several patients said, "I don't want a mammogram unless I can find where Marilyn is."

For three years Dr. Helene Johnson and her midwives Esther Triphan, Cathy McDonough, and Betsy Zech brought energy and lots of new little customers to the Bridgman office.

Elaine Starbuck became acquainted with SWMC in the early 1990s. At the time she worked at Hooks Drug in downtown Stevensville, which involved delivering injectables to SWMC's clinics. Elaine took a position with

SWMC at the Berrien Springs pediatric clinic in 1996. When that clinic was closed, she transferred to Stevensville, then to Bridgman as a receptionist. She has also worked with medical records and insurance referrals. Some of her fondest memories involve parties and picnics. She'll never forget Dr. Schultz sitting on a toilet seat onstage, telling funny Christmas stories. She also remembers potlucks at the Berrien Springs river park, and playing softball with Dr. Brad Ferrari. The family atmosphere at SWMC cemented loyalties.

Staff doesn't forget the accommodations physicians would make to help employees in need. Long after their children are grown, staff can talk about the doctors who invited them to bring their kids to staff meetings and let them play on the floor so the mothers could attend the meeting. When children of staff members were sick, they could hang out for a few hours in an unused exam room while their mom worked. If mothers needed to drop down to part-time, doctors understood. If mothers needed to work extra hours, doctors supported that, too.

Leslie Tate, former Bridgman office manager, once learned of a local church youth group looking for ways to raise money for a short-term mission trip. Instead of paying a professional painter, she hired them to paint the staff's break room.

Cathy Erickson

Cathy Erickson has been a nurse with SWMC since 1991. Susan Newcomer trained Cathy before transferring north to the Stevensville clinic. One day Don Gast brought around a new doctor. Dr. Atkinson walked up and shook the doctor's hand. "Hi, I'm Herb Atkinson. How are you serving our Lord today?"

Just an observer, Cathy was challenged by the question. She decided on that day that she wanted always to be involved in some sort of ministry, to have an answer if Dr. A ever asked her. Another time, Dr. Atkinson told someone within earshot of Cathy, "I'm Herb Atkinson. What did our Lord teach you this morning in your time with Him?" From that moment, Cathy made a point in her morning devotions to learn something applicable to life every day and take that lesson with her into the office.

Dr. Atkinson had not directed those questions to the nurse charting halfway down the hall. He probably wasn't even aware she was listening.

God used those two questions to change how Cathy lives. Another morning Cathy and Penny Vollman, the receptionist, were opening the office for the day when in rushed a pregnant mom. One of Dr. A's obstetrics patients, she was in her third pregnancy. Knowing she was in labor, she'd dropped her children off at a sitter and ran another errand before coming to the office. By then, labor had progressed considerably.

Dr. Atkinson was at the hospital. Clearly, the woman wasn't going to deliver at the hospital. Cathy helped the woman into a room, and there wasn't time for much else. "God delivered the baby. I just caught it," Cathy says.

Cathy found out later that the woman had suffered complications with her second delivery. The next Mother's Day, the baby's mother sent Cathy a Mother's Day card.

This was Cathy's first solo delivery. She wasn't even Dr. Atkinson's nurse at the time; she was working with Dr. Rhodes. That early in the morning she was the only nurse in the clinic. She suggested splitting the delivery fee with Dr. Atkinson — she teased that it would've been fair to get half.

In 1996, the Bridgman office moved from The Cave to a renovated Tru-Value hardware store on Red Arrow Highway. A pole barn in the rear of the property converted into a storage space for missionaries' furniture.

The former plumbing section in the hardware store became the procedure room Dr. Rhodes used for doing vasectomies. One day, mid-procedure, he accidentally set some gauze on fire with the electric cautery. Without raising an eyebrow, he flipped the fiery gauze off the table, and his nurse, Barb Opelt, stomped it out. Not a word was said. The procedure continued as if nothing had happened. The patient never knew a thing.

The Bridgman clinic staffs often start the day with prayer. "It's amazing how God takes care of your day when you start that way," Cathy says. "A patient will come in without any specific complaints. He just doesn't feel normal. Something tells you to do an EKG. Lo and behold, you find out the poor guy is having a heart attack. God takes care of us. He protects and carries the whole clinic. If you're running behind, a patient will forget her appointment and not show up, and you'll actually be ahead of schedule. Someone will walk in with a bloody towel and you have the time to help him without disregarding any scheduled patients. These are the kinds of daily miracles we experience — or maybe notice — because we prayed."

Other miracle stories are often just as subtle. An older gentleman was told a shattering diagnosis. His doctor advised him to get things in order: his life expectancy at that point was six months. Five years later, the gentleman served as primary caregiver for his ill wife. There was no medical explanation for his endurance.

Mary Beth Good, PA-C

Mary Beth Good, PA-C (physician's assistant-certified) heard about SWMC through Drs. Mark and Donna Harrison. She called Don Gast in 1995 to ask about an internship rotation with Dr. Atkinson. Dr. Atkinson was a terrific mentor, and Mary Beth found SWMC a great fit with her passion for missions.

Interestingly enough, while she has not yet taken a short-term mission trip with SWMC, Mary Beth has been to Honduras several times with Great Lakes Eyecare. Great Lakes Eyecare, located on Niles Road in St. Joseph, is not directly affiliated with SWMC, but its founder, Dr. David Cooke, is one of Dr. Weldon Cooke's sons. Mary Beth had lived in Honduras for a year in 1993 when she heard that Dr. David Cooke regularly traveled to Honduras, she asked if he could use her help.

At the time Mary Beth Good formally joined SWMC in 1996, the clinic had fewer than a handful of physician assistants, called in the industry mid-level providers. She says SWMC physicians have always treated her as a colleague and have continued to hire more PAs.

In Mary Beth's view, another of SWMC's inclusive concepts is the counseling department. Counseling services were developed at SWMC in the 1970s. At that time very few medical clinics had their own counseling department, and fewer still offered Christian counseling. Rarer still has always been the camaraderie among physicians and counselors, the sharing of input and referrals that benefit clients.

Dr. Marcia Wiinamaki, PsyD, is the director of SWMC Christian counseling and psychological services at SWMC. She oversees counseling at three locations: Stevensville, Berrien Springs, and Niles. She coordinates six counselors: Richard A. Watson, Mary Frank, Flori Mejeur, Nancy Tripp, Edie Zars, and Ron Phillips.

Dr. Jon Osburn

When Dr. Jon Osburn joined SWMC and began working at the Bridgman clinic in 2002, he inherited some of Dr. Atkinson's and Dr. Holly

Tapley's family medicine patients. One of Dr. Osburn's patients, an octogenarian, has seen SWMC physicians since the group formed. He has kept mementos of the clinic throughout the years and one day he brought an old brochure in for Dr. Osburn to read, featuring a very young-looking Dr. A.

During Dr. A's funeral at Woodland Shores, people shared the many ways he had quietly helped them. The full extent of Dr. Atkinson's influence is impossible to measure. On his way home he would stop to visit patients and former patients. At one house, he trimmed a friend's toenails. At another, he listened and prayed. He poked his head into offices and said hello to many. Every office where Dr. Atkinson ever worked claims him as one of their grandfathers.

Dr. Chuck Pierson is another Bridgman grandfather. "Papa Pierson" is always brimming with stories. When he worked at Bridgman, he always had time to go up front and socialize.

Dr. James Kroeze

Dr. James Kroeze joined SWMC in 2001 around the time Drs. Atkinson, Suzanne Hayward, and Holly Tapley left their respective part-time practices. He has taken a dozen staff, including nurses and secretaries, to the Dominican Republic on three short-term mission trips.

One of Dr. Kroeze's favorite patients is a prayer warrior with a physically weak heart. When they pray together in his office, she breaks out in tongues. He referred her to a heart specialist at the University of Michigan, one of the best heart surgeons in the world. After three heart valve replacements, that specialist told the woman, "We can't do anything more."

"Back at home, my regular doctor prays with me, and that always helps," the woman said. "Can you pray with me?"

"I've never done it before," the specialist admitted.

A Dictaphone sat over in the corner. The woman pointed to it and said, "It's kind of like talking into that Dictaphone."

The doctor shrugged and launched into a peculiar monologue: "Dear God period. Please help insert name period."

Another of Dr. Kroeze's patients was an alcoholic with high blood pressure. Dr. Kroeze talked honestly with him about how his drinking would irreversibly affect his body. The man confessed he'd wanted to stop drinking for a long time, but just couldn't do it. Dr. Kroeze offered the man a double referral: a 12-step program and Jesus.

A few months later, the patient returned to Dr. Kroeze a changed man. The man reconciled with his family and his heart and blood pressure are much improved. "I drank for 40 years, and I feel like I'm out of prison," he exclaimed. "One of the guys in my 12-step group said, 'If Christ has set you free, you're free indeed,' and that's the truth."

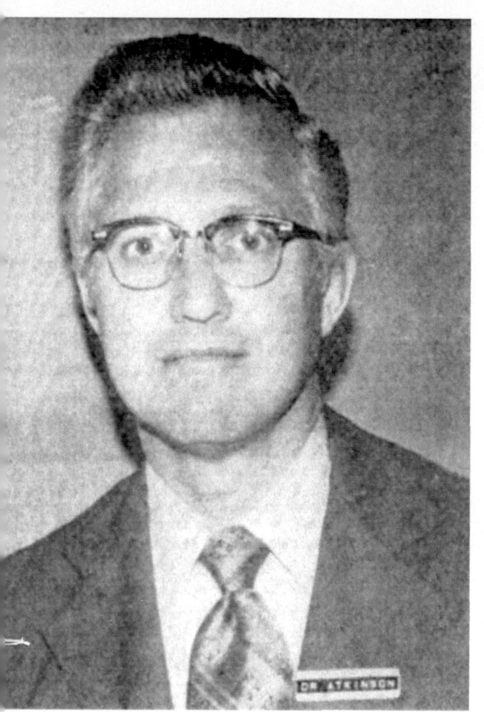

ɫerbert Atkinson

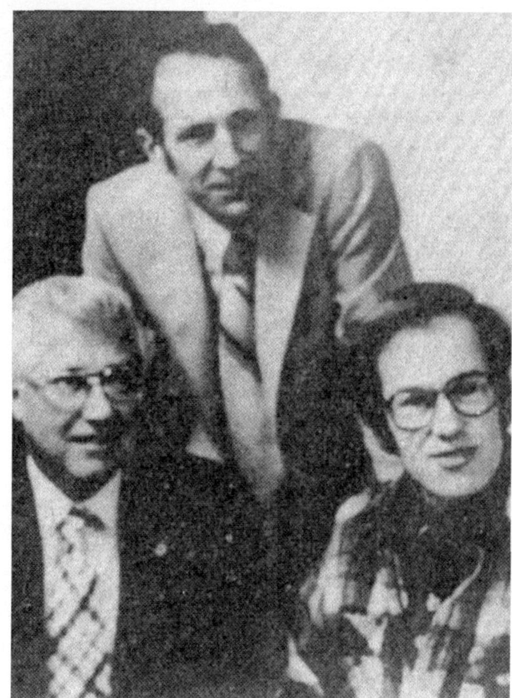

From left: Dr. Herbert Atkinson,
Dr. Roland Stephens, and Dr. Richard Roach

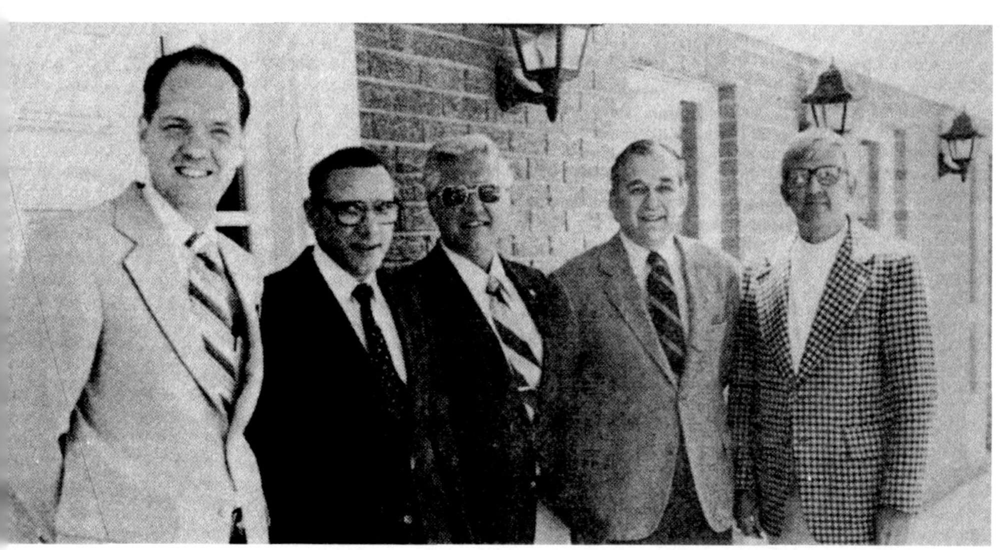

physicians assigned to Southwestern Medical Clinic's new family health clinic opening June 2, 1980 evensville are shown with clinic administrator Don Gast, far right. The physicians, from left are: obert Patton, Internal Medicine and Cardiology; Dr. Charles Rhodes, Sugery; Dr. Herbert Atkinson, ily Practice; and Dr. Robert Schindler, Surgery

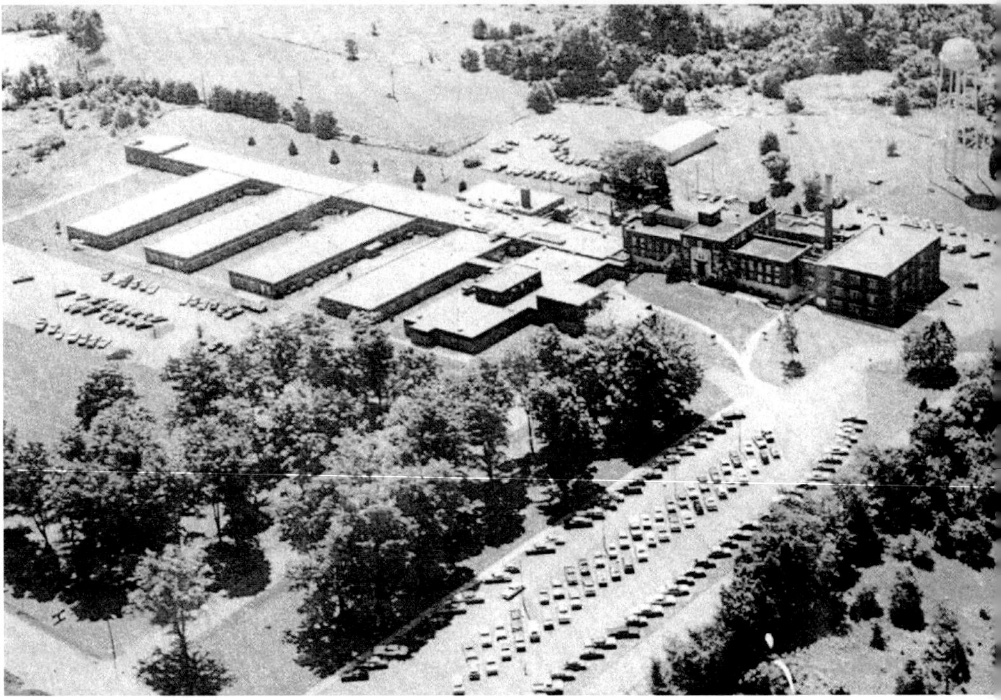

Berrien General Hospital, ca. 1980

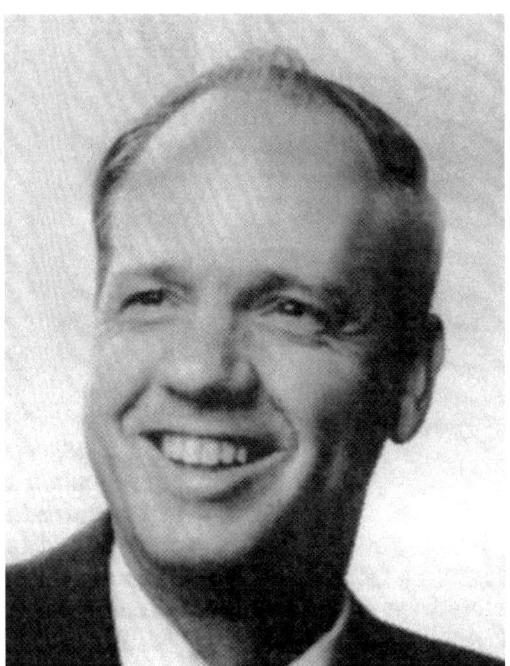

Dr. Robert Patton

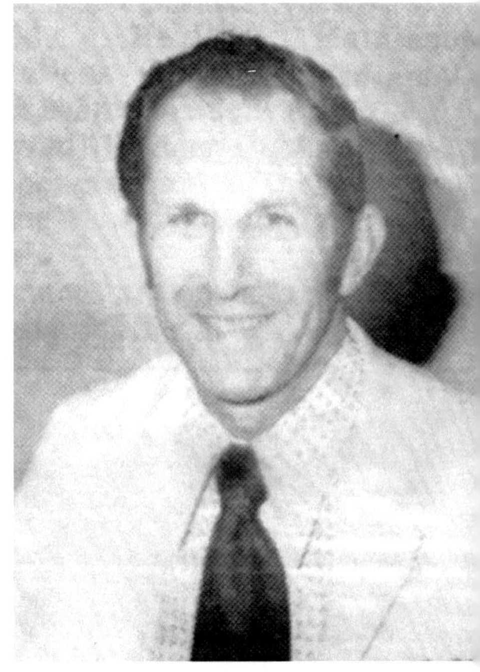

Dr. Roland Stephens

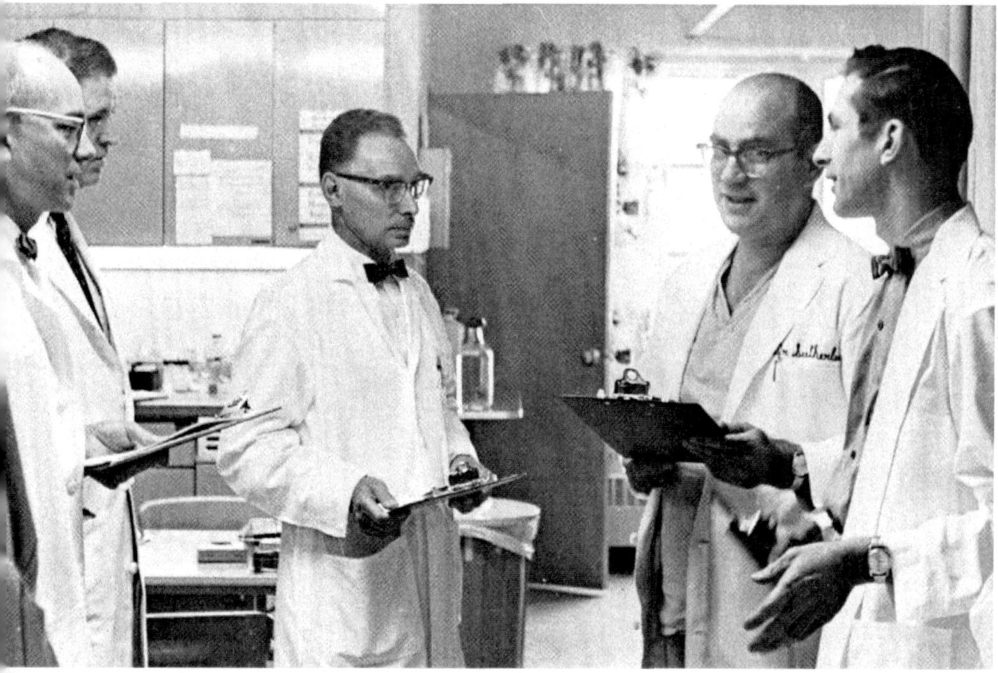

n left: Dr. Weldon Cooke, Dr. Harold Mason, Dr. Doug Taylor, Dr. Burton Sutherland, Dr. Roland Stephens

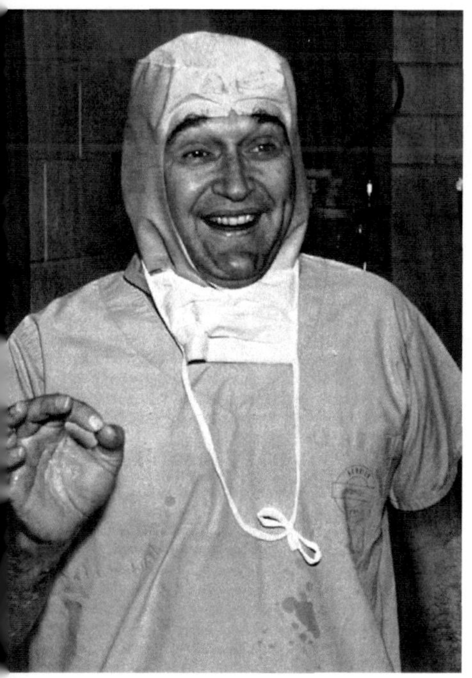

obert Schindler

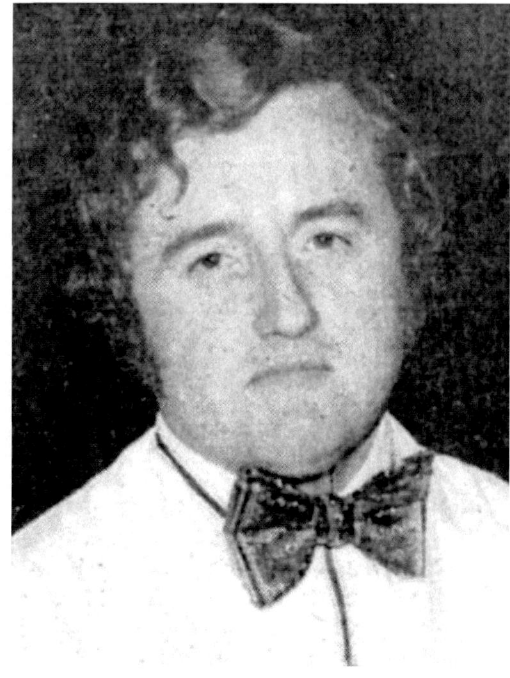

Dr. James Wierman

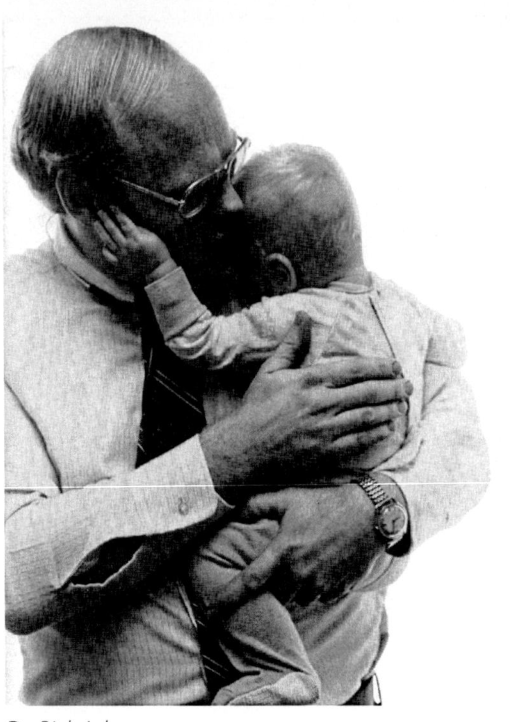
Dr. Rick Johansen

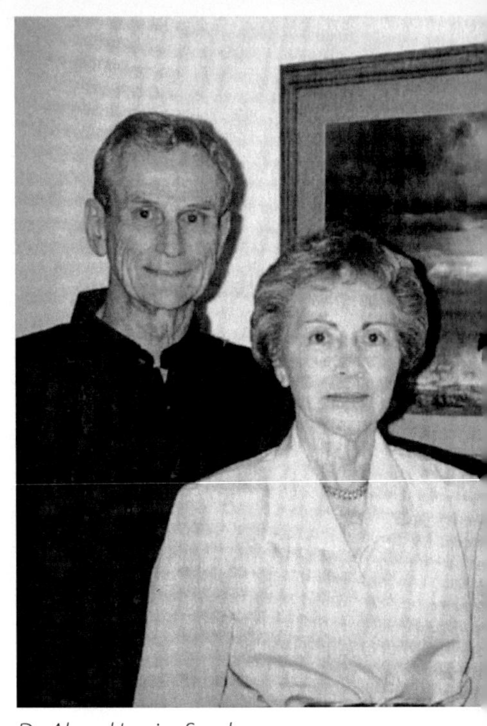
Dr. Al and Louise Snyder

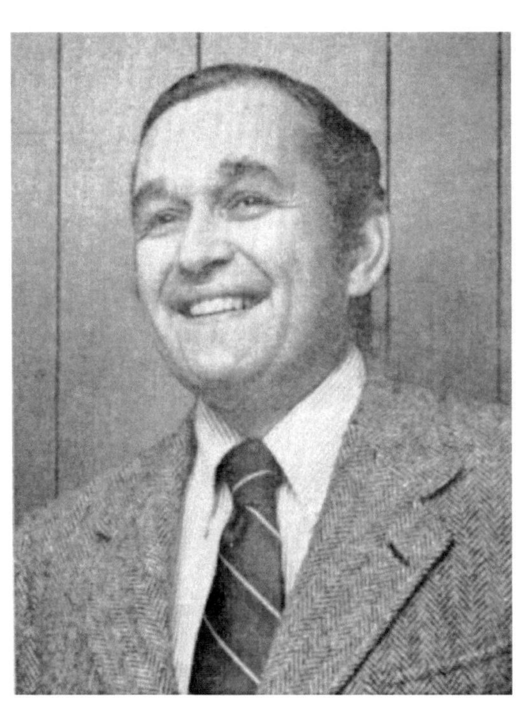
Dr. Robert Schindler

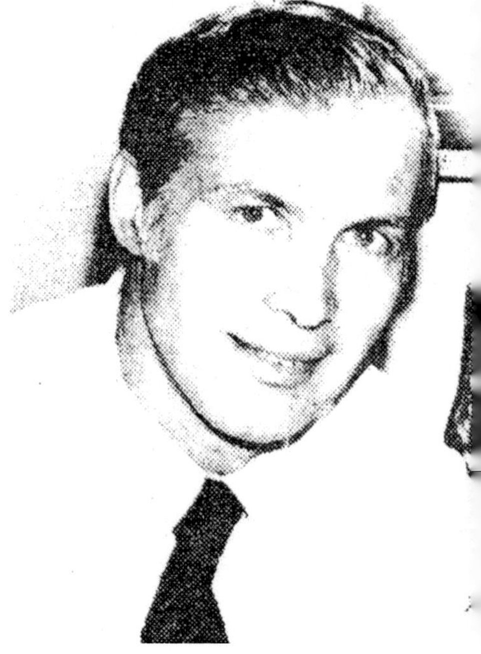
Dr. William Douce

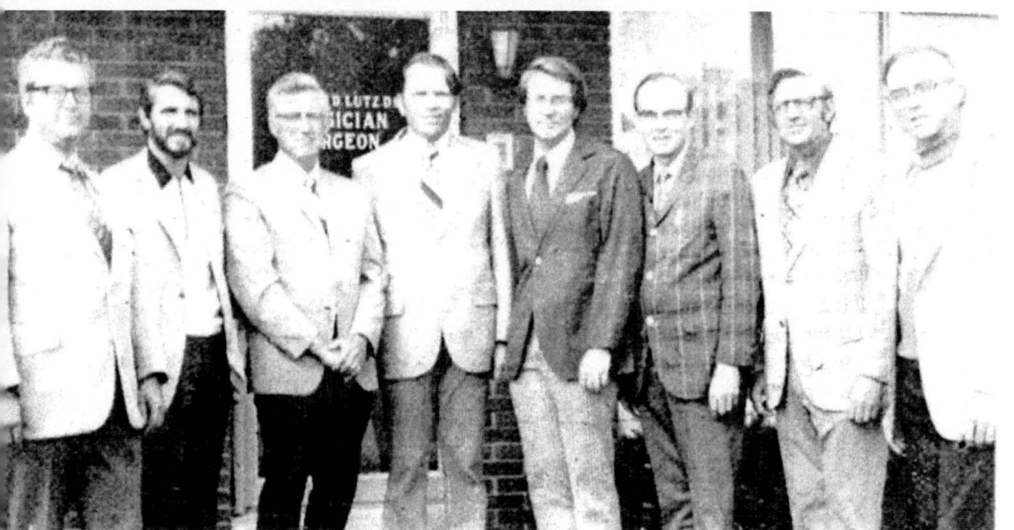

m left: SWMC bought the Berrien Springs practice from Dr. Robert Lutz, on left ; Dr. E. Dewain Silvernale; Herbert Atkinson; Dr. Robert Weche; Dr. Kenley Burkhart; Dr. John Edling; Donald Gast, Administrator outhwestern Medical Clinic; Dr. Weldon Cooke, President of Southwestern Medical Clinic

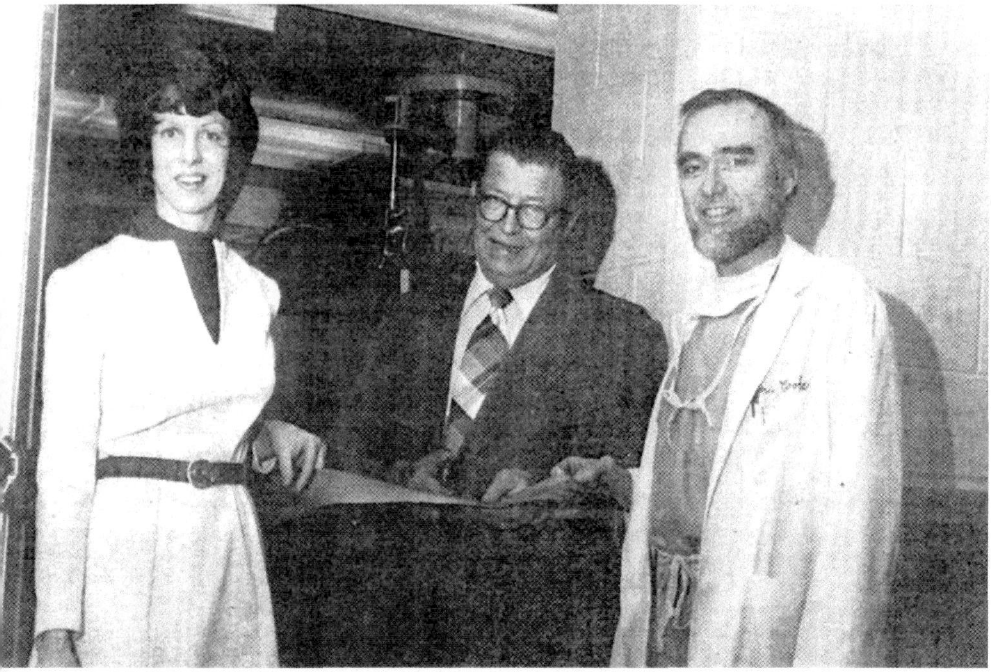

n left: Hospital Administrator Sandra Bruce, Otto Grau, Chairman of the Berrien County Commission ding and grounds committee, and Dr. Weldon Cooke

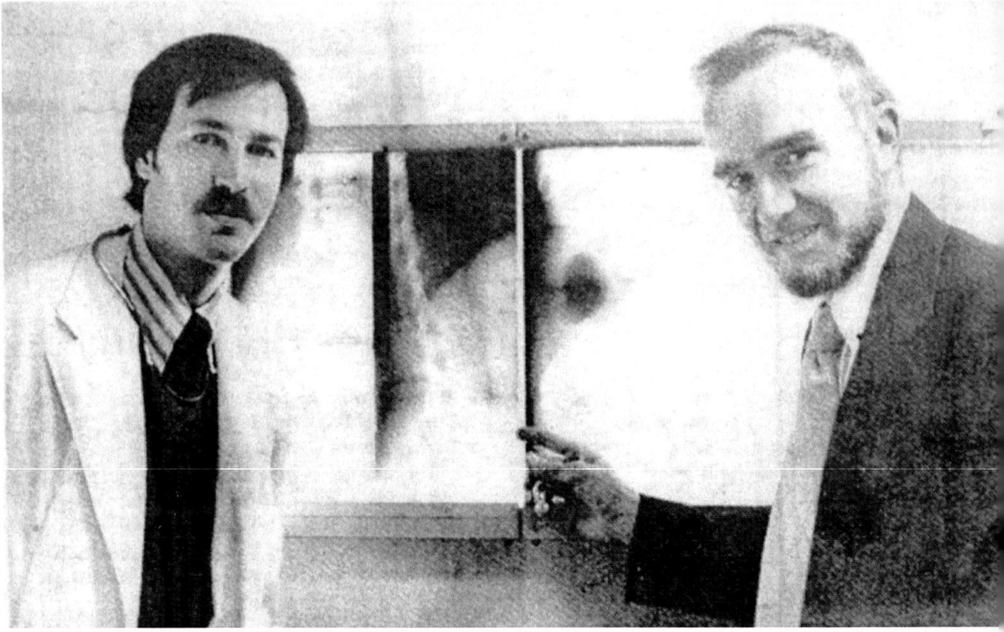

Dr. Weldon Cooke [right], discusses patient care with Daniel Spitters [left], Physician Assistant at Southwestern Medical Clinic, P.C.

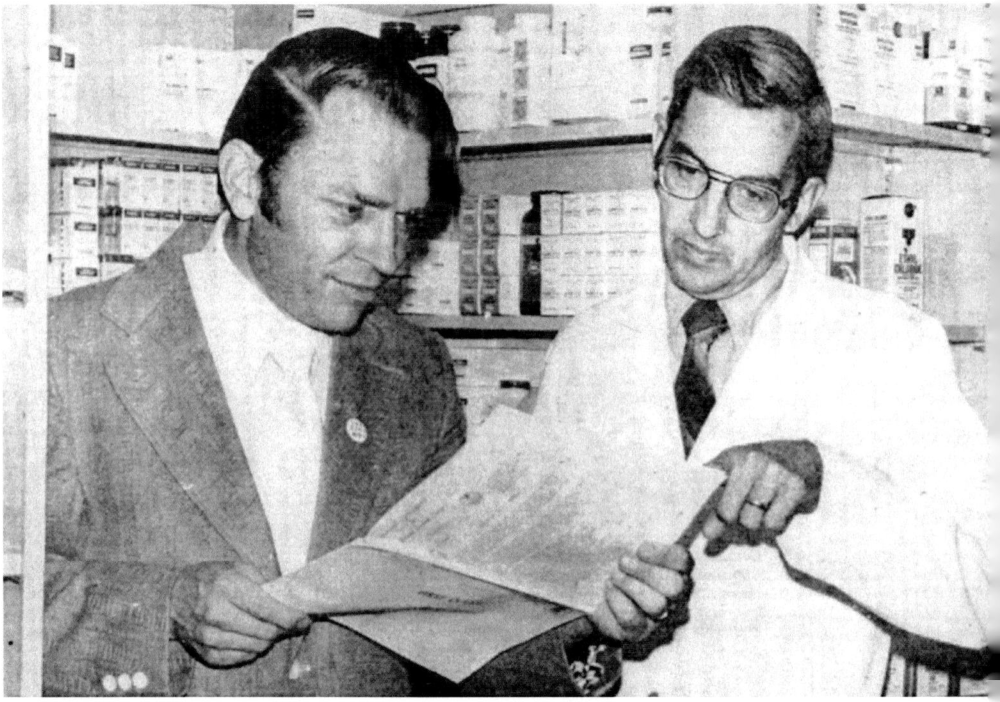

Dr. Robert Wesche and Pharmacist Richard Chaudoir of Berrien General Hospital

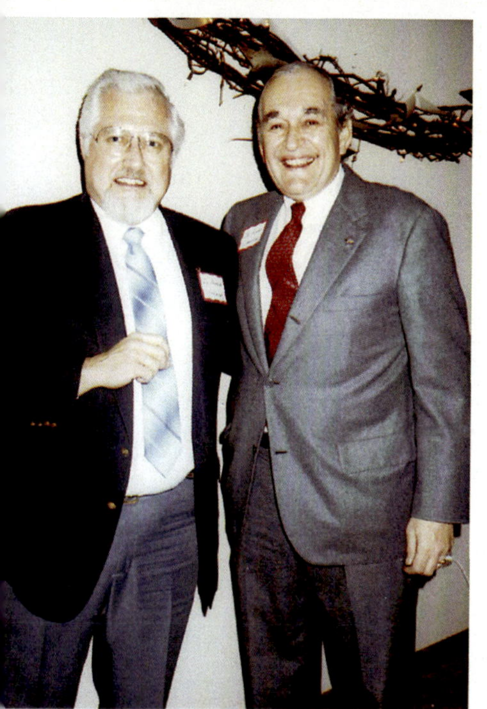

-lerbert Atkinson and Dr. Robert Schindler

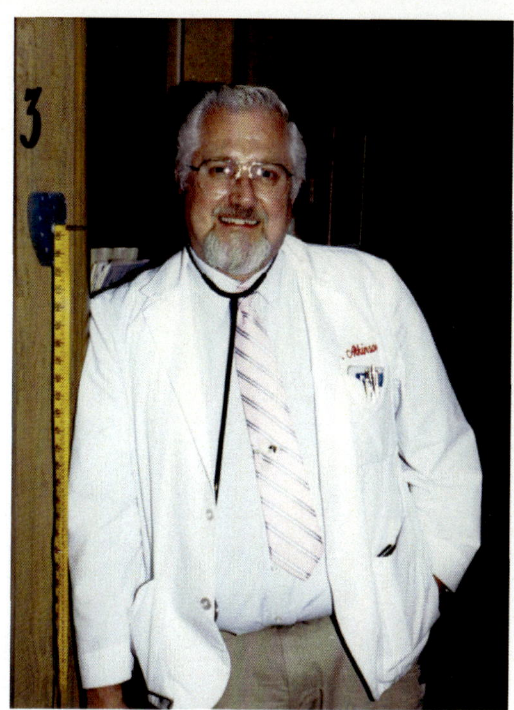

Dr. Herbert Atkinson

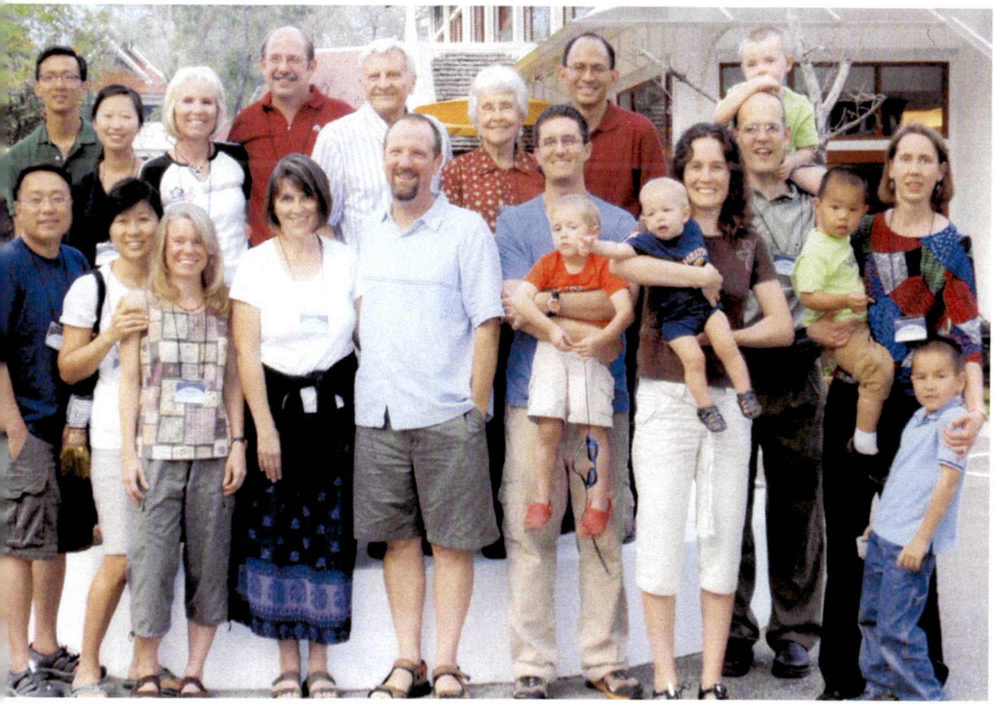

land CMDA Conference 2009 - Front row from left: Dr. and Sandy Burton Lee, Dr. Holly Tapley,
Dan and Suzanne Hayward, Dr. Jason and Natasha Topkins, Dr. Josh and Sherry Underhill.
: row from left: Drs. Paul and Susan Lim, Dr. Dan and Julie Stephens, Dr. Wendell and
jie Geary, and Dr. Rex Cabaltica

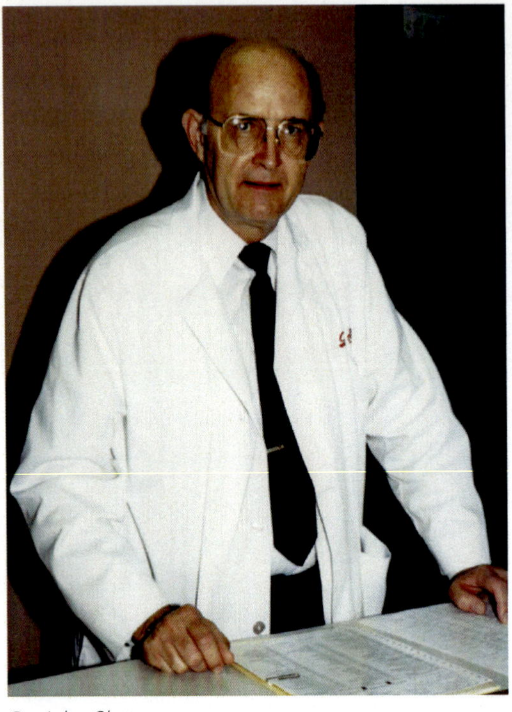

Dr. John Slater

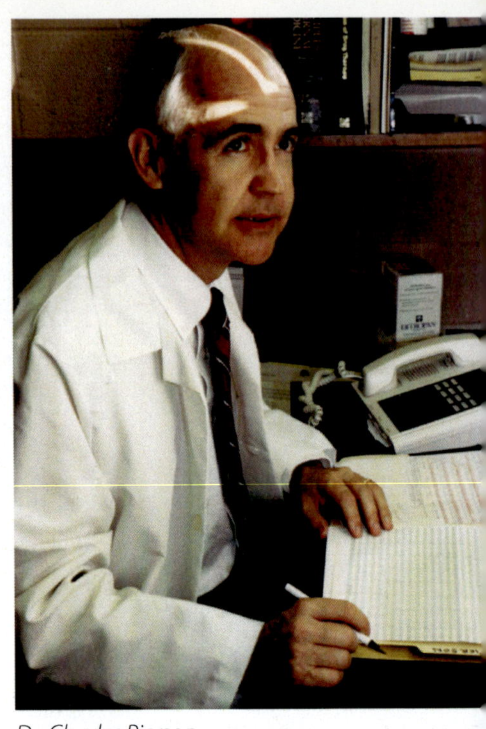
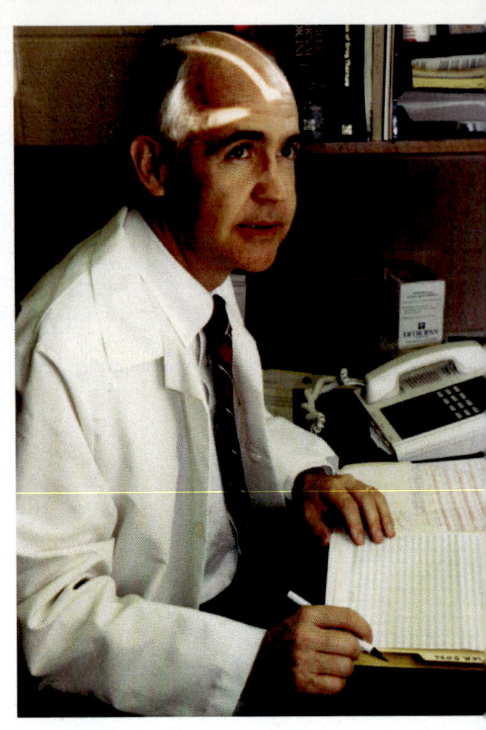

Dr. Charles Pierson

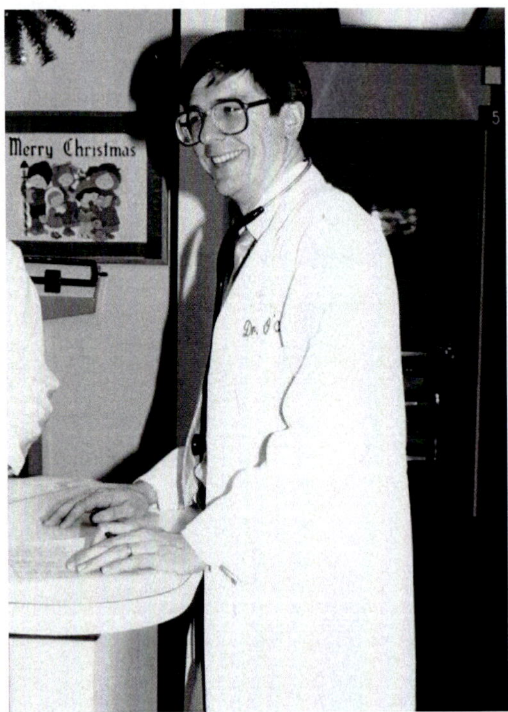

Dr. Kenneth O'Neill

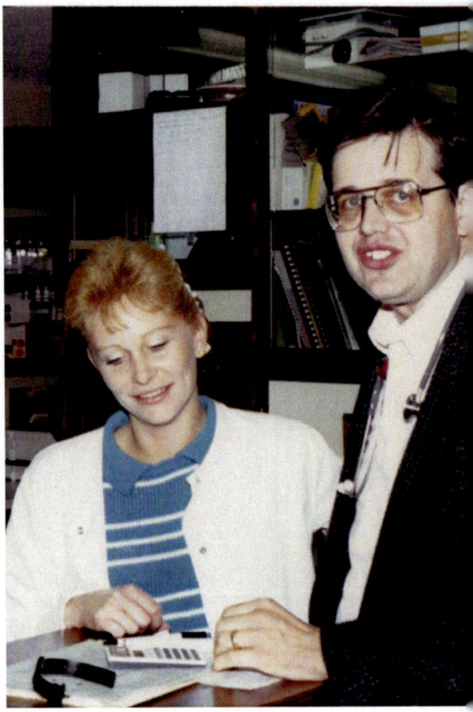

Sharon Gray and Dr. Georg Schultz

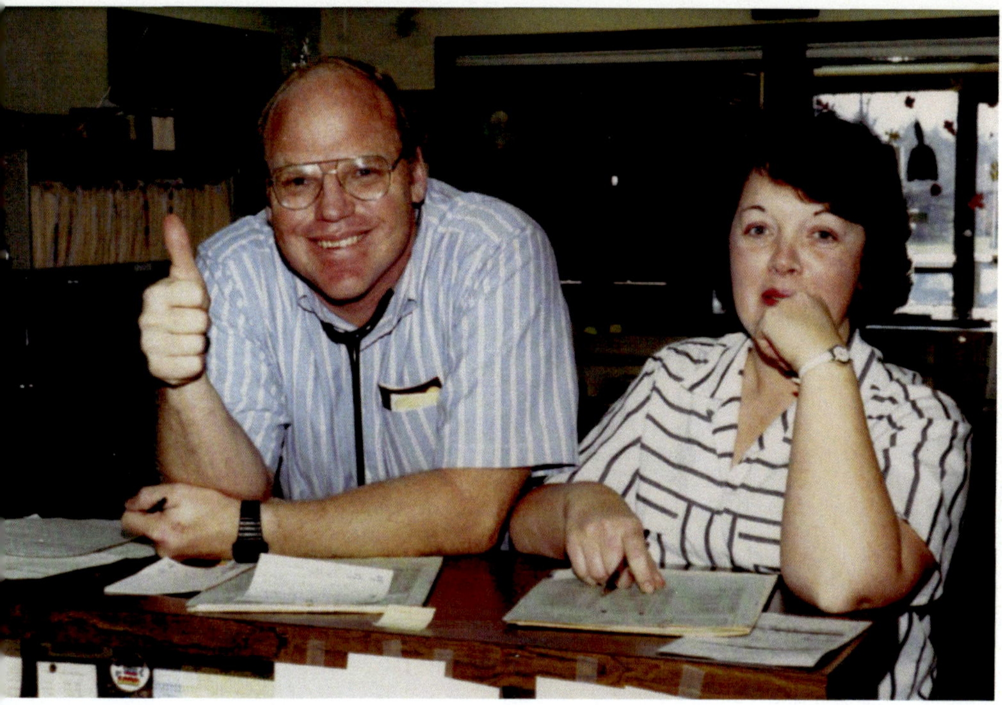

Frederick Johansen and Dianne Warner

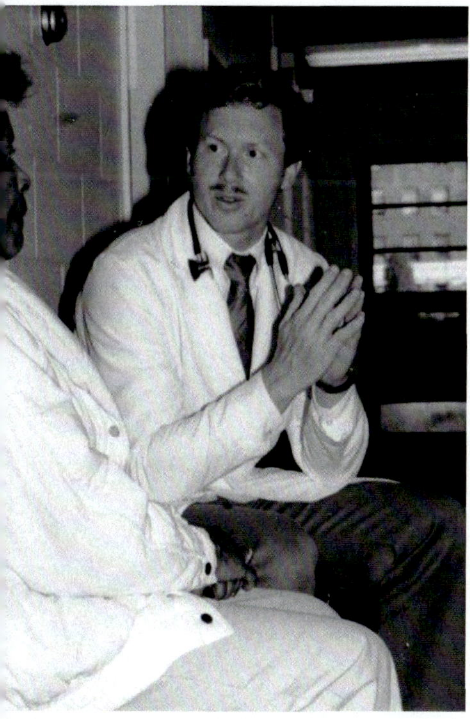

Roy Ringenberg

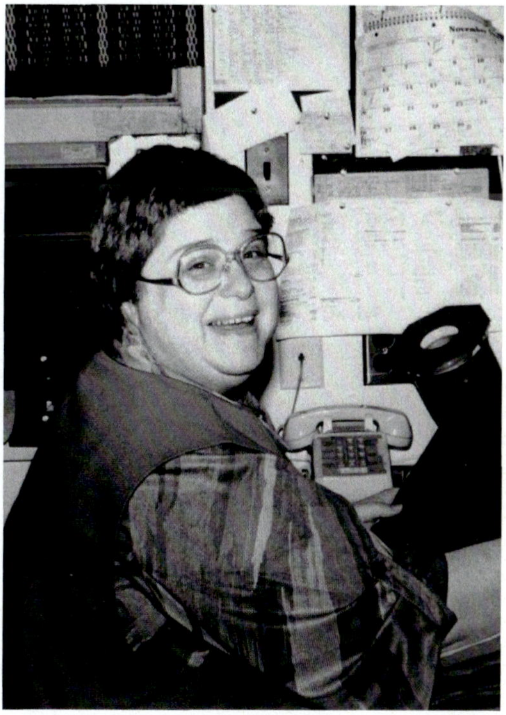

Dr. Janet Frey

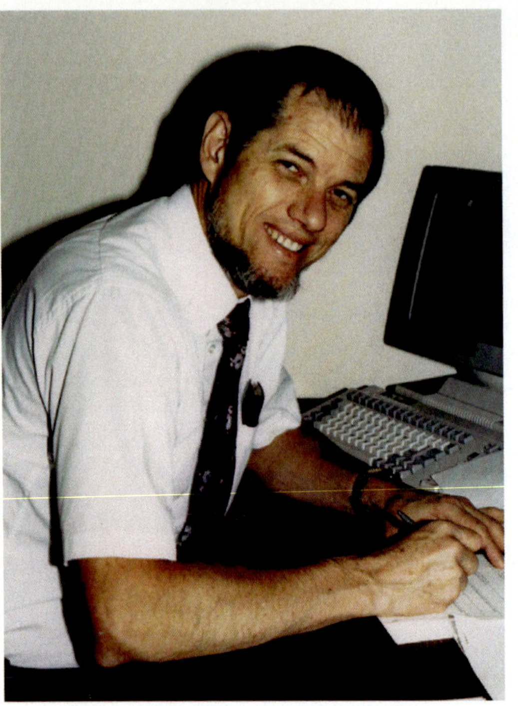

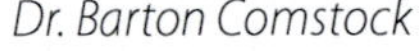

Dr. Barton Comstock

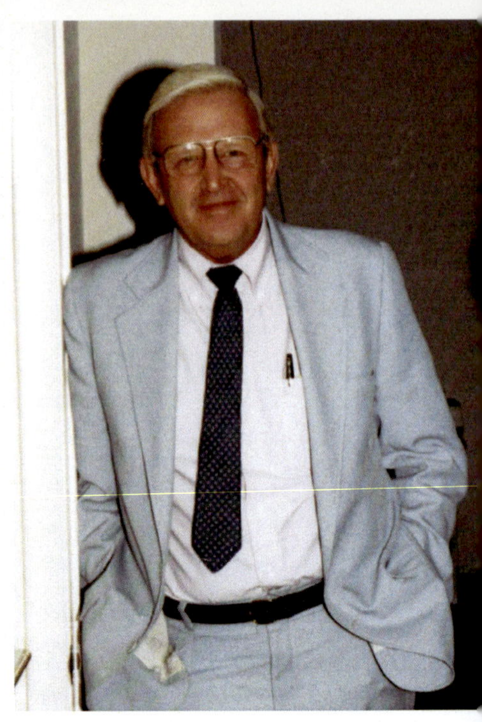

Don Gast

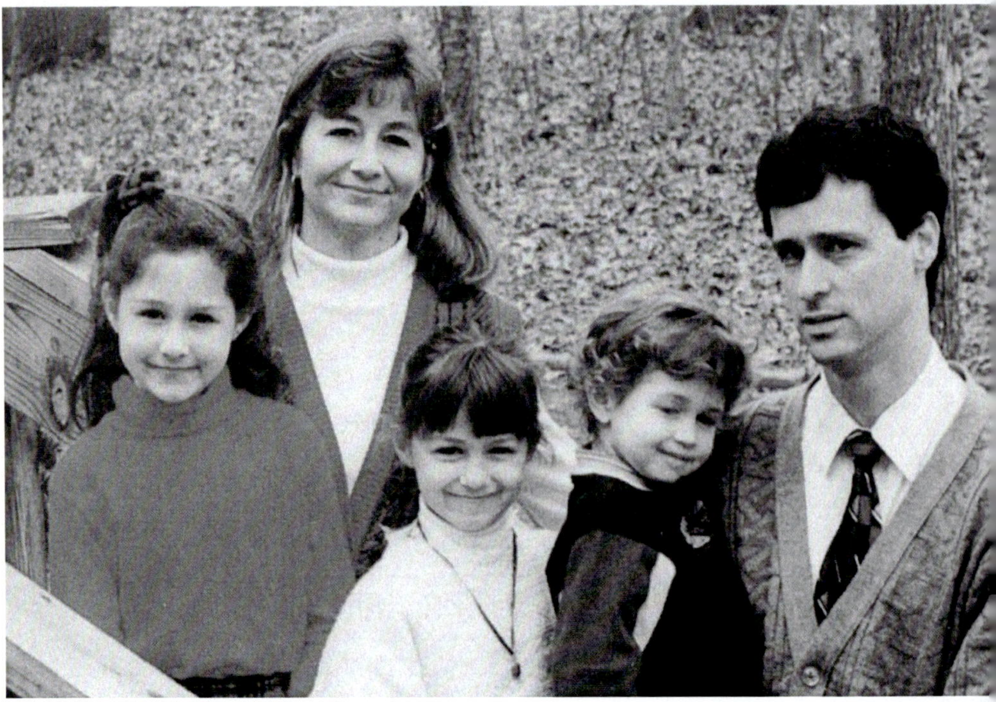

Dr. Dan and DeeAnn (DeeDee) Snyder, Ashley, Rachel and James

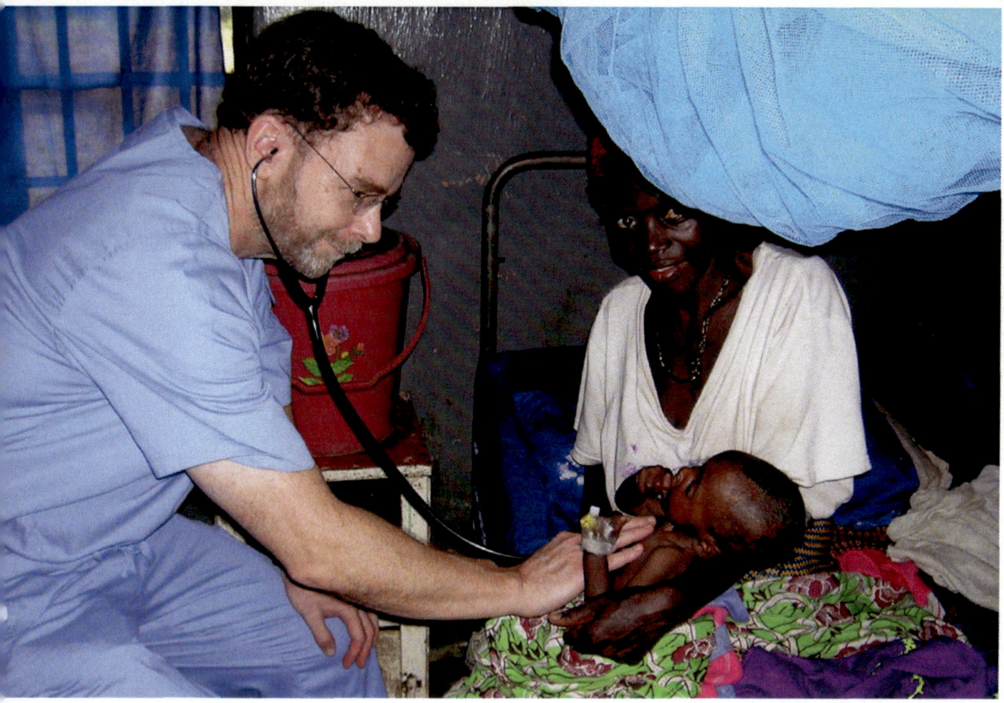

Daniel Metzger 2009

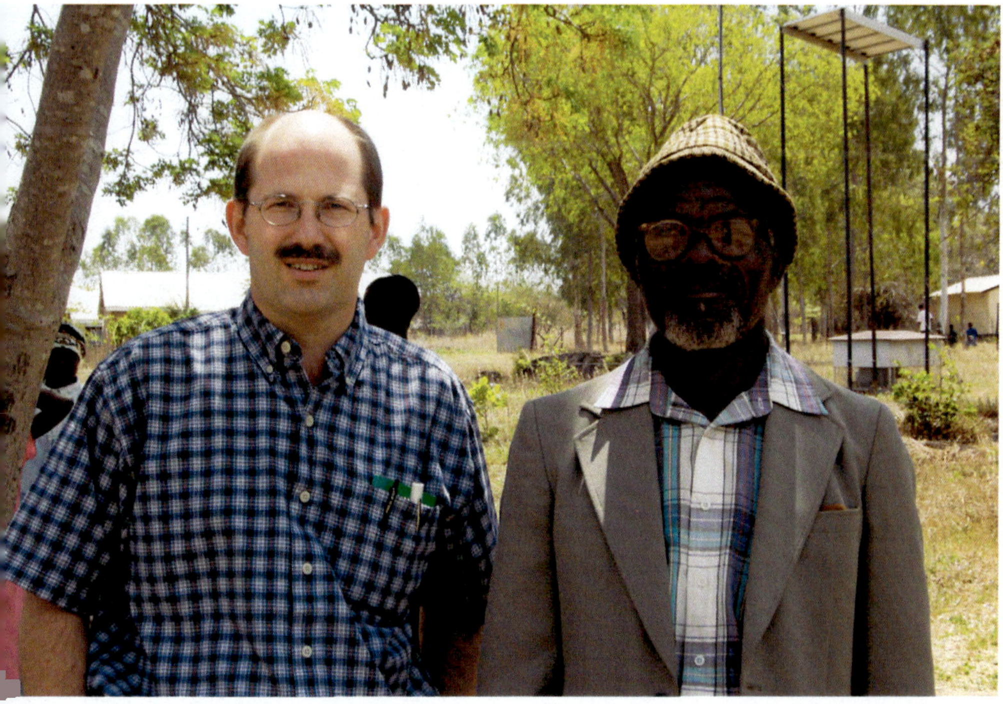

Daniel Stephens and Chizenga - Zimbabwe

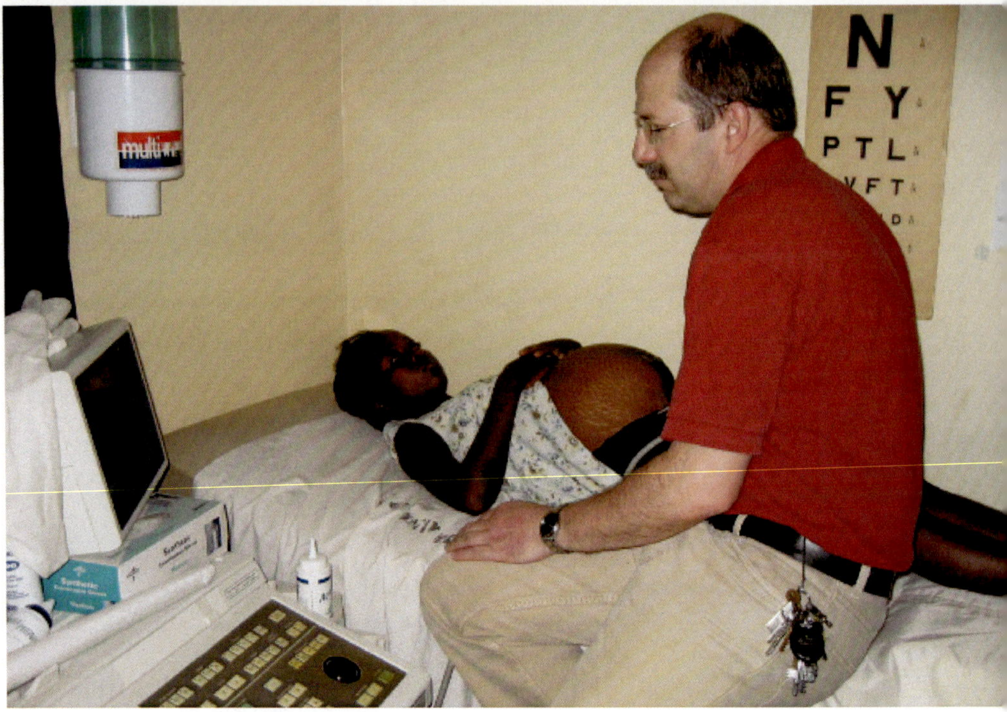

Dr. Daniel Stephens - Zimbabwe

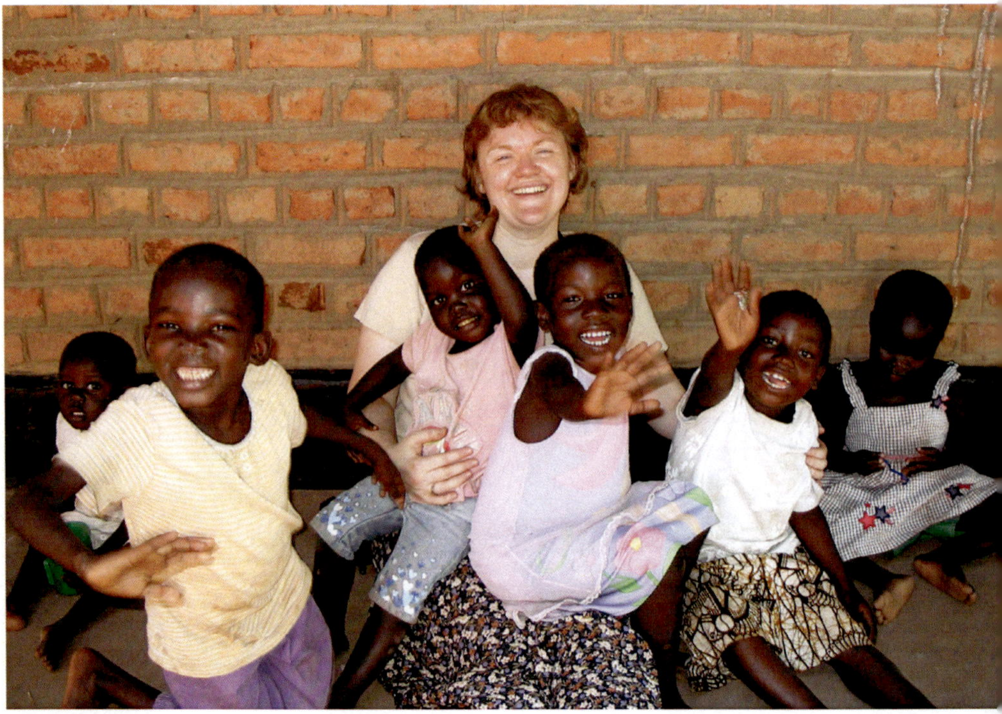

Dr. Heather Marten - Sudan

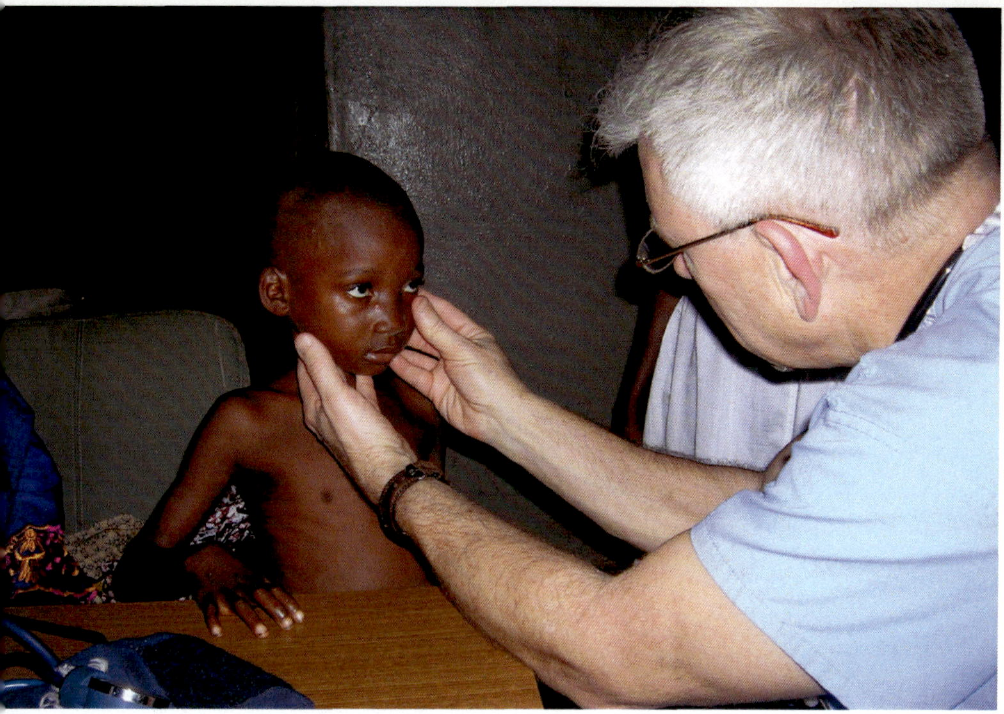

Ronald Baker - Mattru Sierra Leone

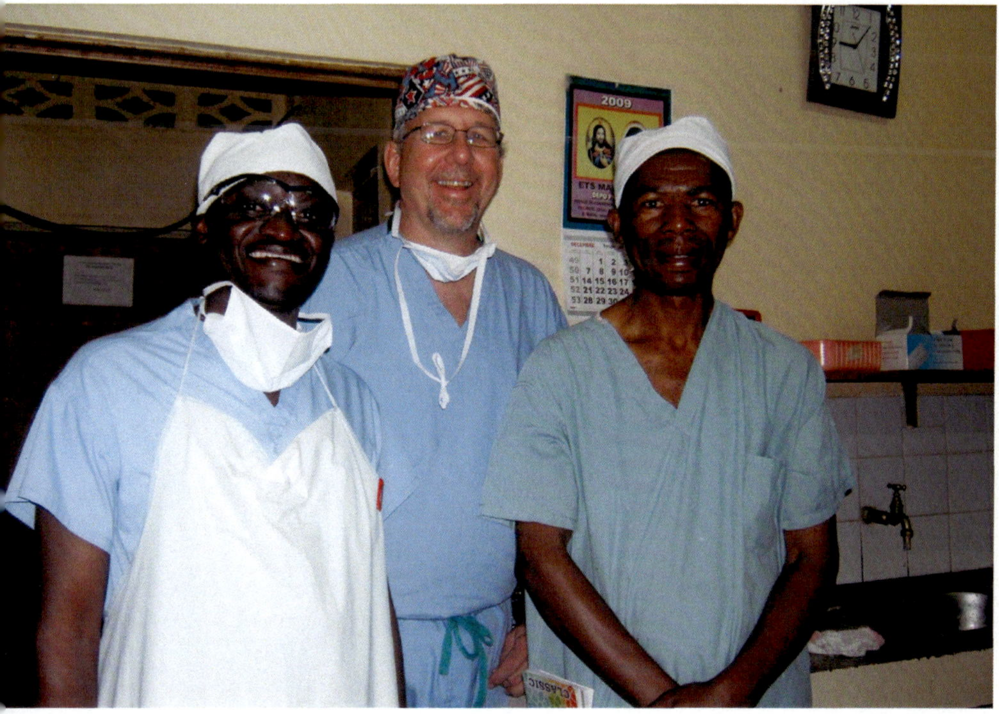

Roy Winslow - Rwanda

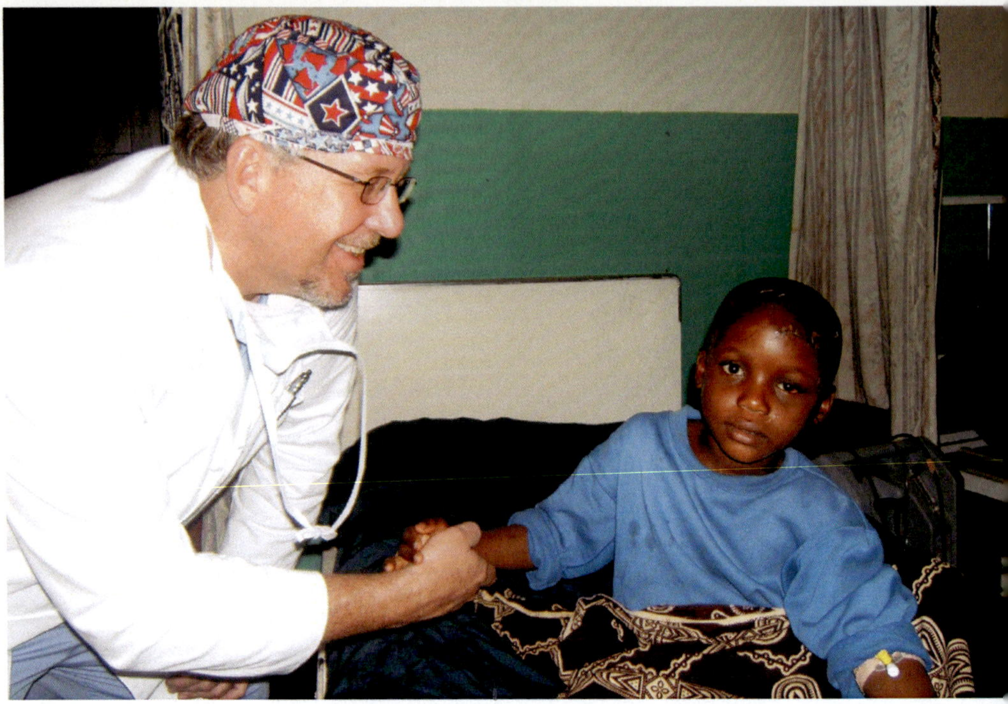

Dr. Roy Winslow - Rwanda

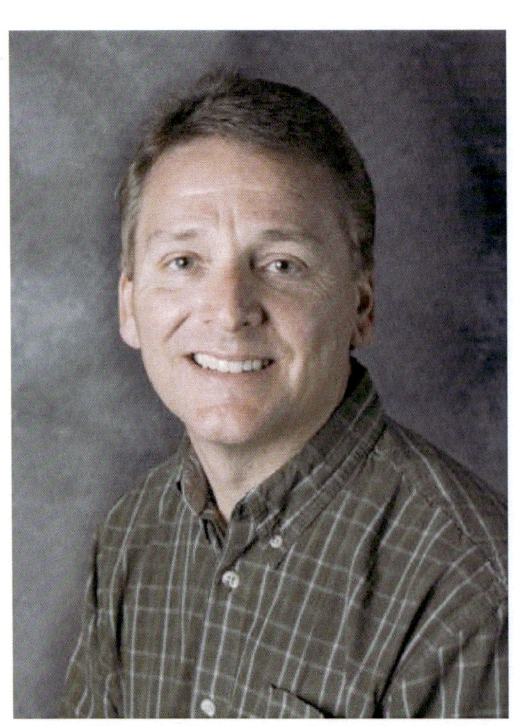

Dr. Michael Chupp

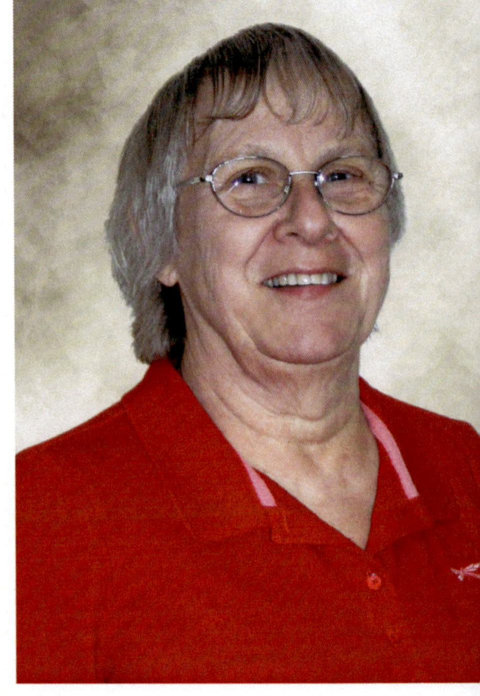

Dr. Helene Johnson

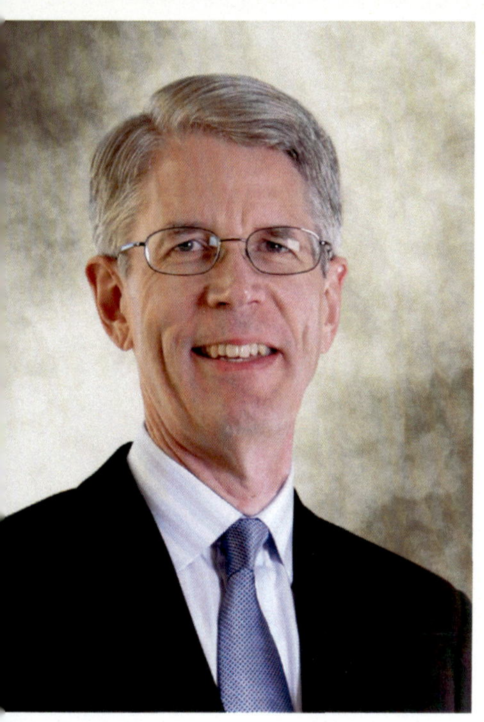

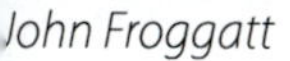

John Froggatt

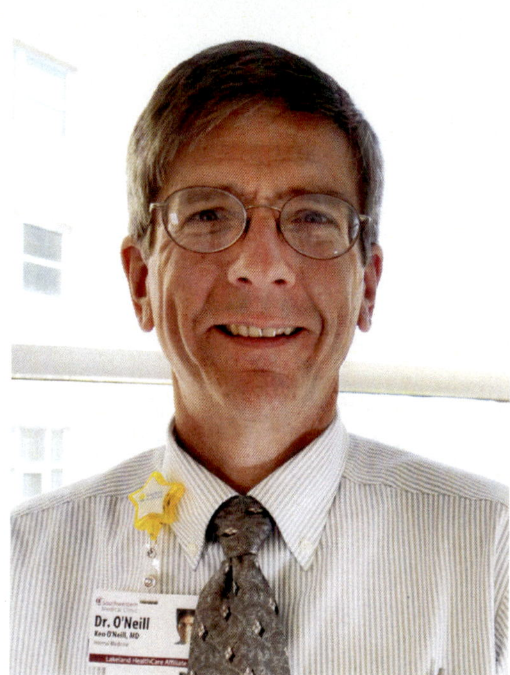

Dr. Kenneth O'Neill

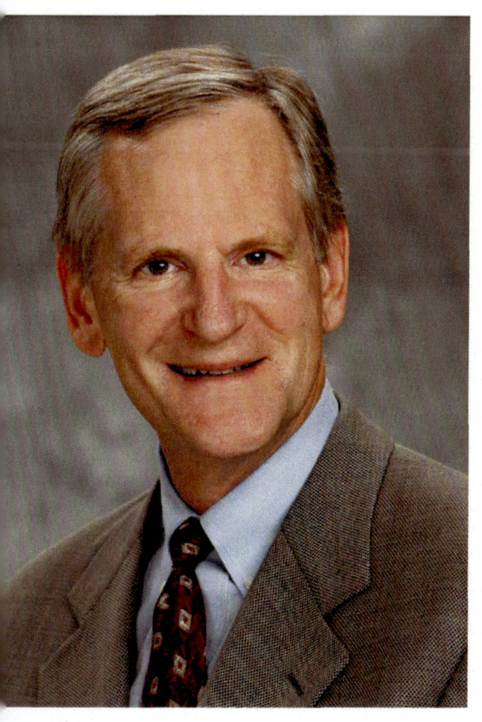

ren White

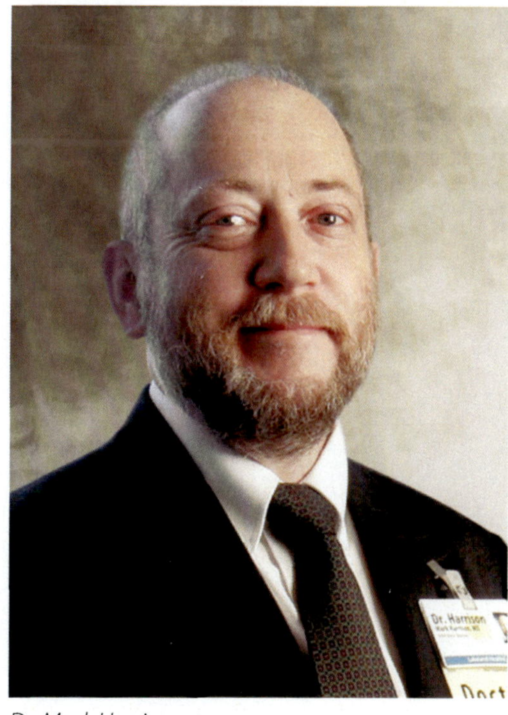

Dr. Mark Harrison

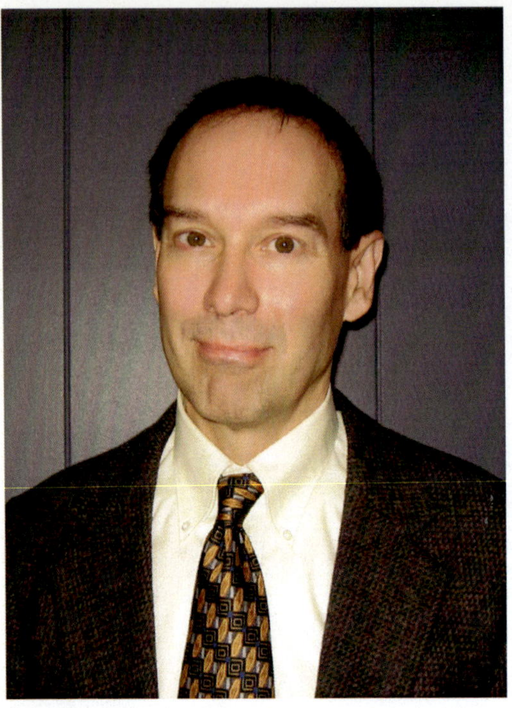

Pat Meyer

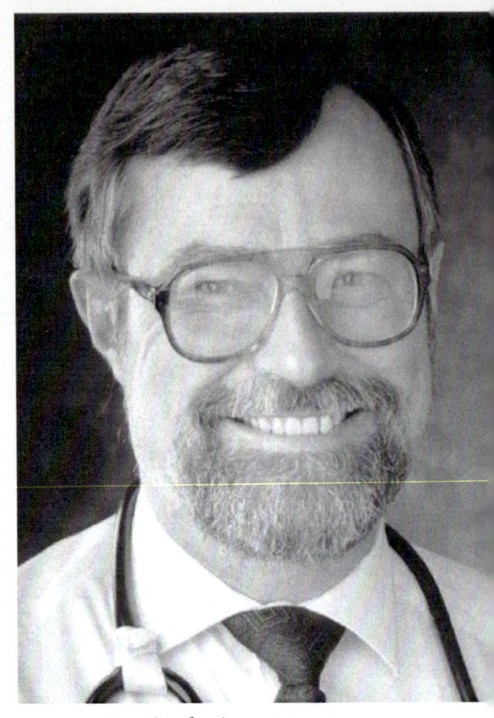

Dr. James Rutherford

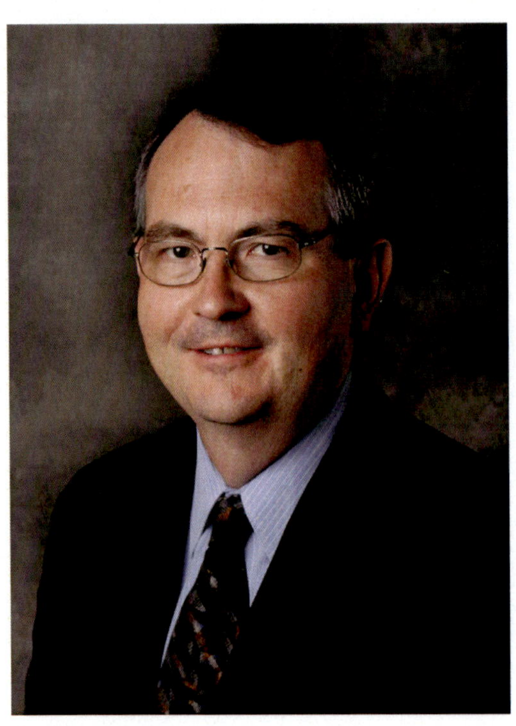

Dr. John Spriegel

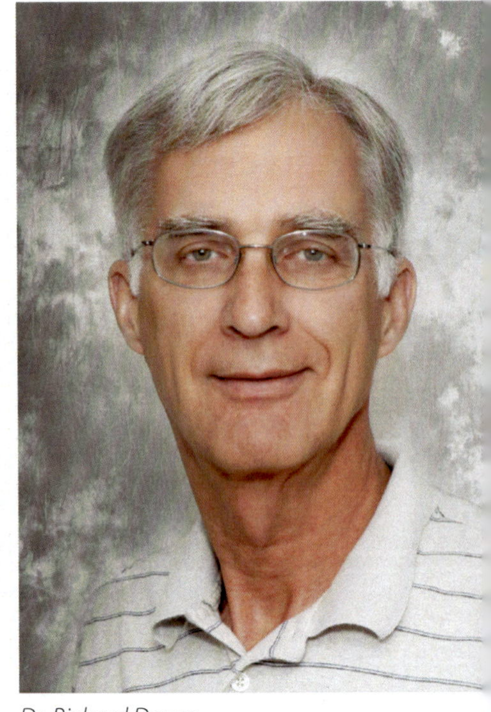

Dr. Richard Douce

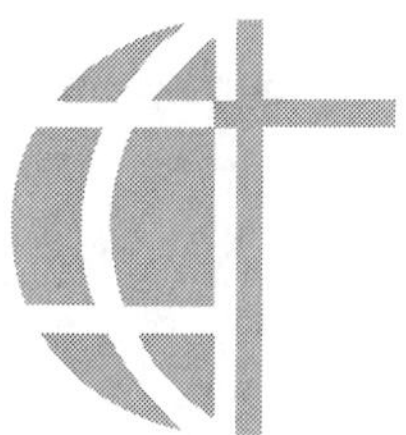

Chapter 20

Stories from the Stevensville Office

Chapter 20

Stories from the Stevensville Office

Newly hired SWMC specialists listened when their patients asked to use Mercy-Memorial Hospital in St. Joseph. The Stevensville office opened in 1980, the nearest SWMC office to the largest hospital in Berrien County. Quickly, the Stevensville office grew into the largest SWMC location. Here are stories about the Stevensville office from the physicians and staff:

Dr. Richard "Dick" Hines

When Dick Hines was attending elementary school in Berrien Springs in the 1960s, SWMC was a little group of doctors who worked at the old work farm, Berrien General Hospital. Berrien General Hospital's reputation had lagged for a bit in the 1950s. It was seen as out of the way and behind the times. People shopping downtown across the river or teaching at Andrews College whispered to each other, "Do they even know what they're doing? Coming back from the mission, don't you think they're all rusty?"

As the 1960s progressed, so did SWMC's reputation. When story after wondrous story began to be told about the fantastic care and amazing results at Berrien General, people began to ask, "What's going on there?"

By the 1970s, when Dick Hines was shooting hoops in the driveway, SWMC was a drawing card for doctors of such caliber as young Dr. Johansen, fresh out of pediatric medical school at Syracuse. He and his wife moved in next door to the Hineses, and he became Dick Hines' physician. Dr. Johansen developed a friendship with Dick Hines. They played one-on-one basketball and had some good talks in the front yard.

Dick Hines knew he wanted to be a doctor. Dr. Johansen talked him into being a pediatrician. When Dr. Hines came back to the area as a young doctor and started working at SWMC in June 1990, he got reacquainted with a co-spelling bee champion from fifth grade, Judy Kubsch. Judy started working for SWMC in high school in 1977. A vital member of the clinic, Judy moved up the ranks through the business office for 35 years.

Dr. Hines also met Marilyn Hurrle, a registered nurse promoted to manager of the Stevensville office. "She helped make our pediatric side what it is," Dr. Hines says. "She's the best of the best."

Susan Newcomer, Don Gast's daughter, started working at SWMC in the 1970s after volunteering for her father's clinic in many ways. She was one of Dr. Hines's research nurses for several years.

In addition to following Dr. Johansen into pediatrics at SWMC, Dr. Hines also sat on the board. He found that, like his early mentor, he enjoyed research. Throughout the years several SWMC doctors offered clinical trials to some of their patients. In 2006 the clinic saw value in building a research department. Doing this, all of the research could be coordinated by a team. Of the SWMC physicians actively participating in research, Dr. Hines had the most patients in clinical trials, so he was drafted as director of research. Karen Styf, RN a long-time SWMC registered nurse became his research assistant.

This research has always been pharmaceutical-sponsored. Most are Phase 3 trials, collecting data from large numbers of patients just prior to the pharmaceutical company submitting the drug to the FDA for approval. By Phase 3, a great deal of information already exists on the safety of the drug. It has been through three or four years of study with animals, then another three or four years of study on healthy human subjects under controlled situations where the pharmaceutical company learns about common side effects and dosage. From there, research proceeds into Phase 2, giving the medication to people who actually have the targeted condition, the disease, under carefully controlled situations. If the medicine is still encouraging, Phase 3 trials are next.

As part of a Phase 3 study, SWMC is one of 50 or 100 sites world-wide participating. Patients can choose to enroll in the study to try this medication for free as part of the clinical trial. Dr. Hines estimates SWMC has participated in about 100 studies. Of 300 people who participate in a study, some studies have only two or three SWMC participants, but a typical number is about 10. Well over 1,000 SWMC patients have enrolled throughout the years.

Patients generally enjoy being subjects in clinical trials. First, they have access to a drug that's not commonly available that might help them feel better. A significant number of patients have had good effects from the drugs and have been helped in the process. Second, because of data collection, doctor visits are more detailed. Third, these studies are free. During the study, patients get free doctor consultation and care they might not have otherwise been able to afford.

Marilyn Hurrle

Marilyn Hurrle, R.N., manager of the Stevensville office at 5515 Cleveland Ave., started working for SWMC "much too late" in 1978. She wishes she could have joined the clinic sooner. Since being Michigan Guernsey Queen prior to 1978, Marilyn has held various titles. One of her most notorious was SWMC's OSHA Queen.

She earned that title partly because she was never afraid to ask the big questions. One day circa 1989, she asked Don Gast, "What is all this hoopla about Hepatitis-B shots we nurses are supposed to be learning about?"

Don said, "I'll have to do some research." Not long afterward he walked into the pediatric office lugging a huge nurse binder loaded full of 1,500 pages. He said, "Here's the Hepatitis- B stuff you were asking about. How about you help me?"

That binder was the beginnings of OSHA regulations. It didn't take long for Marilyn to realize they needed a program. She put the program together and they rolled it into new staff orientation. "We ran a good program as a stand-alone office," Marilyn says.

Marilyn worked in the Berrien Springs adult office both before and after it moved to Ferry Street. She transferred to Bridgman, then also worked in the Berrien Springs pediatrics office, in Sawyer, at Berrien Center, Stevensville's pediatrics office on Fairview, and then to Stevensville's office on Cleveland Avenue.

One legendary event occurred in the Bridgman office, more specifically in the tiny patient bathroom. According to Marilyn, the sink or stool had overflowed, so she dutifully went upstairs and got a wet-dry vacuum from the building owner, Dr. Dale Smith the dentist. Wet-dry vacuum in tow, she knelt on the floor, half in the hall, and went to work on the bathroom carpet.

"It was a busy day," Dr. Rick Johansen recalled. "Several other doctors were there. Marilyn started vacuuming, and the canister was behind her in the hall. She was vacuuming her little heart out, oblivious to the fact that packing peanuts were blowing all over the floor. The more she vacuumed, the more hunks of fiber sprayed out of the back end of the vacuum. The rest of us just slid to the floor laughing."

"I heard Dr. Johansen laughing hysterically behind me," Marilyn confirmed, "and mind you, wet-dry vacuums are noisy creatures. He was practically in tears, he was laughing so hard. All these Styrofoam balls were scattered all over the hallway. Whether a critter had stored them in there or whatever, it was quite a sight."

Marilyn told a story on Dr. Johansen, too. Once at the Berrien Springs office, they decorated for a birthday party with oodles of balloons. Dr. Johansen decided to sit on a balloon and pop it. He sat on it, but it just flubbered. He bounced up and down on it and the staff died laughing. "Gee, this is a tough little bugger," he said. He bounced higher and higher. Suddenly it popped, and his legs flew over his head.

Marilyn and Dr. Comstock had great fun in the Bridgman office. Initially, the office was sometimes slow as they built a pediatrics practice. Throughout the years, Southwestern operated as moneywise as possible, so Marilyn and the doctors cleaned the toilets and changed the light bulbs. The first time Marilyn changed a light bulb, she got out to her car to go home and found a light bulb wedged in her door handle. She rolled her eyes, attributing it to some neighborhood kid's idea of a joke. The bulb was no good. It rattled, so she threw it in the trash.

It took Marilyn about four light bulb changes to realize "our funny guy in the office" had planted them all over. Finally, it clicked. It became a game of who could hide the light bulb better.

Marilyn often said to new employees, "We have an excellent pediatric staff here, but you have to remember, a good pediatrician behaves like a four-year-old a lot of the time." Dr. Comstock is so tall, instead of giving Marilyn a sticky note, he'd put it up on the ceiling light. In the morning, the light might be lined with sticky notes, with Dr. Comstock gone covering ER in a pinch or making rounds at the hospital to build the practice.

Another of Marilyn's titles is The Frog Lady. Her office is overpopulated by frog kitsch. Coworkers contribute to the collection. At home in the early 1990s, Marilyn dug some garden ponds. "I was so excited about it," Marilyn said. "Dr. Comstock had his own pond, too. I told him I was going to go buy tadpoles."

A few days later, she went outside to check on her growing tadpoles and discovered a huge frog in her pond. "Holy cow," she gasped, "my frogs have really grown."

At work she told Dr. Comstock all about it. She was so proud of her healthy frog. "You'd think I'd given it steroids or something," she raved. Dr. Comstock smirked and started laughing. He'd caught a few of his giants and hidden them in her pond.

Marilyn worked with Dr. Bob Schindler in the Bridgman office. She was the second nurse, his support nurse. She was responsible for rooming patients and assisting them in surgeries. Dr. Schindler came in the back door and called out in his big baritone voice, "I'm here, let's move."

He'd come in, look through the charts on his desk and go through his messages, and informally impart wisdom to Marilyn. He coached her about the power of prayer and gave her his famous 72-hour advice. "No matter how upset or angry you are, you go home and pray about it for 72 hours, and then decide what to do with it," he told her. "You'll find out a lot of times, Marilyn, that what you thought was a major issue is just a drop in the bucket. After three days it seems trivial."

Before OSHA, latex gloves were pretty much unheard of. When Marilyn assisted Dr. Schindler with surgeries, he'd have her hold a body part while he sewed on it. Their hands would be red with blood. Even after OSHA, getting Dr. Schindler to wear gloves outside of surgery was a challenge. "He wanted to get on his suture right now, and never thought a thing about it," Marilyn says. Sometimes she laughs thinking about it, and then shudders and thanks the Lord that she never got any horrible diseases.

Dr. Schindler joked, "She's my fill-in nurse. She's a pediatric nurse, and they sent her here to learn what real medicine is all about. We practice real medicine here."

Marilyn joked right back, "Let me see how good you are teaching someone how to breastfeed."

They used to do Sigmoidoscopies right in the office, a colon exam, and some patients didn't prep so well and would not be clean. Dr. Schindler would say to Marilyn, "Come here, take a look at this. See that little spot? What's that?" and when Marilyn leaned down for a closer look, he'd give it a good spray of water and suddenly "that" was gushing all down the front of Marilyn's smock.

Dr. Schindler was known for his impeccable memory. Before entering a patient room, he might pick up the chart and ask, "Where's her surgery we did 15 years ago? I need that pathology report." The nurses tried to keep the charts well-organized and full of all the pertinent information, but inevitably Dr. Schindler wanted something they didn't have in the chart.

Once, in friendly retaliation, the nurses concocted a fictitious patient. In the late 1990s, right after Kathy Harbert started working as a triage nurse, someone brought in a blow-up, life-sized doll. They named it Joe Bleu, laid it in an examining room, and created an elaborate chart and hung it on the examining room door. Dr. Schindler pulled out the chart and skimmed it. Brows furrowing, he gave it a more careful look. "I don't remember this patient," he said quietly.

"Oh, sure, you saw him just a few times," they assured him. "The last time he came in was a handful of years ago," and they coached him on the "patient's history." Looking more and more confused, Dr. Schindler paged slowly through the chart. "I don't think I've ever seen this man," he repeated. His staff clustered helpfully around him, murmuring tidbits of what they "remembered" about Mr. Bleu.

By the time Dr. Schindler was ready to go in he said dubiously, "I think I remember that," and he closed the door behind him.

He was in the room a long time. The nurses lined up outside the door, waiting to see what he would do. When he came out, all deadpan, he had orders written and began soberly advising his nurses about the plan of care. Suddenly, he burst out laughing and said, "You guys got me good."

Several years later, they played a similar prank on Dr. Ron Baker. Not minding blood and guts, he was an avid hunter. They erected a target-practice deer in an examining room. Like with Dr. Schindler, they wrote up a fake chart, named the patient something like Lorraine Dee Rudolph, and described an open wound. When Dr. Baker rushed in to help the patient, he came face to face with the deer, complete with an arrow in the center of the target. When he came out, he'd written "removal of foreign body" as a diagnosis and shook his head, grinning ear to ear.

In the month of January, if anyone left after a long day and found all the snow cleaned off his or her car, no doubt Dr. Baker had done it. Dr. Baker also loved snowball fights. One time, right during the middle of the day, probably 10 or more staff joined in a spontaneous snowball fight. Marilyn announced the event overhead. Laughing pediatrics patients joined them. Dr. Hines needed to pay Marilyn back for something and had his eye out for her. When she didn't come outside, he went in and found her walking down the back hall. Before he could get her first, she hollered, "I was looking for you, too," and she lambasted him on the chest. Snow landed all over the carpet. Wide-eyed, the staff said, "She threw a snowball in the building!" Dr. Hines had quite a laugh.

Southwestern had a reputation for staying open in all kinds of weather. One time Dr. Pierson refused to close the walk-in clinic and got snowed in and couldn't go home. He probably survived by eating a cold can of green beans and ketchup, his classic fallback if he forgot lunch.

Marilyn has worked with Lorene Schlutt, LPN, since way back in the old Stevensville office on Fairview. A patient once called her Laverne, so to this day she answers to Laverne. If Lorene got frustrated with Marilyn, Marilyn turned on polka music and begged Lorene to polka with her. If that didn't work, Marilyn would sit with her back turned and throw paper clips over her shoulder at Lorene. Finally, Lorene would wail, "You're driving me nuts!" and start laughing. Lorene has retired but still works as needed.

Dr. Richard "Dick" Hines worked at the Fairview office. Dr. Johansen brought him in and introduced him, and in mid-conversation they found out Dr. Hines had been a patient of Dr. Johansen's. Dr. Hines went with the flow, not drawing attention until he became a research director around the turn of the millennium. Right after Dr. Hines started, Marilyn went through a divorce and her little girl was in a parochial school. One day the child called and needed a ride home. Dr. Hines offered to go get her. He was driving an old Porsche. Marilyn's daughter to this day laughs about a doctor coming to pick her up in a fancy car. "It exemplifies the family atmosphere." Marilyn said. "We have a good time. Medicine's changed, the environment is much more stressful because of government and insurance changes, but the doctors are like my brothers. Oh, there were moments when we would snarl, because I'm strong willed as well, but through all my trials, they supported me as much as my immediate blood family did," she said.

"Don Gast, the original administrator until he stepped down to be the Senior Vice President of External Affairs, always managed the organization as part of his family. He set the mark," Marilyn said. Don's daughter Susan Newcomer still works in the Stevensville clinic. "The clinic did what it did so well because of his example and his love for the missionaries and the physicians' love for the mission," Marilyn added.

A missionary doctor who'd done some time overseas before joining the Stevensville OB group in 1997, Dr. Dale I. Carroll loved to tell tales at lunchtime. One time a tribal group he wanted to help invited him to their village to be honored. By custom, the village dried a gourd and hollowed it out like a little bottle. Then they half-filled it with cow's milk and let it sit on a shelf in the hut to ferment for a while. As soon as Dr. Carroll arrived, they took the same cow that had given the milk, poked it in the neck, and dripped its blood into the gourd with the chunky milk. With fanfare, they stirred up the concoction and presented it to Dr. Carroll as a tribute to his visit. He had to eat this delicacy in their presence. He survived to tell the Stevensville office all about it over lunch!

In the early days Marilyn heard accountants saying over and over, "We're not making any money," and at first she worried, but the clinic stayed open through the power of prayer. She got used to hearing it. Confident that the Lord had a purpose for the clinic, she became assured that He would keep the doors open.

At conferences throughout the years, strangers would hear she worked at Southwestern and say, "You guys are a Christian group. How do you guys survive?" and her answer has always been, "The power of prayer."

With medicine, Marilyn concluded, there has been much change and turmoil in the past decade. Patients now feel ultra-informed. They come in telling the doctors what they want, dictating care, demanding time. They go home and get on the Internet to compare the information they find to what the physician has told them. That's been harder to make the job fun. But the financial and reimbursement changes have been the toughest factors. The fact that Southwestern has been able to adjust and even grow its impact on the community, Marilyn said, "speaks of the Lord's love for us and the protection he has given us all these years."

Dr. Georg Christian Schultz

Little Georg Schultz' dad was a pastor. His congregation was interested in feeding the hungry. In Sunday school, they collected $50 every year to buy a dairy calf. Georg and his Dad raised several calves during those the years. When each calf was grown, they'd ship the heifer to Mexico. They were cows with great milk production. One Mexican family couldn't support them; a school had to support them. In high school, Georg traveled to Mexico to look for the heifers and their homes. Georg found one of his cows, a light brown Swiss he had named HOPE: Help Other People Eat. "She didn't remember me," Dr. Schultz joked. But he never forgot HOPE or the lessons he learned while raising the cows.

Georg's father was greatly interested in missions. Every September when the crops came in, the church held a Harvest Home Mission Festival. Georg's father brought in an active missionary to speak. Georg watched those missionaries. He talked to them. He listened to their exciting stories about India and other places and was enamored by missions.

Initially, he planned to be a grain farmer. He was going to go help the Mexicans raise crops and be an agricultural missionary. Seeing Georg's love of math and science, his Dad had other ideas. He said, "Why don't you go to medical school." Georg considered that medicine, like agriculture, could also be a mission. When he got to medical school, it was hard. Finally, in his third year, one of the pediatric professors took him under his wing. Under that professor's encouragement, Georg went into pediatrics and God has used him to influence many.

Dr. Schultz and his wife, Liz, started out in a group practice in Missouri. Then they broke off into a solo practice in Cape Girardeau. They became good friends with Dr. Schindler's niece. His grandnephew suffered from asthma. Dr. Schultz took care of them. Dr. Schultz joined a local CMS (Christian Medical Society) chapter and spent two weeks in Jamaica on short-term missions. At the time, he thought that was only the beginning.

One time Dr. Schindler came to speak for their little CMS chapter. Dr. Schultz brought Dr. Schindler home and they talked at length in his basement. Dr. Schultz had been thinking about getting someone to join his practice in Cape Girardeau. But after talking with Dr. Schindler, Dr. Schultz and Liz decided to join SWMC. They packed up. Dr. Schultz said to his church friends, "I'm off. I'll soon be in Africa someday." That never happened until his daughter Sarah went overseas 20 years later.

Dr. Georg Schultz and Liz came to SWMC in 1987. At that time Berrien General Hospital was the hub of SWMC. Back then, as now, a non-compulsory devotions meeting was held weekly at 7 a.m. on Mondays. Dr. Helene Johnson and Don Gast sat in the corner. Dr. Schindler sat in the front, on the right hand of the person giving the devotions. Whoever led devotions sat at the head of the table. Everyone took turns sharing, and if anyone came into town from the mission field, their schedule was priority. After devotions, the focus of the prayer time was to pray for the foreign missions. Now, both foreign and local missions are emphasized.

When Dr. Schultz formed his habit of attending weekly SWMC devotions, he found them to be a great introduction to the core of the clinic. At devotions he met all the missionaries, learned about them spiritually, and heard about their missions. He also got to know the group and sense at a deeper level its purpose. Decades later, Dr. Schultz still gets up early every Monday to attend devotions with his colleagues, and this decades-old habit reminds him of his calling and the purpose of the clinic. It also provides occasional spontaneous humor.

Devotions are held at Lakeland Regional Medical Center, St. Joseph (formerly Memorial Hospital of St. Joseph) now. One morning Dr. Richard Douce came to the meeting, back from Ecuador. He was telling Dr. Schultz about his work at Vozandes Hospital, when midway through a story, Dr. Ringenberg walked into the room. Their eyes widened. "What are you doing here?" they both asked each other. "Wow!" Both worked in Ecuador, but they hadn't realized they were back in Berrien County at the same time. To Dr. Schultz, this humorous moment illustrated the spinning gears of the clinic, bringing together so many international physicians at once.

No less than when he was a boy, Dr. Schultz thrills to hear what missionaries like Dr. Stephens and Dr. Wesche and others have to say when they come to town. When Dr. Wesche came back and talked at length during devotions, everybody got a real sense of what was going on in Kenya. When Dr. Atkinson got some money together for a tractor at Dr. Stephens' hospital, the joy in the room was almost palpable. Dr. Chupp dedicated the new Tenwek Hospital Operating Room to Dr. Wesche, and Dr. Schultz heard firsthand about that during devotions too.

As the years and now decades have passed, Dr. Schultz has not been called to full time overseas missions. So, the personal blessing for him has been to share his excitement and enthusiasm about missions to his own children, and, now, as they have become adults, to see them go overseas. Sarah has been to Rwanda several times and would like to work there full time someday as a surgeon. Jim and Darcy have been to Sumatra.

Dr. Schultz was overjoyed when his daughter came to him and said, "I want to go to Rwanda for a while. Can you come?" He'll never forget riding onto the Kibogora Hospital compound with Sarah and the Winslows crammed in a Land Rover. While the vehicle was still moving, people crowded around them, and Dr. Winslow leaped out of the vehicle. He was so excited he jumped out of the car to hug the pharmacist, Ezekiel. They were deep in breathless conversation before the Land Rover ground to a stop.

Long before Dr. Schultz met Dr. Bart Comstock, he had a brush with the family. Dr. Schultz was arranging his short-term trip to Jamaica with his brother and his EMT friend, with the CMS. Several times he called the CMS head office in Dallas. A very friendly lady always answered the phone and gave him the best help getting the trip arranged. Who was this lady? She was Dr. Comstock's mom.

Dr. Comstock's parents were missionaries in Brazil, and he spent time there as a child. Dr. Comstock was one of the first pediatricians to join SWMC after Dr. Johansen. He helped with migrant clinics before InterCare opened. He was president of the SWMC Corporation for a while. With a real heart for missions both local and abroad, he has taken groups from Berrien Center Bible Church to the Dominican Republic to help at a Kids Alive orphanage. His wife, Marilyn, is similar in temperament to his mom — very gregarious and pleasant.

SWMC's concept with InterCare is that they are friends but not family. With a heart for southern Michigan dwellers who cannot otherwise afford medical care, InterCare is currently more of a governmental organization than a Christian organization. SWMC has helped InterCare without being the main movers. Dr. Bill Wilkinson contracted out at InterCare for years before leaving SWMC to work for InterCare directly. Dr. Barb Boyd went from SWMC to InterCare and now works at Lakeland Hospital. In Berrien County's small-town community, doctors all rub shoulders with each other and become acquainted. In fact, just about every citizen in Berrien County is familiar with the good doctors.

Most everyone knows Dr. Schultz. Dr. Schultz explains two public-knowledge personal idiosyncrasies. "I repeat myself," he says. "All the time, I say things like, 'You're a good mom, you're a good mom.'"

Not long ago, his identity got stolen. Someone downloaded some insurance files over in Detroit, and someone called Fifth-Third Bank in his name and wanted a debit card. However, the person didn't have quite enough information. They called the bank call center three times. Finally, the Detroit call center called the Stevensville branch. Stevensville hadn't heard anything about a request from Dr. Schultz for a debit card. Detroit played the recorded voice, and the tellers over at Stevensville said, "That's not Dr. Schultz. He doesn't sound like him at all. He didn't repeat himself!"

The other idiosyncrasy is that Dr. Schultz eats ketchup on everything. He's even been known to take a packet of ketchup and slurp it down. People have had a lot of fun humoring Dr. Schultz with ketchup.

Dr. Schultz has a community-wide reputation for loving his pint-sized patients and spending time with them. SWMC administrative assistant Carolyn Philip has numerous grandchildren. They all trouped into the office one day. One of them needed shots but didn't need the audience of all his siblings. Dr. Schultz took them into his office for a few minutes. They sat and talked, and soon lots of little kids were climbing all over him. Offhand, he says, "That was just a watchin' the kids kinda thing."

SWMC physicians are heroes in many circles. Dr. Schultz' daughter Sarah attended Hope College, and one day one of her professors brought in a guest speaker, a Holland-area physician. To a wide-eyed classroom, the physician vividly explained the African medical practices he encountered during his mission trip. In colorful detail, he described the bloody wounds and dire condition of a patient brought in after a machete attack. Completely unprepared, the physician's mind whirled: What should I do? How can I handle this?

As the physician was grappling with the case, into the room walked a surgeon who cannot be named here. The speaker described him as a superman: "He walked in and took care of this patient, and all was good." The class sat amazed, listening to the superhero tale.

Sarah said, "Well, I've had supper with him, and we've been to his house!"

In the early 1990s, during Desert Storm, this same surgeon had a momentary temptation to leave SWMC. One day he told Dr. Schultz, "I feel the need to volunteer for the war in Iraq."

With his large, expressive, and intuitive eyes, Dr. Schultz looked at his colleague. They're about the same age — not especially young. Dr. Schultz said slowly, "You need to talk to your wife about this."

The surgeon didn't go to Iraq, but he's a guy for whom a challenge wouldn't turn him back. He dealt with massive machete wounds; he could've dealt with Desert Storm.

Such are the physicians who populate SWMC, who work alongside Dr. Schultz. Dr. Atkinson once told Dr. Schultz his Congo story. Even as the Atkinsons' plane raced along the ground and rose into the air, rebels were firing gunshots at them. The closest Dr. Schultz ever got to that was at Kibogora. The hospital sits on a hill, and the church is sited on the crest of the hill. In front of the church was a concrete slab, about 10' x 10'. The slab marked where some of the bodies were laid to rest after rebels attacked the hospital during the genocide. In 2005 when Dr. Schultz and Sarah stood beside it, the slab was unmarked, stark functionality. A memorial has since been erected.

During Monday morning devotions, Dr. Atkinson didn't claim a special seat. In his later years when they held devotions at Lakeland, Dr. Atkinson sat in the middle, dishing out encouragement to all his colleagues who clustered around him. "He was always encouraging. I wish I'd appreciated this more," Dr. Schultz says. "He'd stop by the office on Wednesdays, after he retired, and want to pray with us for our patients. He wanted to encourage us, and I was so busy, often distracted, but it meant a lot. Now it means even more. With all the changes in medicine, [I want to remember his example and encourage others] to keep doing that good stuff, keep doing that good stuff."

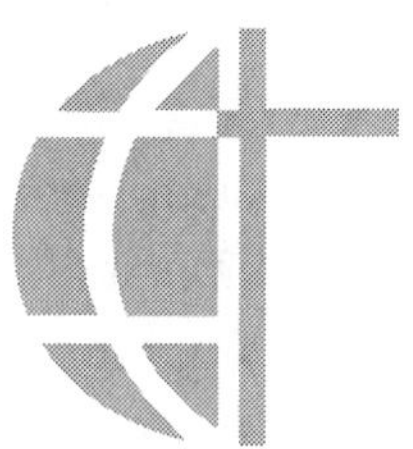

Chapter 21

History and Stories about Southwestern Niles

Chapter 21

History and Stories about Southwestern Niles

One more experiment, "Southwestern South County," started small. SWMC's first Niles clinic faced Grant Street across from Pawating Hospital. It was a little building with two physicians: Dr. Andy Rutherford and Dr. Dan Metzger. Busier than elves, they wanted to expand the clinic but didn't have room.

Around the same time, another well-established clinic in Niles began looking for a buyer. The Four Flags Medical Clinic, later called Michiana Walk-In Clinic, was not located near the hospital, but it sat on the busiest full-access highway connecting southwest Michigan to northern Indiana. SWMC doctors had helped Four Flags/Michiana Walk-In Clinic when short-handed, so they had already informally begun building clients. Also, there was plenty of room to grow.

SWMC prayed about it. As SWMC doctors had done before them in order to launch the other satellite clinics, the Niles-area SWMC physicians banded to form a business association called Niles Business Associates, LLC. They pooled their resources and bought shares of the building.

Joyce Bailey, who had left Pawating Hospital in 1990 to manage the Michiana Walk-In clinic, stayed as clinic coordinator. Dr. Dan Metzger was installed as family practitioner and Dr. Andy Rutherford as a pediatrician — both simply moved across town from Grant Street. Dr. Rutherford took the title of medical director. Diane Smith came from the business office in Berrien Center as business coordinator. The walk-in clinic stayed open through renovations that lasted from mid-1990 to September 1991. At that time, the clinic celebrated its grand opening as Southwestern Medical Clinic — Niles.

Joyce and Diane have worked side-by-side since the office opened. Though their titles have changed — Joyce has been called clinic coordinator, then director, now manager; Diane has been business coordinator and now serves as receptionist and medical records coordinator — they have worked to coordinate both the clinical and business aspects of the clinic.

Don Gast pursued a rural health clinic designation for the Niles clinic, and it was granted in August 1993. This designation provided a supplementary income, a partial reimbursement, which is sometimes several years in arrears. One requirement to become a rural health clinic: hiring a midlevel provider, or a physician assistant. Keith Schierling, PA, was hired. He saw patients and also worked in the walk-in clinic.

Southwestern physicians from "north county," including Berrien Springs, St. Joseph, Bridgman, and Stevensville, traveled to Niles as needed. Some of these included Dr. Dan Stephens, Dr. Jonathan Saxe, Dr. Doug Wilson, and Dr. Bob Wesche.

New doctors who joined SWMC were placed at Niles to reduce the cross-county travel. Dr. Greg Crabill, a family practitioner; Dr. Neil Martin, a pediatrician; pediatric nurse practitioner Claretta Munger; and Dr. David Grellmann all joined between 1992 and 1993. Also by the end of that year, Drs. Mark and Donna Joan Harrison joined. In 1994, PA Fred Kyte came. Drs. Jonathan Saxe and Doug Wilson, surgeons, still rotated to Niles one day a week. Dr. Marilyn Hunter, a pediatrician, came in 1995. Also that year, Dr. Wesche was home on furlough and worked at Niles.

Amid all the comings and goings, Dr. Rutherford was in and out himself on short-term trips overseas. For him, the hardest thing about going away was leaving his desk unguarded. Everyone else considered his desktop an eyesore. He kept every little slip of paper. Sticky notes decorated liberally. It was an avalanche risk. Joyce Bailey and anonymous others would clean it up a bit while he was gone.

He'd come back wearing his favorite brown pants and beige shirt and hurry into his office. Even as he was changing from his outdoor shoes into his loafers, his eyes roved his desk. He could see right away if anything had been "tidied up." This was one of the few things that ever made him grumpy.

Back in the 1990s the clinic was full of charts. Stacks of charts were everywhere, and everyone shared the same charts. The chart world was a black hole. If Dr. Rutherford needed a chart, he'd ask every warm body who walked by to find him the chart until someone brought it.

Niles had its share of tough personal times. Dr. Grellman's three-year-old daughter was diagnosed with a carcinoma in the abdomen. The whole clinic rallied around the Grellman family as the Grellmans tunneled through the miseries of hour-away treatments at Bronson Hospital in Kalamazoo for a year before they lost their daughter.

The Harrisons lost a child, too. Drs. Mark S. and Donna Joan Harrison came to SWMC in 1993 with two young children. Shortly after arriving, Dr. Donna Joan Harrison became pregnant with their third child, Paul, who was born in 1994 and died in 1996 due to a major heart problem. Paul's death marked a turning point for the Harrison family, the Niles office, and the entire clinic.

Since medical school in 1982, Dr. Donna Joan Harrison had been actively involved in pro-life public policy both domestically and overseas. In 2000 she left SWMC to work more actively in public policy and to rear their five children. She spoke to the Michigan state senate, the United States senate subcommittee on partial birth abortion, the FDA, and the United Nations Prep Committee. She was appointed director of research and public policy of the American Association of Pro-Life Obstetricians and Gynecologists and chair of its subcommittee on RU486, coauthoring a citizen petition filed with the FDA to remove RU486 from the U.S. market. She is also chairman of the board of directors of Americans United for Life. She has helped formulate pro-life public policy law in Eastern Europe, Latin America, and Africa.

Equally brilliant, Dr. Mark Harrison is board-certified in infectious diseases, pediatrics, and internal medicine. He serves on the SWMC board, Lakeland medical practice board, has served as Lakeland Hospital chief of staff, and has a reputation for high involvement and high impact in everything he takes on.

While Niles survived tough times, fun times were also frequent. The Metzgers hosted potlucks and Christmas parties complete with caroling, stories, and a gift exchange. Staff collected money to get a gift for each provider, and physicians gave gifts to the staff. A clinic builds a family atmosphere making memories like these together.

From 1995-1996, Niles clinic underwent a major renovation to double the building's size. Dr. Rutherford insisted that the clinic not be interrupted in its service to the patients. Throughout the renovation the clinic was open seven days a week, with the urgent care open on Saturdays and Sundays.

Staff worked under dangling wires, moving their desks into hallways. They cordoned the charts off in the waiting room. During the day jackhammers jolted nurses trying to write in charts; men laid pipelines underfoot; and the clinic worked through it all. In April 1996, they opened the new rooms just in time. That year Dr. Jones, Dr. Dan Stephens, and pediatrician Dr. Lois Lello all arrived.

In 1997, Dr. Bob Spees, an internal medicine specialist, joined; his wife Dr. Annalise Spees worked part-time. Dr. Daniel Joyce joined as a family practitioner. Dr. Paul Lim rotated to Niles as a part-time surgeon. Dr. Donna Harrison came back to work part-time after having another child. That next year as the Speeses left, Dr. Samir N. Rizk came.

Around this time, Dr. Rutherford and incoming SWMC administrator Warren White discussed ways to add more income to the clinic. With Dr. Rutherford's laboratory background, a lab seemed logical. So they took a small back room, brought in some chemistry, and Dr. Rutherford began running some of his own draws.

One day Sally Hanson, a registered medical technologist (med tech) who worked in the Niles walk-in clinic, asked Dr. Rutherford if she could do some quality control on the urine dip sticks and small blood counts. He was all for it. In fact, they soon added a microscope. Next came the fledgling Niles lab's first Coulter, a larger analyzer to perform complete blood counts (CBCs).

Having a lab was a tremendous help to both the walk-in and pediatrics providers to diagnose patients quickly in one office visit without having to wait for results to come back from the hospital.

Diane Baker, also a registered medical technologist, relocated back to Michigan in 1995 to work in Lakeland Regional Medical Center's laboratory. Not long afterward she took a position as lab manager at SWMC's Niles clinic, where she and others started a core laboratory. To say that it soon outgrew the available space at the Niles clinic is an understatement. The lab staff and providers in the Niles clinic were "crunched like sardines." They moved the core lab to Berrien Springs. This was a reasonably centralized location for all SWMC's clinics. Thus, every SWMC location utilized the lab.

As the laboratory grew, SWMC installed a laboratory information system (LIS), which allowed the providers in all of the SWMC locations to access laboratory test results as soon as they were complete. Couriers picked up specimens from each clinic twice daily, so there was rarely a time when test results were not received by the ordering provider by the next day.

Phlebotomy students in the clinics helped both parties. The students learned hands-on skills; SWMC staff learned current trends and techniques in obtaining blood specimens. Also, SWMC hired top-notch graduates.

Sally rose to be lab supervisor while Diane was promoted to lab director. They sensed God working through them to save lives. Since many providers and patients traveled overseas, they sometimes came across uncommon specimens. Once they found a patient with malaria. In another instance, a patient had abnormal blood clotting. They also screened CBCs for infection, allergic reactions, and leukemia. It was rewarding for them to be on the front line to assist in detecting diseases that might otherwise not have been identified.

With God's help, they were able to build a laboratory which they pray exemplified the compassion and excellence required as servants of His. The lab was successful for its entire existence — about two decades.

In 1999 John Kittredge replaced Keith Schierling as PA. Margaret Marsh joined as a part-time nurse practitioner. In 2000 pediatrician Dr. Joshua Underhill arrived. Dr. Samir Rizk helped Dr. VanOosterhaut part-time at the LTACH acute facility in Berrien Center. Dr. Grellman left, and John Kittredge left in June, so Niles took on Steve Smith, PA, full time in September. In 2001 Dr. William Dukes and Dr. Mary Pat McManmon joined as family practice doctors. The next year Dr. Judy Black joined as a new pediatrician just out of school. Dr. Brad Ferrari also joined, as well as pediatrician Dr. Shanna Kautzmann.

Dr. Rutherford, his close friend Don Gast, and incoming SWMC administrator Warren White were always trying to look for things the clinic could keep in the office to reduce outside expenses. One of the more successful ideas was to do bone density exams. The Niles office ran its own bone density exams from 2001-2011. Dr. Rutherford read those for a while, and then talked Dr. Brad Ferrari into doing it.

Niles also participated in research, though Stevensville is the base for the research department. Research involves looking at new drugs and immunizations being considered for market approval. Research interested SWMC for several reasons. Market research brings in revenue. It brings the latest medicine to the attention of both doctors and patients. But more importantly, research means being a part of advancing medicine. Dr. Richard Hines and Karen Styf directed the research department as of 2013.

The Niles clinic has also offered counseling services for more than a decade. Counseling services are coordinated by licensed clinical psychologist and counselor Dr. Marcia Wiinamaki in Stevensville.

Counselors offer services in Stevensville, Bridgman, and Niles. Interns rotate through as well.

Dr. William Dukes left in August 2003. When Dr. Delbert Huelskoetter came to Niles from Illinois, he was supposed to be a part-time, short-term fill; but Dr. Dukes left the clinic a little short. So Dr. Huelskoetter became full time between family practice and the walk-in clinic. He also stayed three years — much longer than he'd planned — which was a blessing in many ways. Dr. Huelskoetter went to Mayo Clinic every year for training and knew many people there. A lifetime friend, he visits SWMC — Niles every time he's in the area.

Also in 2003 nurse practitioner Margaret Marsh, Dr. Kautzmann, and Dr. McManmon left. PA Mary Ramsey came, as well as Dr. Genevieve Peterson for a short time.

The year 2004 was unintentionally a year of change at Niles. Margaret Marsh came back and helped in pediatrics. Dr. Gordon (pseudonym), an internal medicine/infectious disease specialist, joined SWMC and worked in Niles. That changed the clinic in several ways. In the past, Dr. Mark Harrison was the infectious disease specialist working at the old Berrien Center office. When Dr. Gordon came, those patients were routed to Niles. Suddenly, Niles saw a great increase of HIV patients. Dr. Gordon, so young and brilliant and energetic, amazed everyone with his breadth and depth of knowledge.

The following year brought many changes. Pediatrician Dr. Chris Harvey came, and, though young, his old soul reminded everyone of the clinic grandfathers. He understood and lived out SWMC's priorities. He quickly joined SWMC leadership. Also in 2005, Dr. Judy Black was married and moved to Chicago. Dr. Lois Lello returned part-time after having children. Dr. Leanne Miller helped with pediatrics part-time. Dr. Richard Bardin worked part-time at Niles and filled his week at AL-TACH. Dr. Crabill only worked part-time during the wars. He signed up for reserves and got deployed for a month or two. When he returned, he took a temporary leave from SWMC. But the temporary leave was for naught. He joined the military full time.

The Niles lab moved into an old SWMC office in Berrien Springs. Dr. Richard Bardin became medical director of the lab at that time. Dr. Bardin had a background in lab work and also had just gone to school for pathology before coming to SWMC. The lab was very successful in Berrien

Springs and existed until 2010. Dr. Bardin and his wife, Debbie, now work at a hospital in Cameroon.

Niles continued its own point of care lab, operating without a CBC (complete blood count) machine. Niles continues to employ two full time lab technicians who do drug screens, lab draws, mono tests, occult bloods, and influenza tests. Nurses run pregnancy, strep, and hemoglobin tests at nurses' stations.

Niles tried to run its own heart studies with Dr. Rizk. They had a cardio machine for a short time that took pictures of the heart, similar to an ECHO machine. They also ran treadmill stress tests. But these things didn't last too long because the demand wasn't high enough to bring in enough profit to keep them going.

One that lasted longer was an x-ray. Niles clinic had an x-ray machine for years. It became obsolete and they had trouble getting outside radiologists to read their pictures. After a two-year process, Niles and Stevensville clinics have "gone digital" with their x-rays. Hospital radiologists read their x-rays electronically.

In 2006 Dr. Ball (pseudonym) joined SWMC. Dr. Richard Hirschler also worked part-time to full time, helping in the walk-in clinic. Dr. Sterling Thompson joined in 2007. Planning a career in the ministry, Dr. Thompson attended graduate school at Andrews University in Berrien Springs. He already had his doctorate of medicine and wanted to keep up his license, so he worked at Niles several days a week while going to school full time and living on campus. This fascinated staff and patients, and he was very willing to discuss his calling and his plans.

Also in 2007, Jordan Wagner, PA, worked part-time. Dr. Huelskoetter worked through July. In 2011, planning and training for electronic records swept through SWMC, spearheaded by Dr. Ken O'Neill. Electronic records had been talked about since 2005. In 2008 medical records were implemented in segments. One building implemented medical records in March. In April, another building went digital, and so on. Niles clinic was last in June. The workers at Niles got to see everyone else go through it first, so they learned a lot from the other offices.

Dr. Underhill left midway through 2009. Dr. Charlotte Lofgren, a pediatrician, came in the summer after graduating. Dr. Holly Tapley rotated to Niles part-time while in the states, mostly in the walk-in clinic.

In 2010 Dr. Bardin left to work in Cameroon. Dr. Thompson graduated from Andrews University and moved to Texas in a unique position to combine his medical and missions degrees. Late that year, Kate Smith, PA, started part-time in the walk-in clinic. In 2011 Dr. Patrick Holbert, former ER doctor in the Lakeland system, started working two days at Niles' urgent walk-in clinic and one day in Stevensville. Dr. Daniel Margules, a contract physician, rotated to Niles several days a week.

In June 2006, Sandy Criswell, RN, spent a month at Karanda Hospital with Ruth Rutherford to help Dr. Dan Stephens with his AIDS and TB clinics. For years Sandy had heard the stories told by physicians home on furlough. The trip opened her eyes to the need. Right outside the back gate of Karanda Hospital, vendors stack caskets of all sizes: children's little caskets, slightly larger caskets for teenagers. Business is always steady.

When Sandy came home she wanted to continue to help. She started collecting pop bottles and aluminum. Whenever \$50 adds up, she sends it to Dr. Dan Stephens to use at Karanda. In five years she has sent \$1,500. She has also helped arrange for supplies such as catheters and different medicines. Poignant thank-you letters that come back keep the momentum going throughout the Niles clinic to bring in more pop bottles and aluminum. Ten-cent donations, multiplied, can save lives.

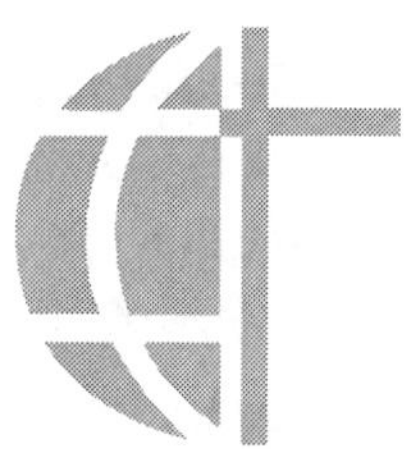

Chapter 22

South County's Heart and Soul

Chapter 22

South County's Heart and Soul

Dr. James "Andy" Rutherford

Dr. James "Andy" Rutherford and his wife, Ruth, were both second generation missionaries. Andy grew up in Ethiopia; Ruth grew up in the Congo/Zaire. But they didn't meet in Africa. They met in Kalamazoo, Michigan.

Ruth was in nurse's training at Bronson Hospital. Andy was at Western Michigan University in the ROTC program, earning his bachelor's degree in medical technology, and he spent time in Bronson Hospital. They hit it off right away. After receiving his degree, Andy went into the military and was stationed in North Carolina during the Vietnam War, working in the lab, handling cases coming back from Vietnam.

Andy had not given up his dream of becoming a medical doctor. But he didn't get accepted into medical school. He had done poorly in organic chemistry and quantitative analysis at Wheaton College, which was reflected in a lower GPA. He did get accepted into the physician assistant program at Duke University or in Trinity's master's program in hospital administration. He chose Trinity, thrived there in San Antonio, and eventually was introduced to a southern Baptist adoption agency. Andy and Ruth's little girl arrived to them from the hospital at six days old.

Now with a young family, Andy completed his second year of a hospital administration internship in Arkansas near relatives. He still wanted to be a physician. Ruth, however, dreaded the lifestyle changes and work schedule. Applying to the medical school at the University of Arkansas at Little Rock, Andy was put on its waiting list.

Ruth can still remember when Andy called her on the telephone with the news. She was in Michigan visiting his parents. Andy said, "They called me, and they have an opening in July. I know how you feel about doctors and the busy life they have. Will you commit to this life with me, through med school and beyond? If not, I would be willing to give up my dream of becoming a doctor."

"Of course I was going to commit," Ruth says now. "But he was wise to ask me that way. That stuck with me all the way through, when his hours were horrible. I had made a commitment."

After Dr. Rutherford's four years of medical school, he still wanted to go to the mission field, so he signed up for a rotating internship and first year surgery abroad. His senior year, in 1973, a son came to the Rutherfords. Also that year, Dr. Rutherford got a Readers' Digest scholarship to go to South Africa for three months. These three fast-paced months would prove crucial in two ways. First, he found TEAM (TheEvangelical Alliance Mission), their sending organization to the full time mission field for the rest of their careers. Second, he met Dr. Doug Taylor at the Mosvold Mission Hospital in South Africa. Dr. Taylor told him glowing stories about Southwestern Medical Clinic. Intrigued, Dr. Rutherford filed Dr. Taylor's comments for later. Instead, after a year of surgery residency, he and Ruth joined TEAM, thinking they were going to South Africa.

But the South African government took over Mosvold Hospital. TEAM asked the Rutherfords if they would consider going to a small mission hospital in the UAE (the United Arab Emirates). "We told TEAM, our hearts are in Africa, but we'll tell all the doctors we know about the need of a doctor in UAE."

They prayed that the Lord would lay UAE on someone's heart and went through all their doctor friends. None were interested. Then Dr. Rutherford and Ruth looked at each other and confessed that, instead of their friends' hearts, the Lord had been working on their own hearts. He wanted the Rutherfords in Arabia.

One evening in 1976 about 10 p.m., the telephone rang. A supporter spoke rapidly, urgently. A baby boy needed parents, and the supporter knew they'd adopted two children already. Would they be interested in adopting a third?

That was tough. Adopting a baby at this time meant road blocks everywhere. They would have to raise extra support, and they'd already had some trouble raising what TEAM said they would need as a family of four. Also, six months after the adoption — when they already planned to be abroad — they would have to go to court to finalize the adoption. The Lord had clearly taught them with their previous adoptions that children are an inheritance from the Lord. But how would it be possible?

Dr. Rutherford and Ruth wrestled with their decision all night. The next day they learned that certain rules could be bent for veteran adopting parents. They could go to court and fill out the paperwork before they left and, six months later, send a letter letting the court know how they were doing.

The Rutherfords called TEAM to try to find answers about the amount of extra support they would need to pull out of a hat. TEAM had already voiced some admonitions to them to raise more support, so they dialed TEAM's number with trepidation. An unfamiliar voice answered the telephone. This affable fellow chuckled and said, "TEAM is all about faith. If God wants you to have that baby, He'll bring in the extra money."

Before noon the Rutherfords called to accept the baby. Later that day, Dr. Rutherford was on call in his surgery residency, but at 6 p.m. for a brief supper break, he and Ruth met a nurse in the hospital parking lot. She passed to them their new baby, less than 24 hours old. Dr. Rutherford held his son, kissed his wife, put their new son in her arms, and ran back in to finish his night shift.

In the fall they went to UAE. Dr. Rutherford helped with hospital administration and launched the lab. Meanwhile, he thought ahead to a residency and debated between ophthalmology and pediatrics. At the TEAM mission hospital in UAE, God settled Dr. Rutherford's debate, and both he and Ruth found their calling.

Jesus had a big heart for children, and in UAE, Dr. Rutherford fell in love with the young patients. One tiny child who tugged his heart was born with a tragic blood flow abnormality. All blood-compatible staff members donated blood. Dr. Rutherford pumped in his own blood for the little one. They did everything they could, but the baby didn't make it. Dr. Rutherford desperately wanted to know how to help kids like that. When the Rutherfords returned to Little Rock from 1981-1983, he completed his pediatric residency, all the while thinking about the babies in UAE.

After returning to UAE, Dr. Rutherford dug out an old address that Dr. Doug Taylor had given him a decade before. He started writing to Don Gast. In 1987, the Rutherfords' next furlough, they came to Southwestern Medical Clinic. Ruth worked as a nurse. That year Dr. Rutherford traveled to a different Southwestern clinic every day of the week. It was hectic, but their colleagues' generosity was remarkable. God used them in many ways to bless the Rutherfords and to show them His providence. One big blessing was housing. The Metzgers were going to Sierra Leone, so the Rutherfords moved into the Berrien Springs house the Metzgers had been renting.

In 1990, after 14 years on the mission field, the Rutherfords made a drastic change. Dr. Rutherford's sister had died of cancer, and he was the only child left to take care of his parents in Decatur, Michigan. Dr. Rutherford contacted Southwestern wondering if a permanent position would be available for him. They asked if he'd be willing to build the Niles office, to stay at that one location rather than traveling to Bridgman, Berrien Springs, Berrien Center, and the rest. Willing? Eagerly they made the Niles office their home mission. It was a settling move for Dr. Rutherford, even though he had planned to live his whole life in UAE.

The 11th Street clinic was still a Four Flags Walk-in Clinic back then. Southwestern Medical Clinic was across from the Pawating Hospital Emergency Room on Grant Street. Southwestern-Niles moved to the former Four Flags Walk-in Clinic along old U.S.-31 the year after Dr. Rutherford came to stay, in 1991, and subsequently put an addition on the building to enlarge it.

Dr. Rutherford worked at Southwestern in Niles the rest of his life, for 14 years. Ruth worked at the same office as a nurse. Dr. Rutherford served on various SWMC boards as well as working full time at the Niles clinic.

Dr. Rutherford was more than a pediatrician. He was a minister and an advocate. His colleague Dr. Dan Metzger said of him, "He was a workaholic but wouldn't call it that, because he was so happy. He loved what he was doing. His whole life was ministry." Other pediatricians outside SWMC would fault him for his two-hour rounds in the evening, calling such time-consuming rounds excessive and unnecessary. But Dr. Rutherford considered his rounds key to ministering to his patients and their families, whether in the states or abroad. He brought his own children on rounds with him in UAE. If a family was bedside, Dr. Rutherford served coffee and fruit and chatted with them, one of his kids sitting beside him.

Due to his work, Dr. Rutherford sometimes got inadvertently pulled into court cases involving children. He would go to court to advise in cases of abuse. One time a prosecutor accused him of having an affair with a foster mother because Dr. Rutherford said he felt the child was better off in the foster home than with his own mother. The accusation was outrageous, and everyone in the court room who knew of Dr. Rutherford understood his compassionate intentions. He loved children and looked out for their best interests, always.

Dr. Rutherford had a knack for smoothing rough waters. Nurses sometimes came to him with an interpersonal problem. Embroiled in the midst of it, it momentarily seemed huge to them. Looking at the situation from his point of view, such matters were trivial in light of the life-and-death physical and spiritual situations he'd lived through. He'd look at his red-faced nurses and start laughing, and his demeanor lightened them up. They appreciated him for it.

Dr. Rutherford and Ruth did not forget their little mission hospital in Arabia. Almost every year they returned for a month or two to relieve the mission doctors in the summertime. In October 2002 the Rutherfords went back, thinking they would stay for two years. Six months later, frustrated with changes, Dr. Rutherford felt compelled to return to the states. It was God's timing. Their kids had that last year with their dad.

About a year later, in 2004, Dr. Rutherford started having abdominal discomfort. At that time he was taking care of pediatric behavioral medicine and thought he was just stressed. He brushed it off. By the end of March he scheduled an ultrasound. Something was spotted in his liver. Another Southwestern-Niles physician, Dr. Delbert Heulskoetter, recommended a liver specialist at Mayo Clinic. Near the end of April, on a Sunday, the Rutherfords made the trip to Mayo. They saw the specialists on Monday, had a biopsy taken on Tuesday, and on Wednesday learned he had a fast-growing cancer and would have surgery on Thursday. The cancer was even further advanced than they had feared. Surgery was long and unsuccessful. By Sunday they'd pumped 27 units of blood into Dr. Rutherford's body. Ruth knew they couldn't keep that up for long. His albumin dropped lower. The staff at Mayo kept Dr. Rutherford comfortable on IVs, but by Monday morning Ruth had to let him go.

It all happened extremely fast. Ruth recalled later, "A couple furloughing we knew well in UAE wanted to come see him, relatives were coming, our pastor and several other pastors were coming. So, we decided we would wait until 7 p.m. to take him off the vent. By then everyone had come. We wanted this to be a glorious home going. Sixteen of us crowded around my husband in the ICU: singing, reading scripture, and praying. All of a sudden, through our worship, his numbers stabilized.

"I said to a nurse, 'I wish I had hugged and kissed him more before surgery,' so they moved his bed and rearranged things so I could lie right beside him in bed. Those last two days I was by his side, as close as I could be. This was all God's work. Before we had left for Mayo, Andy had suggested I not come along. 'I will be right by your side every bit of the way,' I had told him. Sure enough I was, every bit of that long way, much longer than we'd planned, but I was right there. I felt even though he was unconscious, our spirits were together, side by side. He knew I was there."

One time near the end, when she stepped out of the room, his numbers began dropping. She got back in bed and sang quietly again, song after song, for about an hour. Then quietly he was gone.

Southwestern Medical Clinic was devastated by Dr. Andy Rutherford's sudden death on April 27, 2004. Founding physician of the Niles office, the humble pediatrician and staunch children's advocate was a strong leader at SWMC and in the community. They erected a small stone memorial at the Niles office entrance. While they are assured of his eternal joy in heaven, and know they will join him someday, his colleagues keenly miss him years later. They remember his work ethic — his daily ministry — and, in their own ways, hope to memorialize Dr. Rutherford by emulating the traits and habits they most admired in him.

Ruth continued to work at the Niles office until 2011 and has been on more than a dozen mission trips since her husband's death. Rather than being haunted by his absence in these efforts they'd tackled together, Ruth feels comforted and knows he would be proud of all she has finished in his memory.

Dr. Dan and Elaine Metzger

Dan Metzger was the first person in his family to go to college. When Dan was an undergrad, Dr. Herb Atkinson came to speak at the Bloomington, Indiana Presbyterian church Dan had just started attending. Having grown up Catholic, Dan had accepted Christ during a Navigators meeting in college. He was amazed at the stories Dr. Atkinson shared. He prayed, "God, if you want me to do medical missions, get me into medical school," which He did. This was one of the first amazing signs and wonders God performed to build Dr. Metzger's faith.

SWMC did not stick in Dr. Metzger's head, but he remembered the African stories. He completed his residency in South Bend, still thinking about going into missions. He went to the Urbana InterVarsity conference to check out recruiting booths. There, he learned most sponsoring organizations wanted their prospective missionaries to take a year of Bible college and spend a year fundraising before going abroad. Dr. Metzger didn't relish taking a couple years up front not doing any medical work. He was getting deflated.

Then Dr. Metzger stopped at the SIM (Serving in Mission) booth and met Dr. Bob Schindler, who was helping recruit. Dr. Metzger poured out his dilemma. Dr. Schindler broke into a smile. "Not a problem," he boomed. "Why don't you come across the state line and work for us at SWMC for a year? You can take Bible classes by correspondence."

That's how Dr. Metzger came to interview with SWMC six years after hearing Dr. Atkinson talk about Africa. Inside SWMC's front door, Dan Metzger saw the name Dr. Herb Atkinson and remarked, "I remember him! He told all those hair-raising stories."

It was winter of 1982. Michigan weather was brutal. Ice and snow covered the roads. Driving Dr. Metzger and his wife, Elaine, around to all SWMC's offices, Don Gast warmed them with stories. He talked about how Dr. Schindler and Dr. Atkinson were kicked out of their countries and unexpectedly showed up back at SWMC. To make room for everyone, SWMC opened more satellite offices.

Don told a story that might've chilled a prospective partner less committed to missions: the Dr. Wesche tithing legend. At a monthly meeting, when the accountant presented depressing financial information and suggested reducing the tithe to missions, Dr. Wesche as chairman of the board nipped that idea in the bud. "Oh, no," Dr. Wesche said. "In times like these, you give more to God, and then He will bless."

Don's excitement for missions drew in the Metzgers. How many places in the world can claim three core guys who were classmates with Jim Elliot? That was a very special era. The Metzgers started working at SWMC in July 1982. Dr. Metzger traveled to Berrien Springs, Benton Harbor, Bridgman, and Berrien Center — one place in the morning and another in the afternoon — and filled in at the Berrien General ER. Calling it a hassle would be an understatement, in the days before computers and car phones. But every day was exciting, and the missions-minded climate kept the Metzgers motivated to pursue their own international calling.

The Metzgers knew they were being called to foreign missions, but they didn't know where in the world God wanted them to go. When the Metzgers started working in July, Dr. Ron Baker was just finishing his year of furlough. On Dr. Metzger's first day of work, Dr. Baker gave him a tour of the hospital. By "coincidence," SWMC held a picnic with a dual purpose: to welcome the Metzgers and bid farewell to the Bakers. Both times, Dr. Baker talked to Dr. Metzger about Sierra Leone. A month later the Bakers were gone, back to the field. They only overlapped about a month. In that month, the seeds were planted and began to germinate.

During one Monday morning devotion meeting, Dr. Richard Roach had the idea that everyone should write an encouraging letter to a missionary doctor. Dr. Roach knew that the newbie Dr. Metzger had met Dr. Baker, so he suggested Dr. Metzger should write to him. Dr. Metzger wrote a newsy, encouraging little note to his new acquaintance in Sierra Leone.

A week or so later, the corporation got a letter from Dr. Baker telling how the doctor out there with him, Dr. Tom Ritter, was going home that summer and wouldn't be coming back. Dr. Baker was anticipating being at the hospital in Sierra Leone by himself and wondered if SWMC had any doctors wanting to replace Dr. Ritter. Dr. Metzger went home and talked with Elaine about it. "How'd you like to go to Sierra Leone?" he asked.

She said, "Isn't that the little country next to India (Sri Lanka)?"

They found Sierra Leone on the map, and Dr. Metzger sent another letter to Dr. Baker, volunteering his services. Not long afterward a letter from Dr. Baker came in the mail. It was friendly enough; Dr. Baker shared general news but didn't mention anything about Dr. Metzger's offer. Dr. Metzger tried not to be offended. The response didn't roll off Dr. Metzger's back as he'd hoped it would. He was pretty let down. But he tried to tell himself it was perfectly rational for Dr. Baker to hope for someone with more experience.

A week or two later, a second letter from Dr. Ron Baker came, very excited about Dr. Metzger's offer. Their letters had crossed en route. To and from Sierra Leone, snail mail is more like slug mail. Dr. Metzger's hope returned. Of course Dr. Baker would be happy with any warm body.

Sierra Leone didn't require a year of Bible college or a great deal of fundraising. The Metzgers worked at SWMC for a year, as planned, and took off across the globe. With a young child, Elaine did not work as a nurse on the field. She'd been warned by other mother-nurses that it's a black hole: there's no end to how much they need you to work, and she needed to stay home with a young child. They were right. Elaine was never busier in her whole life.

While Dr. Metzger got acquainted with the staff and procedures,

Dr. Baker shared his own story of coming to Mutru Hospital. Dr. Baker grew up in Sierra Leone. His father had started the first two co-ed boarding schools in the country. Leading people in the Sierra Leonean government were graduates of the high schools Dr. Baker's father started. So when Dr. Baker came back to Sierra Leone after medical school, it was like a native son returning home, and his reputation grew. People traveled over from Guinea to see Dr. Baker at the hospital.

The original missionary doctor at the hospital in Mutru, Dr. Pratt, had gotten involved in the wrong side of politics and was not allowed to return. Dr. Baker thought he was joining Dr. Pratt, but he ended up on his own.

When Dr. Baker went on furlough, and Dr. Metzger worked alone at the hospital in Mutru for a year, there was always a shortage of one thing or another. One time they suffered a shortage of milk. They couldn't even get enough powdered milk to feed kwashiorkor kids. Dr. Metzger wrote an appeal to the bishop. The worldwide mission board sent a whole shipping container of powdered milk to the hospital.

A generator ran on Tuesday and Thursday and a few hours in the evening. Fuel was always in short supply. Repeatedly, the hospital nearly ran out of diesel fuel to run the generator. Fuel trucks came irregularly. The hospital never knew when it would get more. One night during an emergency surgery, Dr. Metzger used the last of the fuel. The missionaries gathered early in the morning and earnestly prayed. That same morning the tanker showed up. God's hand has clearly provided in numerous similar situations.

Originally, the hospital staff had to hand-pump water from a stream behind the hospital. By the 1980s, someone had rigged running cold (not clean) water into the hospital. They built a wonderful water tank just before the Metzgers got there. Mutru was about a 60 to 70 bed hospital, depending on how many extra cots were pulled out, or two people to a bed. Capacities were flexible.

The Metzgers did two three-year terms with a furlough. At the end of his second term, Dr. Metzger felt something wasn't quite right. He still felt like a fish out of water and felt maybe he was used better by God in his own culture. The people in Sierra Leone were very sad to see him go. And truly, the Metzgers were surprised by their unplanned decision not to return to Sierra Leone. They felt a little bereft and asked God a few questions. Within months after they left in 1990, civil war broke out in Sierra Leone.

The country was shut down for a decade.

Instead of looking for another foreign assignment, the Metzgers spent that decade in the U.S. rearing their child and hosting foster and exchange students. SWMC had just opened the Niles office. Dr. Rutherford and Dr. Neil Martin were the only two doctors in the office. SWMC offered Dr. Metzger the option of traveling as always or working in Niles. As years passed, Dr. Metzger became the senior doctor in the Niles office.

They did keep asking God if that was what He wanted for them. One nurse whom they had worked with in Mutru went to work with Mercy Ships. The Metzgers kept in touch with Jean Campbell as she climbed the ladder and eventually was in charge of all medical personnel. They sent her an early Christmas letter and mentioned their son was graduating from college in the spring. Right at that time, a Mercy Ship was doing an offshore trip to Sierra Leone. Jean asked Dr. Metzger if he'd join the crew. The commitment was November 3 through May 4...perfect timing.

Before the Metzgers left for the Mercy Ship in 2003, two of SWMC's four Niles family practice doctors left. Dr. Metzger asked Dr. Andy Rutherford if he should back out of the Mercy Ship contract and stay on to help at SWMC Niles. Dr. Rutherford exclaimed, "No, surely not. Things will work out here."

The week the Metzgers left, things worked out for the short-term. Dr. Heulskoetter was that short-term replacement. He loved it at SWMC and ended up staying four years, and happened to factor into Dr. Rutherford's final chapter. Dr. Rutherford unexpectedly died while the Metzgers were on the Mercy Ship.

The Metzgers learned by email about Dr. Rutherford. During their first terms, communication was mainly by numbered air mail — and some mail never arrived. Back then there was no telephone service in Mutru. The hospital had a ham radio to contact the business office in Freetown twice a day. They got into Freetown themselves four times a year to maybe make a phone call home. To make that call, they had to go down to the national telephone office in Freetown, the capital city, and wait their turn to request an overseas phone call. After that, they paid in advance for their minutes and waited hours more to make the call. Needless to say, they had to make big plans by mail with family beforehand for the phone call.

On their return to Sierra Leone with the ship, they found the Freetown market ladies in their rickety makeshift stalls, selling fabric and local produce, jabbering away on cell phones. The market ladies showed the Metzgers how to use their phone card for local calls and a different card for international phone calls. In 2008 the Metzgers went to Mutru again, short-term with Dr. Baker. By that time, cell phones and towers had arrived upcountry in Mutru. Everyone had cell phones.

Hospital care in Sierra Leone, however, has greatly regressed because of the war. They worked on a 50-year-old refitted ocean liner. When the ship docked in Freetown, it was only a six-hour drive to Mutru. They did get to go to Mutru and see a lot of their old friends and colleagues again. But sadly nothing was the same. The hospital, which once had one of the best reputations in the country despite its remote location, never recovered after the civil war.

Years before, Dr. Metzger had written a letter home to SWMC, mentioning how nice it would be to have an x-ray machine. A bunch of SWMC doctors put their money together. Someone arranged a Peace Corps volunteer x-ray technician who trained some local guys. During the civil war, Mutru was ravaged. Raiders stole the x-ray machine from the hospital, intending to sell it on the black market, but it weighed too much for the raiders' dugout canoe, so it's at the bottom of the river.

A surgery technician did a C-section on his own during the war years and kept the hospital going as a clinic. But when raiders came through the area, they did not bypass the hospital. They stripped the water pipes. They even stripped out the electrical wires. They took everything except the concrete walls.

After the war, it was 13 years before the country had any stability at all. When the mission board evacuated all the missionaries the second time, they said no one was going back. The church was nationalized by then. But the national church could not afford to run the hospital. Doctors Without Borders came in and got the hospital going again.

Doctors Without Borders runs like a crisis organization. They come during a short-term crisis time, and during that time they pay for everything and they give everything for free. But they don't make a plan to help the hospital maintain itself when they leave, so then the hospital is left high and dry. Around 2008, eager Sierra Leoneans had started to dig a well again, but didn't know how to finish it. There's still no running water in the hospital. There's also no doctor, only a physician assistant to run it. They have no electricity. Mutru is just a shell, a shadow of what it used to be. Trash litters the compound. A dozen national employees work there, going months without pay.

During a short-term visit Dr. Metzger, Dr. Baker, and another physician were able to do some surgery, doctoring, and help the hospital pay its staff three months' back salary. They made a special ceremony of a gift in recognition of the few still there.

Dr. Metzger's advice to young medical students interested in foreign missions: first, try not to accumulate too much debt. This will keep you home more than any other factor. Second, take short-term medical missions trips on scholarships when you're a student, for as long as you can and as many times as you can. He recommends two-to-three-month stints. Of course, consider coming to SWMC. Above all, keep God foremost in every area of your life, and He will faithfully organize and reveal your life's journey, one step at a time.

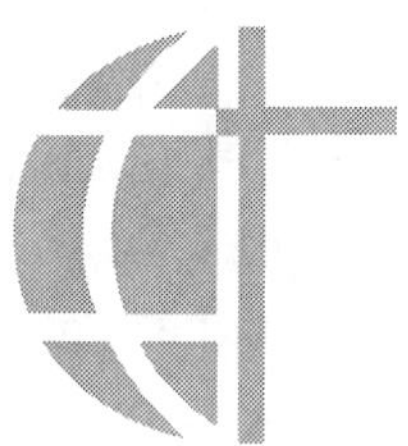

Chapter 23

The Mission Hospital at Mount Darwin

Chapter 23

The Mission Hospital at Mount Darwin

What does a career missionary doctor look like? Is he dressed in traditional African garb? Does he wear an old-fashioned black suit and carry a leather Bible in one deeply tanned hand and a gator-skin medical bag in the other?

Certainly one expects a career missionary doctor to be a man of stature, one who by his very nature stands out in a crowd because of his high calling and unique lifestyle.

Dr. Dan Stephens defies all stereotypes. An unassuming man, neither deeply tanned nor sporting a festive Rhodesian nhembe, he walks quickly, jingling a giant ring of keys on his belt. For all anyone might know, he could be the director of maintenance at a medical facility.

He blends well into his surroundings and could easily be overlooked, and he is fine with that. His fascinating accent and his command of vocabulary only hint of his education and of the significant figure he is in African medicine and Southwestern Medical Clinic history.

Preparations

Dr. Dan Stephens has the distinction of being a second-generation member of Southwestern Medical Clinic. His father Dr. Roland Stephens came to Berrien County Hospital in 1960, when Dan was about five years old, and was one of the four signers of the original incorporation papers. Dan was the young boy who explored Berrien General Hospital and found in the basement Dr. Meyers' white mice.

The young Stephens family lived in southwestern Michigan a couple of years before going to Gunderson-Horness Mission Hospital in Rhodesia, now named Karanda Hospital, 30 miles northeast of Mt. Darwin in Mashonaland Central Province, Mt. Darwin District, Zimbabwe (same location), in 1962. Dan grew up in Africa and considers himself a global citizen.

As a teenager in Rhodesia, following in his father's footsteps was unthinkable. Dan watched his father grow old under the heavy responsibility of serving as the only doctor at the hospital. "I was furious at the mission; I thought Dad was so overworked. I wrote them a letter: 'You're killing him. He needs more help.'"

He says with a crooked smile, "Eventually I answered my own letter."

"At age 12 I decided if the Lord would allow me to be a doctor, I'd be a missionary for Him for 10 years. Ten years!" Dr. Dan Stephens laughs at himself.

In August 1991 Dr. Dan Stephens returned to Zimbabwe — as a surgeon. He went into surgery because, as he learned growing up watching his father, surgical skills are handy and indeed necessary. In his view, surgeons by their training are able to handle most every emergency that comes into their clinic: wounds, problem deliveries, colectomies, the works.

In 1989, when Dr. Stephens signed on with SWMC, about a dozen other SWMC doctors worked stateside at the time. SWMC didn't have enough work for a fourth surgeon, so they sent Dr. Stephens out to rural migrant clinics in Eau Claire and Cass County and the like.

Additionally, when he returned for his first two furloughs, he moonlighted in ERs and clinics. While the work was intense and not specific to his area of expertise, he feels it was the perfect continuing education. "It made me comfortable with almost any patient and medical problem," he said.

He valued these experiences, but has been quick to add that nowadays this kind of experience in the U.S. is unlikely because of insurance regulations. In the late '80s and early '90s, he often worked alongside a seasoned SWMC surgeon. Rubbing shoulders with mentors helped further prepare him to return alongside his father in the remote Karanda Hospital. For reimbursement purposes, two surgeons don't typically scrub in together now.

The timing of his arrival in the late 1980s and early 1990s coincided with countless changes at Southwestern, both because of industry changes and because of Southwestern's quick growth in that decade.

The Benefits of Returning to SWMC as Frequently as Possible

Dr. Dan Stephens has known most of the doctors at SWMC throughout the years, because he tries to return for a month annually. In addition, he makes an effort to spend a year in the states for every four years abroad. These are practices he's learned watching predecessors struggle.

"Dr. Smith (pseudonym)…stayed away eight years before having to practice in the states, and it was very difficult," Dr. Stephens says, because of the incredible changes: new meds, new information programs, new policies and procedures due to changes in insurance and medical knowledge.

Dr. Charles Paine, Dr. Stephens recalls, spent awhile afield. When he finally came back, "they put him in long-term care. The poor man was faced with fifty or so new drugs. He lasted a month and retired. It was too much."

Learning from Dr. Paine's experience, Dr. Stephens says one of the first places he visits at SWMC every year is the medicine closet. "I go down and just look in there at all the new drugs and get familiarized with them."

Another reason he likes to return annually for a month is because, "This maintains my privileges at the hospital so I don't have to reapply every time."

Except for the one month annually in the states, he spends four years abroad, then one year in the states practicing at SWMC. "As Schindler used to say, 'You need to be a global surgeon.' He encouraged functioning in both worlds, and that's what I've tried to do. Dad functioned globally, too, almost to his detriment."

In the states, Dr. Dan Stephens's father tried to treat patients for all their problems in much the same way as he treated patients at Karanda. Rather than referring to specialists, Dr. Roland Stephens performed orthopedic surgeries himself. "Dad was faced with a number of lawsuits and had to be forcibly told not to [do orthopedic surgeries] here," Dr. Dan Stephens recalled.

Working at SWMC has given Dr. Stephens and his colleagues invaluable insights as they watch each other succeed or fail at the numerous intricacies of globe-hopping and global practice.

Funds

Many SWMC doctors have served at Tenwek Hospital in Bomet, Kenya, so it was altogether understandable that they had Tenwek's needs in sharp focus. "[Dr.] Mike Chupp came back here and raised half a million to build a wing on Tenwek." A lot of money came from SWMC, Dr. Dan Stephens remembered.

Not long after, "[Dr.] Atkinson went over there and [Dr.] Chupp gave him a whole new laundry list. So, [Dr.] Atkinson wrote a letter to the group, strongly urging everyone in the group to give more to Tenwek."

Over at Karanda, feeling somewhat overlooked, Dr. Stephens said, "Wait a minute. I want a tractor."

"[Dr.] Atkinson and Don Gast got me a tractor," Dr. Stephens remembered with satisfaction.

Karanda Hospital has used the tractor to haul river sand, pit sand, and stone for the hospital's numerous building projects. Daily, the tractor pulls the trailer that is used to pick up all the trash from the hospital and the 35-odd homes in the hospital compound, as well as the nursing and primary schools. The tractor also mows 20 acres of grass, repairs roads, hauls pipes and engines for the wells, hauls water from the river when needed, regularly tows vehicles stuck in the river crossing, and plows staff's fields. The tractor also off-loads shipping containers from trucks. In short, Dr. Stephens writes, the tractor is used all day, every day.

And SWMC has stepped in with further assistance. According to Dr. Stephens, one of the benefits of SWMC's huge growth in the 1990s was that funds were spread around. For the past decade or more, SWMC has sponsored a different major mission fundraiser every year.

Karanda Hospital

In addition to being a second-generation SWMC physician, Dr. Dan Stephens is also a second-generation surgeon at Karanda Hospital in Zimbabwe.

Karanda Hospital was founded in 1961 and its nursing school in 1964. Located 30 miles northeast of Mt. Darwin, Zimbabwe, in a tiny, remote village on a dirt and gravel road a long way from the nearest city, it would seem an unlikely spot for a hospital or nursing school. But both were desperately needed in the 1960s and are even more today with the country ravaged by three nightmares: violence, famine, and AIDS.

With two or three full time doctors and a dozen staff, the 120-bed hospital sees 300 surgical cases per month. This is enormous for such a staff, but so much more is needed. Karanda needs more personnel in every area from maintenance to nurses to administrative to doctors.

Zimbabwe's AIDS incidence has dropped from a high of around 27% of the population to about 15%. The hospital's population with AIDS remains high — from 30% to 50% — but due to education, the use of condoms, and male circumcision, the hospital has seen a drop in AIDS-infected mothers from 30% to 15%. Karanda treats about 5,000 people per month in its HIV treatment program using antiretroviral drugs.

Karanda has also founded a home-based care system formed to help the chronically ill at a far less cost at home than in a hospital. Karanda has begun a nursing school to help fill its chronic staff shortage and to supplement the education of its own staff, improving nursing care at Karanda and elsewhere. Churches are planted and grow quickly.

Zimbabwean national hospitals have provided erratic service due to political upheaval. This turbulence has made remote Karanda Hospital a hub of activity, drawing patients from as far as 130 miles. But this chaotic situation provides increased opportunities to share the Gospel. Karanda staff sees miracles every day.

Patients can only pay a small fraction of the cost of their care. Zimbabwe's government used to carry the burden of the cost, but now the government can provide very little. Karanda is operating on a shoestring. It can provide its patients with only a subsistence diet while there, and the protein shortages are evidenced by longer healing times after surgeries. Outside the hospital, 50% of the population faces severe hunger and starvation during dry years.

Karanda is one of the busiest hospitals in the country. The national hospitals in the capital city of Harare often send their difficult cases to Karanda, more than a two-hour journey by bus or oxcart. In times of war, such as in 2008-2009, the national hospitals close, forcing more Zimbabweans to bush hospitals for emergency care. Beyond this, Karanda is one of the only hospitals in Zimbabwe able to treat hydrocephalus — water on the brain. Some patients travel six hours by car or days by foot for treatment. Dr. Dan Stephens and his father and a new national doctor treat 90,000 patients per year, deliver 2,000 babies, and perform 3,000 surgeries. In difficult times, Dr. Dan Stephens turns to quick-witted proverbs such as, "Chin up, knees down."

Every morning, Drs. Dan and Roland Stephens, their staff, and 55 nursing students begin the day with devotions in the hospital's little chapel. The students serenade with Zimbabwean hymns, and each person asks for strength and wisdom to meet unexpected challenges through the day.

As hospital supervisor, Dr. Dan Stephens is completing the process to apply to the Pan-African Academy of Christian Surgeons (PAACS). Receiving certification from PAACS would enable Karanda to keep long-term national doctors and train them in surgical skills that would be recognized in the U.S. and Africa. Karanda's national doctor, Dr. Maphios Siamuchembu, has qualified for the surgical program.

Any help that finds its way to Karanda Hospital is like a welcome rain shower during growing season. Short-term mission teams and healthcare students come through Karanda and leave their mark. Then they go home and spread the word about the hospital, its amazing aid, and its poignant need for resources.

Short-termers sometimes tell tall tales about the initiations the Stephenses put them through. One athletic, male medical student blogged about such an adventure — a Sunday morning hike. The destination was the top of a megalith named Pulpit Rock. It turns out the "hike" was a 200-foot natural climbing wall.

When the initiate was unable to ascend the sheer rock without aid, Dr. Dan Stephens brought out the African equivalent of rock-climbing gear. "I know this gear works," he said. "We've used it for women and children making the climb in the past."

So saying, the Stephens men ascended like cats and helped their rope-equipped visitor scrabble up to the top of the huge boulder jutting out of the Zimbabwe bush. The view was magnificent. After an almost equally arduous descent, they jogged full-speed to the hospital to begin their rounds.

Drs. Dan and Roland Stephens, who draw patients from across Zimbabwe because of their excellent reputations, do not zip around in sports cars. Their wives don't shop on Fifth Avenue. The Stephenses and multitudes of other missionary physicians around the world do not measure their success by what they own. This may seem surprising, but they don't even measure their success by whose lives they've spared in those desperate hours in the OR. Instead, one day they anticipate God saying to them, "Well done, good and faithful servant," and that is their measure of a successful life.

Meanwhile they live quietly, unobtrusively. They run to keep fit, for speed and health are necessities to continue their work. And they walk quickly from bedside to bedside, jangling keys that open doors to save lives physically and spiritually for God's glory.

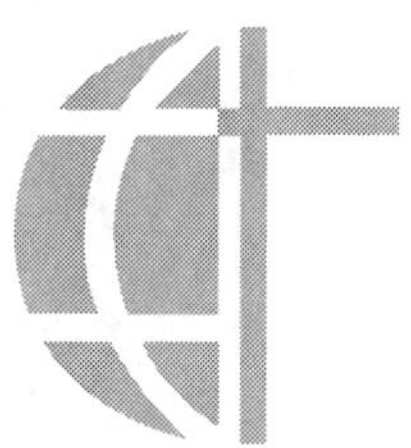

Chapter 24

Insights on the Tenwek Ministry Outreach

Chapter 24

Insights on the Tenwek Ministry Outreach

Bomet, Kenya might seem a remote corner of the world. But Tenwek Hospital caught the attention of missionaries, physicians, and others, worldwide. Franklin Graham, son of the evangelist Billy Graham and CEO of the Billy Graham Evangelistic Association and Samaritan's Purse, said, "Tenwek Hospital is one of the greatest evangelistic outreaches I know of anywhere in the world today."

Franklin Graham further said that Tenwek Hospital *"is widely recognized as one of the premier mission hospitals in the world…[and] has one of the most effective evangelical outreaches of any hospital I have ever visited…The medical ministry of Tenwek Hospital and its many outreach programs impact the lifestyle and health of hundreds of thousands of people throughout the highlands of southwest Kenya and eventually became a model for medical missions around the world."*

Tenwek Hospital was already three decades old when Dr. Bob Wesche joined one other full time doctor in the late 1960s. The little 50-bed hospital up in the hilly tea plantation region of western Kenya hummed with activity day and night, serving the needs of Bomet and the surrounding area. It seemed as though Dr. Wesche never slept. He performed surgeries around the clock in Tenwek's one little surgery room.

Everyone at Tenwek worked hard. Dr. Wesche's wife, Dora, helped in the community health office. Short-term help rotated in and out, and every little while a long-term physician or staff member was added. In 1985, Tenwek Hospital built an addition to accommodate 300 patients. In 1987, the hospital opened the Tenwek School of Nursing. In July 2001, fulfilling a long-term goal, the hospital appointed Steven Mutai as its first Kenyan executive officer.

The hard work and dedication to God paid off. Tenwek Hospital is now one of Kenya's largest mission hospitals. It serves a local community of 5,000 to 6,000 and an extended referral base of 4 to 5 million in a three-county area surrounding Tenwek. Tenwek employs over 600 national staff, treats more than 14,000 inpatients and 130,000 outpatients annually, and performs over 3,000 major surgeries and 2,500 deliveries each year. While being treated or while visiting family members, over one thousand people per year find Christ as Savior.

Tenwek Hospital has a medical library, laboratory, x-ray, and ultrasound capabilities. The hospital and training school prepares medical students, interns, nursing students, dental technicians, laboratory technicians, pharmaceutical technicians, and chaplains. It also provides advanced training for doctors in family practice and surgery.

In 2005, the hospital opened a new surgical complex complete with five surgical suites. They named it the Dr. Robert Woodford Wesche Surgery/Medical Education Building. Dr. Wesche learned of this honor when he and Dora traveled from Arizona, where they had retired, to celebrate the building's completion with their hospital friends.

Dr. Wesche received a 2008 Ageless Heroes Award from Blue Cross Blue Shield of Arizona. During an interview at that time, he stressed the need for more medical personnel in Africa. He said:

> *Twenty-four percent of the world's burden of disease is in Africa. But only three percent of the world's doctors are there. The challenge is to have adequate facilities to do the work, and to learn to do with what you have. We do have donated supplies from the United States, and donated medicines and medical staff... My current focus is to train local Kenyan surgeons.*

With a surgery department faculty that includes four long-term surgeons as well as visiting and volunteer staff from World Medical Mission, Tenwek began a general surgery residency program in 2007. In 2012, 10 residents in the program included several chief residents. These chief residents entered their final year of the five-year training program in 2012. Upon graduation from residency, Tenwek graduates will be surgery-certified across Africa.

Tenwek Hospital also trains family medicine residents. In 2012, four family medicine residents were training at Tenwek in collaboration with Moi University. Moi is Kenya's second largest medical school.

This program fulfills the vision of pioneer missionaries to Africa in the early 1900s; the longing of a series of Tenwek physicians from Dr. Wesche to Dr. Chupp who have dedicated their lives to meeting the desperate need;

and the dream of Africans to learn and provide for their own communities. God has been at work.

SWMC has played a behind-the-scenes but significant role in Tenwek's advancements. Tenwek's recent acquisition of a CT scanner is just one example. Tenwek Hospital operated without a CT scanner until September 2011. The closest CT scanner was a difficult four-hour journey away. For many of Tenwek's patients, this journey was just not possible.

Tenwek's assistant medical director, Dr. John Spriegel, learned of an opportunity to obtain the CT system through a generous donation offered by Toshiba America Medical Systems, Inc. It was a dream come true. But getting the CT system required a lot of planning and work. The hospital needed to raise approximately $700,000 in just a few months to make all the changes required to accommodate and contain the large CT equipment, complete construction to nearby departments impacted by the arrival of the scanner, to train staff, and to build a radiologist's house. To gain perspective, Tenwek Hospital runs on a budget of from $4 to $5 million per year.

The Spriegels launched a desperate campaign to raise this money. They came home and talked to SWMC, other local colleagues, churches, and anyone who would listen. They earnestly sought the Lord's providence in order to raise what seemed an impossible amount of money.

The money came. A refurbished Aquilion 4 CT system was carefully transported and installed. Kenyan leadership in the town of Bomet called the acquisition and installation of the system "nearly impossible" and "miraculous."

Physicians can use the CT system to perform neurosurgical, thoracic, and orthopedic studies. They'll also provide training to future neurosurgeons. In addition to the CT system, Toshiba donated a spare x-ray tube, considered vital in the extended use of the equipment.

Dr. Spriegel's fundraising was pivotal in the acquisition of the CT system. And SWMC was key in Dr. Spriegel's work at Tenwek.

Dr. John And Linda Spriegel

Dr. John Spriegel came into medicine the long way around. He majored in chemical engineering at Princeton and worked for the Amoco Oil Company for a year as a process design engineer. Then he completed a fellowship in occupational medicine and earned a master's degree in public health at Berkeley. He lived for two years in St. Louis working as an occupation physician for Monsanto Company at a high-tech biotechnology research center. Later, he spent three years back near his childhood home of Evanston, Illinois, completing an internal medicine residency at the Evanston Hospital program of Northwestern University. The summer before he interviewed at Southwestern Medical Clinic, he visited missionaries of the Evangelical Free Church in the Congo (now Zaire). Working at Tandala Hospital, he fell in love with the field chairwoman, Linda Gustafson. They came back to the United States, planning to return to the Congo full time. In the meantime, they looked for work in the states.

When Dr. Spriegel interviewed at SWMC, he was engaged to Linda. Perhaps love made him forget about the time change from Chicago to Michigan. Regardless, he arrived an hour late to one of his interviews. SWMC forgave him and took him on anyway. He started at SWMC in the fall and married Linda that November.

Physicians were sometimes in short supply — along with offices and office staff, pencils, and computer terminals. However, grindstones were one thing not in short supply at SWMC. Sometime later Dr. Spriegel remembers asking Don Gast, "What would it take to adapt my practice into working only 60 hours a week?"

Don smiled faintly and said after a moment, "I don't think that would be possible."

Of course that comment would only be fair coming from a fellow grinder. Don took SWMC home with him and even solved SWMC conundrums in his sleep. His heart and mind were always actively pursuing solutions for the missionary physicians and their families and for the practice that employed them. Long after the work day ended, Don was running around pulling together many loose ends.

One time when the Spriegels were preparing to go overseas for a two-year missionary service, Don knew that they were looking for renters for their house. Coming upon a potential renter, Don tried to get into the Spriegels' house to give the visitors a tour. The Spriegels were out of town visiting family in Nebraska. Not knowing how to get a key to their house, Don called a local locksmith. Don convinced the man to break into the Spriegels' house so he could give the tour.

During a high-stress time regarding a personnel issue at the Benton Harbor clinic, Dr. Spriegel once pushed for a meeting with Don as mediator. Don wasn't too pleased by the whole issue, but he agreed to meet...in a church pew at 11:00 a.m. on Sunday morning. The issue eventually sorted itself out.

For Dr. Spriegel, one key meeting typifies the priorities of the clinic even during times of high financial stress. Dr. Bob Wesche, Dr. Spriegel's predecessor at Tenwek Hospital, sat near him at the tense meeting. Finances were very tight, as usual, and the future of the clinic seemed in jeopardy. A factor was Medicaid reimbursement. At the meeting, the physicians discussed whether to cut back on serving Medicaid patients. Dr. Wesche said gravely, "SWMC should only take care of those patients for whom Christ died."

What could anyone say in argument? Dr. Wesche's words hung in the air for several minutes as discussion died. In fact, his words hung in the air for years afterward, reminding everyone of their missions in Berrien County, as well as around the world. Any time someone suggested cutting back on Medicaid or non-paying patients to improve reimbursement ratio, the echo of Dr. Wesche's wise words took away further dissention.

Early on, Dr. Spriegel learned never to complain too loudly. Otherwise, a story of the early doctors at SWMC would always make the point that his predecessors had sacrificed far greater than he. Lessons such as these re-inspired Dr. Spriegel to serve wholeheartedly for Christ in all things, in all places. Sixty-hour weeks were nothing compared to the lifetime of service Christ had planned for him.

The Spriegels did return to Tandala Hospital in the Congo, but not for long. Shortly after they returned, the country erupted in civil war. The Spriegels relocated to Tenwek Hospital in early 1997 due to the conflict. They worked at Tenwek for a year, grimly watching the grisly details unfold in the Congo. When or if they returned, nothing would ever be the same. At the same time, Dr. Spriegel meshed quickly with Tenwek's leadership and staff. Tenwek needed Dr. Spriegel. He told Linda he felt called there permanently. Though Linda's heart still yearned for the Congo, she saw that God was directing them to stay at Tenwek.

God had plans for Linda in Kenya, too. Linda began a Bible study in her home in 2005. What began as a quiet time with two or three women grew into a ministry transforming lives in a radius of several hours' walking distance. Today, more than 1,000 women attend weekly Bible studies around the area of Bomet. This ministry's success is in part due to the prayers and financial contributions of other doctors' wives and women's Bible studies Linda met through SWMC.

At Tenwek Hospital, by 2007 Dr. John Spriegel had accepted simultaneous responsibilities as the Medical Superintendent, AIDS Programs Coordinator, and a consultant on the Medical Ward and the ICU, in addition to his regular full time physician duties. Tenwek has faced financial issues, shortages of supplies and staff, and momentary lapses of priorities during times of stress. Dr. Spriegel's experiences at SWMC have come in handy.

Drs. Dan And Suzanne Hayward

Tenwek Hospital played a major role in another SWMC family's careers. Drs. Dan and Suzanne "Sue" Hayward met at Tenwek Hospital before either had joined SWMC.

Still in school, Dan worked short-term at Tenwek Hospital from March through May 1992, midway through an "international year." He'd taken a year off from residency to do missions work. He'd been to Haiti, where some college roommates had gone. He'd also spent time in Sierra Leone, where his aunt had been a missionary. Kenya wasn't his last stop. In every place, he kept bumping into certain doctors from Michigan. He also met someone else. She was a fourth-year medical student just completing her semester at Tenwek. Their time overlapped, and they quickly became friends. Suzanne returned to Virginia and started her residency. Dan continued to China for a few months before going to Kansas for his final year of internal medicine residency. They missed each other and wanted to live closer.

Dan sent a Christmas letter to Dr. Chuck Pierson whom he had met in Sierra Leone. Dr. Pierson called Dr. Dan Hayward on the phone and said, "Come to Southwestern."

"I know what you guys get paid," Dr. Hayward said. "I have a lot of bills."

"Can I give your name to Don Gast?"

Ten minutes later, Don called Dr. Hayward. During that conversation Dr. Hayward knew SWMC was the place for him. He didn't even interview anywhere else.

Suzanne transferred to South Bend. Dr. Dan Hayward started at SWMC in the summer of 1993. Dating was much easier.

When Dr. Dan Hayward was at Tenwek, he had met Dr. Mike Chupp. Dr. Chupp was full time at Tenwek, but not part of SWMC yet. They joined

SWMC around the same time, part of the legendary crop of eight new doctors. Shortly after the Haywards were married in 1995, Dr. Suzanne Hayward joined the staff of physicians at SWMC, too.

Before the wedding, Dr. Suzanne Hayward had spent time in Sierra Leone. The Haywards planned to work at SWMC for three years and then move to Sierra Leone, but then that country "went bust." The Haywards took a month off, planning to go to Haiti, but then Haiti had a coup and closed up. At that same time Don Gast got a call from Dr. Al Snyder, facing indescribable work in the aftermath of the Rwandan genocide. He begged, "Don, can you find anybody to come help us out?"

Dr. Dan Hayward had already canceled his month of clinic, thinking he was going to Haiti. So he said he'd go help Drs. Al and Dan Snyder in Rwanda instead. It was so unstable, he couldn't get into Rwanda. He spent the month at the Zairian border to Rwanda and worked with Dr. Dan Snyder's brother. Along that border, 1.2 million helpless Rwandan refugees camped. Dr. Hayward and Dr. Snyder tried to help a few thousand at one camp. Despair and abject need oppressed Dr. Hayward. He left weary, praying that God would not call him to more refugee camp work.

The Haywards were still thinking of returning to Sierra Leone, but every door slammed shut. As it became clear Sierra Leone would not be their road, the Haywards looked for other opportunities. They took several short-term trips to India with their church. Dr. Dan Hayward went to Zimbabwe with Dr. Dan Stephens. They plugged into what their SWMC colleagues were doing everywhere.

Having met at Tenwek, the Haywards always wanted to go back. When God gave them four sons, including twins, they waited until their boys were "old enough not to eat dirt and enjoy the experience." Finally, in 2008, they packed up and made it good. The plan was to spend a year. In early planning stages, they'd thought they would join the Chupps and Spriegels. As it turned out, both came home on furlough. Initially, the Haywards were disappointed. But soon things began falling into place. The Chupps moved into the Haywards' Michigan house. The Haywards moved into the Spriegels' Bomet house. They all swapped vehicles. "Okay, God, that's how you want to work this," they said.

Not everything worked out perfectly. Their visa paperwork was messed up, and at the end of six months the Haywards had to leave Kenya. But somehow this was God's plan, too. The very week they had to leave Kenya, a medical missions training conference was held in Thailand. Attending it led to special memories and non-coincidental friendships. They returned to SWMC having been forever enriched by the whole experience.

The conference is one of several large Christian medical missions conferences worldwide. One motivation for these conferences was to provide missionary doctors a stress-free opportunity to earn all their continuing education credits at one time — the continuing education is required to maintain American medical licensure. Beginning in the 1970s, Thailand formed one conference and Africa formed its own in Brackenhurst, Kenya. The conferences alternate years.

It so happened the year the Haywards were in Tenwek, it was the year of the Thailand conference. Typically, African missionaries don't go to the Thai conference. But in December 2007, riots tore Kenya apart. The Brackenhurst conference of February 2008 was canceled because of all the fighting. So in 2009, Thailand allowed the missionaries from Africa to come. At that 2009 Thai conference, 17 past and present SWMC doctors converged for the only time. The Haywards were able to participate because, as Suzanne put it, God had said, "You're going to go."

Here's another aside to illustrate the interconnectedness of medical missions: In fall 2008, an ophthalmologist and his family landed at Tenwek Hospital. They'd wanted to return to Indonesia, but their visas fell through. So they stayed at Tenwek waiting for the paperwork to get ironed out. While there, they trained the hospital staff about ophthalmology. The Haywards didn't know of Dr. Wendell Geary's history with SWMC then. But in February 2009 — just months later — they met Dr. Geary and his wife again at the conference in Thailand.

Often, SWMC doctors "cover" for their colleagues during these conferences. Teams of short-term SWMC doctors generally travel to Tenwek and Karanda so that the doctors working there can attend the Brackenhurst conference. This precedent started from the very first conference in the 1970s, when Dr. Rick Johansen covered at ELWA so the Schindlers could go.

A year after their six-month trip to Tenwek, the Hayward family went back to Tenwek Hospital for a month to help cover for the Brackenhurst conference. They went again for the same reason with a group of SWMC doctors in 2012. While the Haywards are not currently living their original full time mission dreams, after so many return short-term trips, they still consider Bomet a kind of second home.

The Haywards found out that this second-home kind of living is what Dr. Bob and Dora Wesche had done since the '60s, traveling back and forth to Tenwek in its infancy. Despite what their impact on Tenwek might make it seem, the Wesches were never career missionaries. They never raised long-term support. They were always just under short-term status.

Throughout the years, perhaps 25 or more SWMC physicians have volunteered at Tenwek Hospital. This cumulative gift of time and expertise has been an immeasurable benefit to the hospital surrounded by tea fields in Kenya.

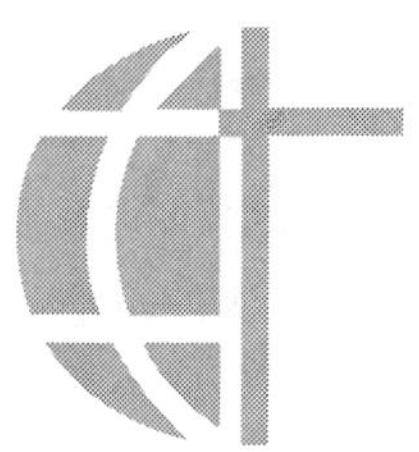

Chapter 25

The Rwandan Massacre and Stories of Survival by God's Grace

Chapter 25

The Rwandan Massacre and Stories of Survival by God's Grace

Dr. C. Albert "Al" Snyder's father worked endless hours as an orthopedic surgeon in Grand Rapids, Michigan. Upon entering college after serving in the Philippines in World War II, he wasn't wearing rose-colored glasses when he talked about being a missionary physician. He interned at Butterworth Hospital in Grand Rapids and entered a surgery residency.

By the end of his schooling in the mid-1950s, he married Louise and they started a family. Instead of a high calling and great adventure, missions work now clearly meant fewer educational choices for their boys; health concerns with minimal medical availability; political turmoil; financial challenges; distance from family; and leaving everything and everyone they knew.

God did not let Dr. Snyder forget his call. By the fall of 1957, the Snyder family embarked to Kibuye, a Free Methodist hospital in Burundi. A skilled surgeon with a nose for a challenge, Dr. Snyder traveled to other African hospitals as well, including Kibimba Hospital, to help with complicated cases.

Word got around of his skill and sense of adventure. In 1968, Dr. Snyder transferred to Kibogora Hospital, Rwanda. This tiny new bush hospital had been merely a dispensary until 1964. When the Snyders arrived it had 40 beds, but by sharing cots between two or more patients, the hospital sometimes counted about 100 inpatients. Under Dr. Snyder's watch, Kibogora earned a reputation for quality, cutting-edge surgery. Sited on a beautiful rise above Lake Kivu, the hospital was nicknamed The Hill. The Hill grew to 175 beds with three satellite dispensaries. It served an immediate population of 100,000 with a referral population of half a million.

Kibogora developed a medical school, which now is beginning to produce national doctors. Also, doctors from around the world preparing for missions can go to Kibogora for part of their training. All of this amazing, foresighted leadership training has taken place in a structure that still functions with oversized wards and outdoor latrines.

For a while, Dr. Snyder returned to Grand Rapids during furloughs to work alongside his father in the ER. But as the U.S. medical climate changed, the ER wanted someone who had been formally trained with an ER residency. At this point, roughly 10 years before retirement, Dr. Snyder joined SWMC. It was God's timing. Dr. Schindler and Dr. Al Snyder worked side-by-side and became close friends. Dr. Snyder was ordained by the Rwandan church, so SWMC colleagues nicknamed him "The Bishop." Children of the other physicians referred to them as "Uncle Al and Aunt Louise."

By the time the Snyders came to SWMC, their children were off to college. Back in Africa, like many other African countries, Ruanda-Urundi had more than its share of political upheaval. Eventually, the land divided into Rwanda and Burundi. During this time of unrest, Dr. Al Snyder's son Dan graduated from medical school. He was unable to go to Kibogora so he went to Haiti instead. He and his father helped each other short-term.

In July 1990, Dr. Al Snyder retired from medical missions. But as is so often the case, a need arose at Kibogora. Less than three years later, the hospital, which had survived an invasion by Tutsi exiles, was without a surgeon. "Friends tried to persuade us that this was not the type of retirement we should consider," Dr. Snyder wrote. Swallowing their misgivings and trying hard not to listen to the news, the Snyders went back. Dr. Snyder kept a journal of their dramatic experience during the Rwandan Genocide of 1994, published by Family Christian Press in diary form in the book "On a Hill Far Away".

Dr. Roy Winslow

Dr. Roy Winslow's connection to Dr. Al Snyder went back many years. Growing up, he was interested in medicine and wanted to be involved with missions. Dr. Snyder spoke at his church from time to time, and young Roy considered him a hero. "He was hilarious, with tongue-in-cheek humor, but he was also very practical. I identified with him. He was an early role model for me."

When Dr. Winslow and his wife, Bev, were in medical school they felt a strong leading from the Lord to pursue missions. They took a short-term trip for three months in 1979 to Kibogora Hospital. It was a dream. Dr. Al Snyder served as Dr. Winslow's mentor and overseer, and Dr. Winslow worked with him directly. An RN, Bev worked in surgery alongside her husband.

In 1979, even at Kibogora Hospital, one of the best hospitals in Rwanda, there was no telephone, only ham radio. A local generator produced the hospital's electricity to run lights and basic medical equipment. The electricity sometimes went out without warning.

Rather than spook Dr. Winslow, these kinds of challenges spurred his interest in medical missions. He saw the huge need for good doctors. Although Dr. Winslow did not become a career missionary, he returned to Rwanda and frequently traveled to other foreign fields short-term throughout his life. He kept in contact with Dr. Al Snyder. When Dr. Snyder joined SWMC, Dr. Winslow contacted SWMC, too; but in an uncommon turn of fate, SWMC had no more room for a surgeon. Dr. Winslow ended up in Pennsylvania for 13 years, working at a four-man surgery group where it was not difficult to take off for short-term missions.

Around 1984 the Winslows had another opportunity to come to SWMC. By this time they knew Dr. Al Snyder pretty well. He happened to be in the states on furlough. Dr. Snyder warned Dr. Winslow, "I'm a general surgeon, but I'm doing rounds in the nursing home."

Sure enough, when Don Gast answered Dr. Winslow's inquiry, he admitted uncharacteristically, "We know you and love you, but we have no room for surgeons in Berrien Center." That year several surgeons came home from the mission field at the same time. At that point, SWMC surgeons weren't yet working at Lakeland.

Meanwhile, the Winslows took many trips to Kibogora Hospital but also went to Haiti, Kenya, Swaziland, and South Africa with Samaritan's Purse World Medical Mission, WMM. At Tenwek Hospital in Kenya they worked with Dr. Roland Stephens and Dr. Wesche. They kept hearing about SWMC coming and going.

SWMC had actually been on the Winslows' radar for years. The first time Dr. Winslow and Bev met Dr. Bob Schindler was while Dr. Winslow was a surgery resident in Cleveland. He was involved in the local CMS chapter. Dr. Schindler was very active in CMS, and he told Dr. Winslow about SWMC. Also, SWMC pediatrician Dr. Bart Comstock, though a man of few words, led a medical student retreat at Gull Lake in Kalamazoo when the Winslows were in medical school. The Winslows just kept encountering SWMC wherever they went in the world.

When Dr. Winslow happened to be serving at Kibogora Hospital with Drs. Al and Dan Snyder in 1994, Dr. Winslow was not yet part of SWMC. Kibogora was roughly the size of Lakeland Hospital in St. Joseph,

Michigan – the largest hospital system in Berrien County. But whereas Lakeland had a whole staff of surgeons, Kibogora had no trained surgeon in 1994. "Consider a hospital that size with no trained surgeon," Dr. Winslow explained. "The situation was pretty desperate."

In the spring of 1994 the Winslows and their 11-year-old son were living in a cottage on a hill overlooking Kibogora, when the Rwandan President's plane was shot down at the airport. "Chaos erupted immediately," Dr. Winslow recalled. "We were hearing of neighboring killings, rampant death squads, and we were in the middle of it."

When you're living it, moment by moment, you don't have a clear perspective of the situation, Bev said. The U.S. ambassador was scheduled to come to Kibogora for a dedication ceremony of a new hospital wing. He cancelled. While disappointed by the ambassador's absence, the hospital went on with the dedication, kept its daily routine, and hoped the violence in the capital would wane.

Rather than settling down, the situation worsened. The Winslows and other foreigners at the hospital thought of fleeing to the embassy, but by this time the embassy was under attack and roadblocks had been erected along the route by warring factions.

President Clinton instructed all U.S. citizens to leave Rwanda, without escort, and flee to the border which would be open for one day. "Do you bunker down and wait it out, or do you risk your life to get out while you can?" Dr. Winslow asked.

On the Winslows' last day at Kibogora, Rwandans brought many slaughtered victims. "Whole families. It was a horrible experience making the decision whether to stay or leave. We had to leave patients behind untreated. We didn't know what would happen."

Fearing for their lives, the Winslows and Snyders and other families decided to make the wild trip to the border. Packing just one bag each, the Winslows and Snyders gathered a caravan of 12 vehicles. "Those dear people lined the roads singing and saying goodbye," Dr. Winslow related with a catch in his voice. "We had a place to go. They didn't. They had to stay and endure."

The Winslows and Snyders never saw many of their Rwandan friends and colleagues again. The next day, militants killed 150 people on the hospital compound.

Meanwhile, the caravan drove across desolate mountains prickling with armed militants. They rolled through villages populated with mobs swinging banana cutters and machetes. At one point the caravan was halted by 200 angry men. In the Winslows' vehicle crouched a Belgian doctor and his Tutsi wife, certain the militia would target them. They prayed fervently.

Out of nowhere, a little red Toyota truck came rattling over the hill. It screeched up to the first vehicle in their caravan. They asked Dr. Snyder why the caravan was traveling without an escort. Someone said to the Toyota, "Why don't you be our escort?" So the Toyota took the lead and directed them like Peter's angel, Dr. Snyder wrote, past roadblock after roadblock.

Reaching a pile of logs or stones, the red Toyota halted and conferred with gang leaders.

Sometimes a bribe of ball-point pens was sufficient. Other times, the friendly Toyota escort simply talked the way through. The conversations may have saved the lives of the people in the caravan.

After several hours, the red Toyota pulled off and waved the swelling caravan on. They had no more problems at roadblocks. The caravan grew to 72 vehicles before reaching the Rwandan border.

Even after crossing the border into Burundi, the Winslows and Snyders and their colleagues remained in harm's way. Burundi was also in the middle of a civil war. An escort to the U.S. embassy advised them not to travel into the capital because the city was under gunfire that night.

U.S. Marines en route home from Somalia flew the Winslows and Snyders to Nairobi. There, they could contact praying and anxious friends and family back in the states and learn the scope of the genocide they had just fled. The Rwandan genocide was accurately portrayed in the movie "Hotel Rwanda."

After flying to Nairobi, the Winslows and Snyders were stranded a week because there were not enough flights. It was a forced vacation, a little decompression time. They decided to visit a wild game preserve. They hired a driver and a guard, as suggested, for protection from thieves. It was rainy season. The first night going out to the game park, they got stuck in the mud. They couldn't even roll their windows down because the lower-elevation countryside was malaria-laden. But it was stifling, so they opened a window just a little bit to get fresh air. In the evening they heard a loud snorting. The guide told them a hippo was just beyond the Jeep. So they sat in the stifling vehicle by the snorting hippo for several hours, listening to the guide advise them why they shouldn't get between a mother hippo and her kids, or between a thirsty hippo and a watering pond.

After nightfall, one of the youngsters in the Jeep piped up and said he needed to go to the bathroom. The guard said he'd take him behind a bush. So the little guy was out in the dark with a man with a gun and a snorting hippo. He was so nervous he couldn't even go to the bathroom. Meanwhile, the adults waited in the Jeep, holding their breaths, listening to the hippo and fearing for the boy's life. Just a few days before, God had protected them from genocide, and to think that now they could have been killed by a charging hippo! About then, another vehicle saw the Jeep's headlights and sent a truck to pull them out of the mud. The rest of their time in the game park was tame.

Another time in Kenya, a bridge was out, and again Dr. Winslow and Bev got stuck in the mud. Bev steered the vehicle while Dr. Winslow tried to dig the vehicle out of the mud with several limber Kenyans to help him. A lion let out an earsplitting roar. Dr. Winslow ran for his life and fell into the mud. The Kenyans all laughed at him. "That lion's probably a mile away, Dr. Winslow," they assured him.

In 1995, despite the continuing volatility, Dr. Winslow returned to Kibogora alone. He helped as much as he could, reported the devastation, and grieved for 280 friends and neighbors interred in a mass grave on the hospital grounds. Rising from the ruin, Kibogora Hospital is now a Rwandan-maintained district hospital — a transition that fulfilled the founders' dream 50 years before. Now foreigners such as the Winslows typically come as educators or financiers, not full time staff.

Dr. Winslow and Bev still travel to Kibogora once or twice a year. Electricity is still unreliable. In 2007 Dr. Winslow, along with SWMC pediatrician Dr. Georg Schultz and Dr. Schultz' medical student daughter Sarah, stood in Kibogora's operating room over a young woman with life-threatening fluid on her heart. "We were preparing to insert a fairly large needle, with the help of a simple ultrasound machine," to remove the fluid, Dr. Winslow related. "All of a sudden the power went out in the room."

The ultrasound machine now sat useless beside them. While Dr. and Sarah Schultz held flashlights, Dr. Winslow utilized basic methods of palpitation (feeling) and percussion (tapping) manually to locate and monitor the fluid. "I drew the fluid out basically blind," Dr. Winslow said. "Half an hour later the lights came on."

In a typical letter home, the Winslows wrote,

As we say our goodbyes to new friends and old at Kibogora, we also gaze over the mountainous horizon one more time. We love our Lake Michigan sunsets at home, but we will miss this lofty elevation, the clear skies devoid of pollution, and the breathtaking constellations vivid in jet-black skies. Having just reflected on the shepherds on their hillside on That Night, we can only imagine the heavens ablaze with the glory of God. The closest we come to a heavenly host is the local army regiment, singing heartily in unison at 5:30 a.m. outside our window. Bev and I are eager to head home, but still feel that strong tug of emotion, from our long relationship here with the Rwandans since 1979.

The men's English class enjoyed a final session with an outdoor party complete with Fantas, Cokes, and cookies. My last day in the hospital brought two emergencies in the afternoon. I had to drain a nasty infection of the neck, of unknown origin, in a young lady. An elbow dislocation also could not wait. Earlier in the week, I had a man with leakage from the small intestine due to typhoid fever and an older lady with leakage from an advanced cancer of the colon. Severe fractures — one of the knee joint and shin, and another in the forearm bones — were managed with an open textbook nearby, for guidance on techniques I have only read about. This is my version of a textbook case. If you know anyone with some sharp drill bits and a full array of bone screws, send them my way. It is tricky to piece bones together with dull instruments and sets of screws with several lengths missing.

We will soon depart on Saturday from Kigali, the capital, for our flights to Entebbe, Uganda, then Brussels, Belgium. From there, we fly to Chicago, landing this Sunday at 1 p.m. Central Standard Time.

At home in the states after their survival of the 1995 genocide, feeling change coming, he and Bev prayed for guidance. On a weekend not long after that, Dr. Winslow got a phone call from Dr. Glenn Snyder, Dr. Al's oldest son. While Dr. Glenn Snyder had never been part of SWMC, he met with one of his father's SWMC colleagues, Dr. Spees, at the International Conference of Medical Missions in Tennessee. "Glenn, we need a general surgeon," Dr. Spees said to Glenn. "Do you know of anyone who might be interested?"

Glenn prayed and then called Dr. Winslow. This time, it was right. "It was so interesting to come to SWMC in that way, with a Snyder after all that," Dr. Winslow said.

Dr. Schindler, head of SWMC surgery department, had decided to cut back on hours. Coming to SWMC, Dr. Winslow actually had fewer opportunities for short-term missions than in Pennsylvania. But meeting with Dr. Ken O'Neill and manager Don Gast in the fall of 1996, he saw their passion for Christ and missions and wanted to be a part of SWMC's mission. He was excited and challenged to support a practice that allowed other surgeons to be full time missionaries. He could establish a permanent surgery practice in Berrien County so that Drs. Chupp, Stephens, and Wesche could come back for furlough and keep their licensing current.

By the time the Pennsylvania practice recruited Dr. Winslow's replacement, it was June of 1997 when the Winslows came to Berrien Center. Finally, their numerous encounters with SWMC fell together. They felt like they had come home.

At the same time, SWMC hired a brand new surgeon, Dr. Paul Lim, right out of residency. He was a sharp young man who stayed with SWMC almost five years and then left for a permanent mission.

Dr. Winslow developed a great respect for Dr. Schindler and listened to his wisdom. Dr. Schindler used terms for toning muscles — isotonic and isometric — to describe the tension of doctors' comings and goings at SWMC. At times SWMC was shorthanded, all its physicians overloaded while their colleagues served overseas. Other times, there were more physicians than needed. The freedom of SWMC doctors to go and serve created this tension and elasticity.

Dr. Schindler's illness and passing were tough times for the international CMDA community, and for SWMC, and especially for Dr. Schindler's surgery department. Dr. Schindler was those surgeons' lead man, and they looked up to him as a father figure and a mentor. Seeing him slowly become weaker and eventually pass away from prostate cancer was a big challenge. The rest of the surgeons felt they had to step up to lead the department, but Dr. Schindler's shoes have never really been filled.

Dr. Winslow rides his bicycle down to Dr. Schindler's gravestone at the cemetery on Cleveland Road and remembers his leader's deep voice reverberating, his great laugh. Dr. Schindler's marker reads, "The greatest privilege in the world is to serve Jesus Christ." Dr. Winslow recalls, "He'd say that, whenever things were tough or when there were disagreements. It's a great reminder to see that on his marker. He left that with us."

Dr. Wesche probably started this phrase, but Dr. Schindler used it, too, and it's a part of SWMC's heritage: "If there's anybody you meet that Jesus Christ didn't die for, you don't have to take care of them." This adage is always in the back of Dr. Winslow's mind when he deals with someone who is challenging. God loves everyone.

Dr. Winslow doesn't force his faith down anyone's throat, but he feels free to express his faith. Since he is a SWMC physician, patients expect and know that he is a believer, and some ask to pray with him in his office or in the holding area before surgery. "I'm not a counselor or pastor, but people trust us for big things during surgery," Dr. Winslow says.

One woman facing breast cancer was sent to Dr. Winslow by Dr. Rick Bardin in Niles, who is now teaching doctors in Africa. Dr. Bardin sent Dr. Winslow the patient for surgical management. The morning of her surgery, she asked the anesthetist if he prayed that morning and he blew her off. Deeply religious and very nervous about the surgery, she asked Dr. Winslow if he prayed that morning. He told her he had prayed, and then he asked her, "Would you like to pray together now?"

He asked her if she was a believer, and she said yes. She told him about playing piano in her church. They prayed behind the curtains in the holding area, and then they had the long process of office visits after that for several months.

The woman wrote a memoir of her cancer survival and produced a book titled, "My Story". She presented a copy of the book to Dr. Winslow several years later during a Christmas party she and her husband held for all of her physicians, nurses, and therapists. She wrote that after Dr. Winslow's prayer, her fears left. Also, still remembering the prayer a week after the surgery, she played a medley of songs at church and credited her strength to do this to the pre-op prayer. "I could pat myself on the back, but I think God ordained that moment," Dr. Winslow says.

At corporation meetings, often a SWMC physician will share a similar faith story or God moment. Sometimes, people decide to trust Christ for the first time while talking with their doctor. Dr. Herb Atkinson had the opportunity to lead many patients to Christ.

After Dr. Atkinson retired, he and his wife, Frieda, supervised the in-office prayer support program. He and Frieda trained others to pray with people who had needs while they sat in the waiting room before being seen by a SWMC physician. Dr. Atkinson regularly sat in Dr. Winslow's waiting room on Monday mornings, praying with patients. At the end of the morning he would tell Dr. Winslow, "God's a miracle-working God. I've been able to pray with so many, and more than a hundred people accepted Christ."

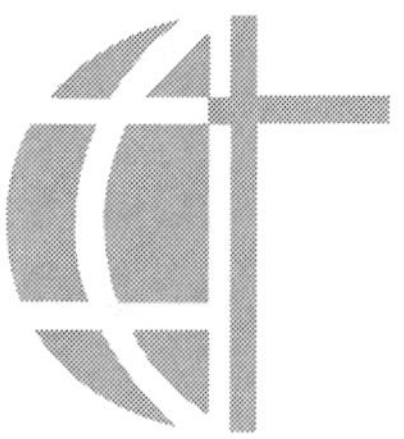

Chapter 26

Modern Missionaries in Haiti and South America

Chapter 26

Modern Missionaries in Haiti and South America

Dr. Dan Snyder

It was a case of house-sharing before island-sharing. Dr. Dan Snyder's parents joined SWMC while he was in college. In 1973, the Silvernales let the Snyders live in their house on Indian Lake for a year while they served in Haiti. Dan Snyder had grown up in Africa. He'd always thought he'd return after medical school. But God had other plans for this son of Dr. Al Snyder. God was preparing, even then, for Dr. Dan Snyder to serve in Haiti.

Two decades later, Dr. Dan and Dee Ann Snyder and their young family began serving with Free Methodist World Missions in 1993. They started out in Rwanda for 10 months, with Dr. Dan Snyder assisting his father in surgery. Dr. Dan Snyder worked night shift while his semi-retired father did daytime surgery, and they performed many C-sections. But war broke out in 1994 and they had to evacuate with the Winslows and couldn't return, so they were reassigned by their mission organization. The location: Dessalines Hospital in Haiti.

Dr. Dan Snyder was not yet a part of SWMC. The first time he joined SWMC in 1998, he needed help paying a $6,000 malpractice insurance premium, so he called up Don Gast. Don said the foundation would pay the bill, and he also offered storage in the basement of the Stevensville office. One time, Dr. Winslow helped them move. The clinic needed the storage moved out of the Stevensville office, so it was moved it into a garage.

Also in 1998, around the time he spoke with Don Gast, he met incoming SWMC administrator Warren White, medical director Dr. Ken O'Neill, and head of surgery Dr. Schindler. They got together at a little pita sandwich restaurant not far from the administration building. "The extent of my early association with SWMC was a couple of lunches and moving furniture around. No money changed hands for six years," Dr. Dan Snyder recalls. "They just assumed I had signed a contract. This was a throwback, a classic Don Gast arrangement."

In 2002, Dr. Dan Snyder was working at a tiny clinic in rural Haiti, minding his own business, when some important doctors came in for a tour.

One of the doctors was teaching at an ethics conference. Dr. Snyder looked at him once, twice, and said to him, "You look so familiar, I think we've met."

The U.S. doctor stared back at Dr. Snyder owlishly and said, "I don't think so."

Dr. Snyder pored through his memory bank of U.S. doctors in Haiti, racked his brain and couldn't figure it out, but he insisted he had met the man before.

The visiting doctor said, "I've never been to Haiti before. I can't possibly know you."

The brief tour was almost over. The hospital was really quite small. Dr. Snyder asked, "Do you know a Glenn Snyder? He's my oldest brother. He's about your age."

"No, but I know Al Snyder."

Dr. Dan Snyder relaxed. "Oh, yes, surely you're familiar with Dad. He's been in missionary work for decades."

"Familiar with him?" The other doctor sniffed. "He works at my clinic back in Michigan."

Suddenly, it clicked. Dr. Dan Snyder exploded, "Oh, good grief, you're my boss!"

Dr. Ken O'Neill certainly had plenty of time to get acquainted with Dr. Al Snyder's son the next year, when he came home on furlough and finally began working at SWMC.

Paperwork can be like a rabbit in technique and like a turtle in speed. Long after Dr. Dan Snyder began working there as a hospitalist, midway into 2004, someone in charge of records called him and said, "We can't find your contract."

"You have to have one," Dr. Snyder said, "because you've stored my furniture for seven years."

The poor records manager tore up the office and the database and the files in storage and never found a contract. She was actually quite surprised not to find one, because by the late 1990s, they'd been tightening things considerably since the days of Don Gast's handshakes and yellow legal pad scribbles. According to the contract they drew up at that time, Dr. Dan Snyder has been associated with SWMC since 2003.

Dr. Snyder attributes SWMC's longevity to Don's abilities, and then to Dr. Ken O'Neill and Dr. Mark Harrison creating the hospitalist program, and foremost to the founders' and leaders' dependence on God. He knows of no other physician group like SWMC in the world. Some of his friends work at a very small, five-member, missions-minded clinic in Wichita – about the size SWMC was when it formed. Other SWMC physicians know of similar small clinics. Throughout the years, various physicians have come to SWMC to learn how it was formed, and grew, and flourished. Most left shaking their heads at the sacrifices of time and pay required to grow and sustain SWMC.

Don Gast was one of Dr. Dan Snyder's heroes. Don was an All-American athlete at Baroda High School and Wheaton College, setting records and having his name engraved on the walls at both schools. But Dr. Snyder didn't just admire Don's basketball prowess. Don helped him and Dee Ann find their house which, with their budget, was no small victory.

The Snyders moved into a house right behind Dr. Herb and Frieda Atkinson's house. Dr. Snyder had known Dr. Atkinson's kids from Africa. Dr. Atkinson gave the Snyders a key to his garage in case of emergency. It seemed he gave most of his neighbors keys, both to his garage and to the kingdom. Scores of neighbors came to Christ and then kept coming back to the Atkinson home for Bible studies. Who more than the Snyders could boast of such inspiration in view out their kitchen window?

Dr. Janet Frey had gone to Rwanda years earlier to help the Snyders. She and her husband, John, also went down to Haiti. The car broke down between the airport and the hospital in an unpleasant area. John Frey wanted to go back to the airport and find different transportation. Dr. Frey said, "Keep going! We might make it!" She determined to keep going forward, and they got to Dessalines. He painted and she taught the radiologist. Dessalines never forgot their fun-loving generosity.

The Snyders became good friends with Dorothy Abrams. A Jewish woman who never converted to Christianity, she ran a clinic in Benton Harbor for many years with a doctor. She and the doctor were getting ready to close the clinic, tired and discouraged, and the way she told the story later, a good-looking, suave guy came in and talked her into handing him the keys. Guess who she was referring to? The don of SWMC, Don Gast. SWMC's Benton Harbor clinic began with Dorothy Abrams and Don Gast's new friendship.

One time Dorothy Abrams was ill in the hospital. Dr. Dan Snyder was sitting on her bed visiting with her when Jule Gast happened to telephone up to her room. Dorothy said, "Jule, guess who I'm in bed with."

Shocked, Jule exclaimed, "Who!"

"Dan Snyder." Big chuckle. That was Dorothy Abrams.

A surgeon walked in later and, according to Dr. Snyder, said something unprofessional. The next day, flowers came to Dorothy from Lakeland CEO Joe Wasserman, some from the surgeon, and some from another Lakeland administrator. Everybody knew Dorothy. Don Gast was asked to speak at her huge Jewish funeral.

Dr. Al Snyder created Central African Healthcare Organization (CAHO), and Dr. Dan Snyder began organizing the same thing in Haiti. Mission hospitals became so formidably expensive that mission boards could not support them anymore. Medical missionaries saw that in order to survive, they must unite. Dr. Dan Snyder wrote Dr. Ken O'Neill, asking if he was interested in developing a hospitalist program at SWMC.

In 2003, Dr. Dan Snyder came home and joined Dr. Matt Ling to start the hospitalist program.

In the hospitalist program, physicians hired by SWMC worked out of one hospital, such as the Lakeland hospitals in St. Joseph or Niles, with SWMC holding the contract. This worked well to fill a staffing need at the hospital. It also worked well for SWMC: by the turn of the millennium, it became fiscally unfeasible to hire physicians short-term into a practice; but they could work in a hospitalist program.

In 2005, Dr. Dan Snyder came home for three years, avoiding Haiti's political upheaval. A few weeks after he returned to Dessalines in 2008, Hurricane Hanna flattened what was left in the wake of the hurricane of 2003. What Hurricane Hanna left behind was submerged in flooding. It was a mess. Then, in January of 2010, the Snyders experienced Haiti's 7.0 earthquake. No building codes protected the impoverished country from widespread destruction.

The hospitalist program became key to Dr. Dan Snyder's sanity — and career — after the hurricane disasters in Haiti. He was able to fly in and out of Berrien County for a week at a time if need be. He was also able to spearhead a number of short-term medical missions trips to assist the overloaded, near-bankrupt Dessalines hospital.

SWMC helped monetarily. It sent supplies. It also sent a short-term medical missions team. But without the hospitalist program with Lakeland, Dr. Snyder would not have been able to go back and forth. SWMC's priority to missions motivated the Snyders to join SWMC, and its flexibility has kept them there.

Dr. Chuck Pierson

Dr. Pierson dedicated his life to Christ in Haiti as a medical student in 1968. While there, he met two SWMC physicians: pediatrician Dr. Silvernale and general practitioner Dr. Edling. Dr. Pierson studied and worked at a family practice in Kalamazoo from 1980-1982, and in the last month of that — June 1982 — he called over to SWMC and arranged a one month externship with Dr. Herb Atkinson. At that time, he arranged to come back and work at SWMC from 1985-1986.

Already involved in medical missions to Sierra Leone, West Africa, he was impressed by SWMC's willingness to make a place for him, as well as eagerness to help him get caught up on stateside medicine. At SWMC he got a grasp on the latest techniques and recommendations for drugs. This seemed particularly true when he came back from overseas in 1989, for much in medicine had changed while he had been gone.

Dr. Pierson visited the Stephenses at Karanda Hospital in Zimbabwe. He visited Dr. Chuck Paine in southern Zambia. He visited Tenwek Hospital in western Kenya. Doctors visited him in Sierra Leone. SWMC is a family, and family members visit and help one another. SWMC is "not like most business organizations," Dr. Pierson says.

Dr. Pierson found Dr. Atkinson an affable optimist. He joked and laughed his way through every difficult situation, a tremendous influence on his patients, coworkers, nurses, office staff, and everyone he met. He shared Jesus Christ with most people he talked with. His influence widened daily. Dr. Herb Atkinson was such a conversationalist, one time he and Dr. Pierson were on their way to Iowa and ended up in Kansas City, 50 miles out of their way. The detour only gave them a chance to finish the conversation properly.

Dr. Pierson emphasizes the importance of prayer. "Prayer has always been a part of all of SWMC's meetings. They prayed over the clinic's finances, missionaries' finances and work, prayed for staff and family members, and for patients. They've had meetings that were primarily in prayer because they didn't see the way out when things didn't look good," he said.

From 1989-2005, Dr. Pierson went overseas again to Sierra Leone, and he has not been in full time practice since then. He is doing deputation again, getting ready to go overseas. "The clinic has never been super flush with cash. It's always been a struggle of our own making: giving for missions, taking people aboard we knew were not going to be productive, but the Lord has always provided," he said.

Dr. Richard W. (Dick) Douce

Dick Douce went forward many times at church revivals throughout his childhood, attended church, and idolized his Uncle Bill, who left to go to Ecuador on the mission field when Dick was seven years old. He kept trying to get Christianity to stick. Finally, at age 14, he attended a Billy Graham crusade and became born again. He read the Bible faithfully, but didn't know Christian fellowship until he joined the Navigators at Ohio State University.

His dad's brother, Dr. Bill Douce, had a wonderful testimony and loved people, and they loved him. The Lord used him to attract Dick to the Lord.

His senior year of college, September 28, 1972, he was drafted. He spent two years in the Army in Germany and decided he would go to medical school. He did not get accepted his first year out of the Army. His parents did not know how to advise him. Spending time alone with the Lord, he began to consider Plan B: reapply, but meanwhile start studying to be a medical technician. A guidance counselor suggested he retake the Medical College Admission Test. He retook it, raised his scores, and was accepted into three medical schools the next year.

He visited his aunt and uncle in Saraguro several times while he was still in college, around 1970. He stayed several weeks, watched his Uncle Bill working in the little clinic and figured, "I could be a missionary if I wanted to."

During his last year of medical school, he took an international rotation in Shell, Ecuador. It was the most positive experience he'd ever had. He left Ecuador certain he should be a missionary. While Dick was in residency in Youngstown, Ohio, Don Gast started asking him to come to SWMC for an interview, prompted for sure by Dr. Bill Douce. He interviewed at SWMC. Around the same time, he attended a CMDS leadership conference in Ohio and talked with Dr. Ken O'Neill, urologist Dr. David Terhune, and several others who eventually came to southwestern Michigan. But another missionary from Ecuador advised him to get more academic experience first. He made up his mind to pursue a fellowship in infectious diseases, so he told SWMC about it. During his two years of fellowship in the University of Cincinnati, Don Gast kept calling and inviting him to come back to SWMC.

It was a no-brainer to interview at Youngstown at the end of his fellowship and residency. He asked them, "What would you think if I told you I plan to be a missionary in two years?" They frowned; that was not consistent with their goals.

He asked Don the same thing, and, of course, Don said, "That's why we're here!"

In July 1985, Dr. Dick Douce and his wife, Marian, and their sons moved into Uncle Bill and Aunt Ilene's house in Berrien Springs while they were in Ecuador. Dr. Dick Douce hired into SWMC as its first subspecialist and found himself the first infectious disease specialist for an hour's drive in any direction. "I probably worked too hard," he said during an international January 29, 2011, telephone interview. "The kids were often still asleep when I left in the morning, and asleep when I came home. I wouldn't see them awake for two weeks at a time."

He worked at Mercy Hospital in Benton Harbor, Memorial Hospital in St. Joseph, Berrien General Hospital, and Pawating Hospital in Niles, and sometimes he worked at the hospital in Dowagiac as well. Looking back, he figured they didn't know how to bill for a subspecialist. Things improved in that area after the arrival of Dr. Mark Harrison, who successfully developed the hospitalist program.

In his early medical career, Dr. Dick Douce had solid interaction with only a few Christian physicians. "You latch on to whatever brand you're around," he says, "and you tell yourself that's how you're going to be." At SWMC he has seen the whole spectrum from quiet, subtle types to Dr. Bob Patton, whose goal was to lead 150 people to Christ per year and who witnessed boldly to everyone who came through his door. Dr. Douce was inspired and encouraged by everyone in the spectrum.

Dr. Douce plays a role in the life and death of a patient. Sometimes he gets to save lives. He has learned to look for opportunities to impact others, as well. "Most surgeons, when they get done with a difficult surgery and see 30 family members clustered around, they run and hide," he says. "I loved watching Dr. Bob Schindler. He'd come out and ask each person how they were related to his patient. He tried to figure out if he knew them. He saw each one as a special connection. It was great to see that kind of model."

In 1987, Dr. Dick Douce was the first keynoter at Jornadas Medicas, a medical conference at Hospital Vozandes in Quito, and he felt called to full time service at Vozandes. First, he had to sell his wife, Marian, on the idea of living in Ecuador. They bought tickets and made the trip, and he excitedly prepared to roll out the country's exquisite beauty for her like a magic carpet. He showed her the gorgeous clean blue sky, the mountains, and the smiling people. She saw graffiti, trash in the streets, homelessness, and misery…and then they experienced a major earthquake. A town was destroyed, gasoline shortage became nightmarish, and when they were stranded in Cuenca, Marian ate some berries that weren't washed and got bacterial dysentery. The sales job couldn't have gone any worse for Dr. Douce.

Despite everything, Marian saw the needs and knew her husband was called to Ecuador. She felt God saying, "If you don't come, I will find someone else to do My work here." She nodded solemnly and told her husband to take the job.

They started the procedure to join HCJB in 1988. By August 1989, they were accepted, so Dr. Douce, Marian, and their sons Dan and Tom moved to Costa Rica to study Spanish for a year. Moving to Quito in 1990, Dr. Dick Douce quickly fell into step alongside Dr. Roy Ringenberg. Dr. Ringenberg had just started a family practice residency there two years earlier. In the beginning, three residents came to the hospital per year. Demand has increased. They've graduated 120 residents since the program started and now host eight residents annually. Some of the best medical residents out of Quito, and now from around the world, have come through their residency program. Dr. Ringenberg and Dr. Dick Douce stimulate residents to join Bible studies and many have become evangelical Christians.

The residency program is also producing short-term Latin American medical missionaries. One mission trip organized by a Vozandes resident to Malawi included family practice medical assistance, HIV/AIDS-specific medical records software and training for the hospital, and weekly Bible studies for the Malawians.

The little medical conference Dr. Dick Douce keynoted in 1987 has continued to grow each year. In 2010, Jornadas Medicas gathered as many chairs as they could find. They set up 500 chairs, but more people kept signing up, shrugging off the seating problem. "No problem, we'll stand," they said. About 800 paid attendees crowded into the conference, plus many more who weren't able to pay. In addition, 21 virtual classrooms around Ecuador filled up. The next year, Jornadas Medicas grew to an estimated 1,200 paid attendees.

Old friends turn up in odd corners of the globe. Dr. Greg Adams and Dr. Dick Douce sat next to each other in medical school. They reconnected when Dr. Greg Adams joined on as a pediatrician with SWMC more than a decade ago before moving to North Carolina. One of Dr. Douce's chief residents at Hospital Vozandes spent time working at the cholera treatment clinic in Haiti. She came back to Hospital Vozandes with a photo of the physician she had to sign out to. "He says he knows you," the resident said. She held up a photo of Dr. Greg Adams.

It's surprising how many people drop into a hospital in Quito, Ecuador. In September 2006, Franklin Graham toured Vozandes. Dr. Douce met up with him at a nurse's station and exclaimed, "I received the Lord with your Dad. So welcome!"

Every four years, the Douces return to Michigan to work at SWMC for a year. During his first furlough, Dr. Douce went right back into infectious diseases. When he came home for his second furlough, new recruit Dr. Mark Harrison had built up an AIDS clinic and, in turn, recruited a series of three or four infectious disease specialists. During the next decade, many moved on to medical missions. Other SWMC physicians who have influenced Dr. Dick Douce have moved on or passed away while he's been in Ecuador. "When you leave the states, things are frozen in your mind," Dick says. "I still miss all the people who have left."

Marian Douce developed SWMC's computer department in the 1980s and during a couple of furloughs. In Ecuador, she solved international technology questions for HCJB and stayed busy as a mom and Bible study leader. They interacted some with Dr. Bill and Ilene Douce, although the senior Douces were in rural Ecuador and Dr. Dick and Marian were in Quito.

The Douces look ahead to career retirement, but like their family members, they won't slow down. It'll be more like spreading out. They have many more goals for Christ's glory, many more people with whom to connect and reconnect. Even as they design the next 20 years of their lives, the Douces look to SWMC — the Atkinsons, the Schindlers, and others who modeled "retirement" before them. "We have a wonderful heritage in SWMC," Dr. Dick Douce says. "You run into other groups trying the same thing, but they don't seem to last as long. It's a privilege to be a part of it and see God's hand."

Dr. Dick Douce emphasizes the importance of the SWMC doctors who remain stateside. "They keep the whole thing floating," he says. "I'm grateful for their service."

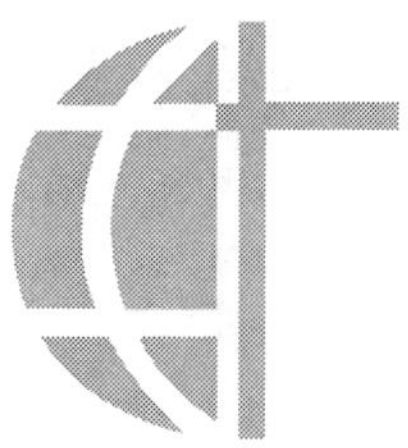

Chapter 27

SWMC's Ripple Effect

Chapter 27

SWMC's Ripple Effect

SWMC Doctors Unwittingly Inspire The Next Generations

As a youngster, Roy Ringenberg hung onto every word of Dr. Schindler's amazing stories about Liberia. Roy's father, Reverend Ralph Ringenberg, pastored in the Missionary Church for more than 50 years. At Grace Missionary Baptist Church in Mooresville, Indiana in the mid-'60s and early '70s, they met Reverend Ray Delahay and his family, who had spent time at Elwa Hospital in Liberia with Dr. Schindler. The Ringenbergs, Delahays, and Schindlers all became friends.

Listening to Dr. Schindler's dramatic storytelling, Roy imagined himself saving lives in Africa. By age 12, he already had designs on following Dr. Schindler's footsteps. Just a decade later, Roy Ringenberg himself would inspire a young man in his parents' church, Mike Chupp.

Roy Ringenberg did not realize his impact on young Mike, whose "peripheral observation" of Roy fueled his own desire to pursue medical missions. "Mike was maybe 8 or 10 years younger than me," Dr. Ringenberg recalls. "Marabeth and I lived in student housing at the IUPUI campus, where the medical school is located, and we attended Grace Missionary [Baptist] Church. We had contact with the youth. I think we went over to the Chupps' for dinner and were able to interact there, and we may have had a couple of conversations where Mike asked specific questions and for guidance between 1975-1979 while I was attending medical school. Mike looked at me as a role model, watching my choices."

Roy consciously planned every educational decision, thinking ahead to missionary service. A year before completing medical school, doctors in training decide on what specialty to take. Roy saw two practical choices for a medical missionary: family practice or surgery. The way he saw it, on the field, a family practitioner could do some surgeries; surgeons could do everything, but they wouldn't be as focused on the general medical side. He was ready to choose one of those specialties to prepare for whatever he might face as a sole physician in a hospital such as Elwa.

But Roy's mentor and advisor, Dr. Charles Kelly, suggested a different route. He said, "God has given you real skill in internal medicine: solving problems, figuring out difficult cases. Even though right now you don't see internal medicine fitting in, pursue that and God will use it."

Likely Dr. Ringenberg talked about Dr. Kelly's advice at the Chupp house: "Use the strengths God has given you. Be obedient in that, even if it does not seem the most logical choice at the time."

After suffering through that decision, and coming to terms with pursuing internal medicine, Dr. Ringenberg began praying about where to train: Indiana University or other places, maybe Mayo Clinic. He visited several great programs. Mayo Clinic began to stand out — in a rather unexpected way.

He remembers, "I went to Mayo and saw how they dealt with patients. All the doctors are good, solid clinicians at Mayo. Other programs boast some excellent researchers, administrators, other strong areas, but not necessarily excellent clinicians. Relating to patients [is important to me]. If I want to reflect Christ, I want to see role models who help me understand and relate to patients. Even though I considered other more renowned internal medicine programs in the country, I went there for the role models. I shared while raising support how I came to that decision. I think Mike heard those stories."

Finding SWMC... on the Other Side of the World

Following Dr. Ringenberg's training at Mayo Clinic, he and his wife spent 1982-1983 in Ogbomosho in Nigeria. They learned about the nine-month-long opening at the Baptist Medical Center in Ogbomosho through Mayo psychiatrist Dr. William Carter Gaventa. Nigeria! Surely, God was showing the Ringenbergs the straight and narrow path that their lives would follow. Surely this nine-month assignment indicated the beginning of a lifelong adventure in Africa.

The Missionary Church raised $4,000 to pay for the Ringenbergs' trip to Ogbomosho. At Ogbomosho, the Nigerian government paid young Dr. Ringenberg's salary as a full professor of internal medicine.

Not long after having arrived, and thinking ahead, the Ringenbergs began to consider where God might want them to work long term. They looked at Jos University Teaching Hospital in Nigeria and also Kamakwie Wesleyan Hospital in Sierra Leone, at that time associated with the Missionary Church.

It just so happened that three SWMC doctors — Dr. Chuck Pierson, Dr. Charles Bruerd, and Dr. Charles Payne — were all working in Sierra Leone at the time: two at the hospital in Kamakwie and one in Freetown. Dr. Pierson and Dr. Payne suggested that Dr. Ringenberg visit SWMC and consider joining the clinic.

A place like SWMC wasn't even in the back of his mind. He planned for more training. He had been thinking about the practicality of earning a master's degree in public health, getting some training in tropical medicine. Another more remote possibility was helping a doctor in New Orleans while working with Tulane University's medical program. But certainly not some little farm-community, work-to-the-bone medical clinic miles away from a good medical school.

So, Dr. Ringenberg laid aside Dr. Pierson and Dr. Payne's advice. When he and his wife and two small children returned to the states, they stayed with his parents. Incredibly, all the study options began to dry up. His parents remarked, "You know, Dr. Bob Schindler works up at that great Christian clinic in Michigan. Maybe you could look him up."

The three Charleses from Sierra Leone reared up in Dr. Ringenberg's mind. At least two of them had told him to visit SWMC. And Dr. Schindler had inspired Dr. Ringenberg to pursue medical missions in the first place. Dr. Ringenberg dialed the phone and made an appointment with Don Gast.

Dr. Ringenberg drove up to Berrien Center and walked into the office across the parking lot from Berrien General Hospital. When Dr. Ringenberg came in, Dr. Schindler happened to be talking with Don. Don explained to Dr. Schindler that Dr. Ringenberg was there for an interview.

"Oh, Roy Ringenberg," Dr. Schindler boomed. "Any relation to Ralph Ringenberg? I know Ralph. That's a great family." He turned to Don. "You should hire him."

Dr. Ken O'Neill had just started at SWMC in internal medicine, and another internist, Dr. Richard Roach, was also there. They didn't need another internist. Nevertheless, they took Dr. Ringenberg on and let him work in the ER.

He might not have even signed a contract at that point. They paid him for working night shifts in Berrien General Hospital's west wing ER or seeing patients in long-term care. Dr. Schindler let Dr. Ringenberg do sutures for him in the OR when there was no one else to help, which was new for him in the states. He'd helped a little at Baptist Medical Center in Nigeria.

Instead of a yawn, Dr. Ringenberg found a bustling hospital at the end of the long driveway off Dean's Hill Road. At that unlikely place, surrounded by Christians of every denomination and theology and background, he learned very much, indeed, without getting a master's at Tulane. At that time SWMC was the largest missions-minded Christian physician group in the United States, if not in the world, and God saw fit to send Dr. Ringenberg there to be a part of their adventures.

Hair-Raising Motorcycle Accidents

One night not long after Dr. Ringenberg started solo ER shifts at Berrien General, a gruesome motorcycle accident happened almost within earshot. A fellow traveling 70 miles per hour on his motorcycle slammed into another vehicle broadside. Though wearing a helmet, he suffered terrible multiple injuries.

Dr. Ringenberg got to work trying to manage the motorcyclist's double lung collapse, high level spine fracture, and neck fracture causing paraplegia. In a blur he was asking for anesthesia to come in, calling desperately for surgeons to come in, and laboring over the man to keep him alive. Several hours later, a Berrien General surgeon flew out in a helicopter with the patient to the University of Chicago. The hospital was impressed that despite Berrien General's limited resources, the man survived. Dr. Ringenberg said the man survived to God's glory.

Another night, a different fellow came in from a bad motorcycle accident. He'd flayed off the front skin of his knee all the way to the kneecap. Dirt and gravel were embedded into the kneecap. A surgeon was backing Dr. Ringenberg in the ER that night, but was tied up with something else. Getting guidance over the phone, Dr. Ringenberg cleaned out the kneecap and stitched it closed. He ordered antibiotics and physical therapy. Over the course of several days and weeks, the patient complained of pain and kept off his knee and ankle. Dr. Ringenberg kept telling him to move around and listen to his physical therapist, but the least amount of pain wasn't tolerable, so the patient found some specialists out west.

Lawyers paid Berrien General Hospital a visit. In the only case where Dr. Ringenberg ever had lawyers come about a patient claiming bad care, the lawyers took a formal deposition from Dr. Ringenberg and examined the patient's chart. When they were through, they threw up their hands. Dr. Ringenberg had documented from the start how carefully the hospital had tried to care for the patient. The lawyers could see that even though Dr. Ringenberg's specialty was internal medicine, the hospital had done a fine job, and the fault rested on their client, who wasn't willing to show up for appointments or cooperate.

Dr. Ringenberg believes God showed the lawyers a testimony of excellent care. They dropped the case, with no settlement. God used that stressful situation to show SWMC's quality and compassionate caring to those lawyers and to the community.

Working feverishly and gaining invaluable experience and skills at Berrien General, Dr. Ringenberg continued to investigate missions. His colleagues at SWMC rallied around him, and several encouraged him to pursue opportunities in their own far-flung neighborhoods. Dr. Schindler was one of those. Another was Dr. Bill Douce.

Not Africa, But Ecuador

Around May 1984, Dr. Ringenberg and Dr. Bill Douce had a memorable conversation in the second floor Berrien General Hospital library. Dr. Douce asked Dr. Ringenberg what he'd enjoyed most about his time in Nigeria. Teaching, Dr. Ringenberg told him. Dr. Douce advised that before making a definite commitment in Africa, Dr. Ringenberg might look into the teaching program at a hospital in Quito.

In fact, in typical Dr. Douce fashion, he whipped out his worn billfold, fished out a small sheet of paper inscribed with a telephone number, and said, "Why don't we call Quito now and see if you can get down there."

He made the telephone call right there on the spot and in less than a minute was talking to the right people in Quito. Dr. Ringenberg couldn't have been more amazed by the whole incident, especially the accessibility and availability of Quito. In Africa just a year before, he'd driven an hour to a telephone. Once at the irregularly functioning phone, he could not make an international phone call but had to wait for his parents to call him — which, of course, had to be carefully prearranged. Often, static interfered with the conversation. In Africa, the ordeal to make one international phone call was costly and might take the better part of an afternoon. By comparison, Quito was surprisingly cutting edge!

Dr. Bill Douce handed the telephone to Dr. Ringenberg, and he talked to Dr. Gil Wagner.

Dr. Wagner told Dr. Ringenberg honestly that his partner, Dr. Brechner, was leaving the mission in just a couple of weeks. Additionally, Dr. Wagner had to be gone for the summer. "If you want to talk to us, you need to get down here before the middle of May," Dr. Wagner said.

That was a scramble. Dr. Ringenberg didn't have the money or time to travel to Ecuador on short notice. A family friend got a $15,000 gift from her parents on her birthday. After tithing, she paid travel expenses for Dr. Ringenberg and his wife, Marabeth. SWMC arranged Dr. Ringenberg's time off. By May 21, they were in Quito. In six days, they toured Vozandes Hospital and School at Quito, visited Shell, and quite a few other places.

Dr. Ringenberg had an opportunity to talk with Dr. Brechner as he packed his books, getting ready to leave. Dr. Brechner was not brimming with optimism. He shook a finger at the window. "See that mountain up there?"

Dr. Ringenberg peered outside at indescribable beauty.

Dr. Brechner threw Dr. Ringenberg a dark look and slung another book in his box. "One day that's going to explode and shower ash all over Quito."

It turned out he was right. But Dr. Ringenberg did not spend much time mulling over Dr. Brechner or his bleak predictions. Instead, he looked around at the opportunities and the miracles. He met a former university Communist Party leader who had somehow found her way to study at Vozandes Hospital. Though not initially eager to hear the Gospel, God had spoken to her, and she'd become a Christian. She was on fire for the Lord, a real leader in her class. Dr. Ringenberg wanted to be a part of a program that could be used of God in such a way.

Coming back to the states after those six whirlwind days in Ecuador, Dr. Ringenberg and Marabeth were uncertain about what to do. In June, they invited Dr. Bob and Marian Schindler over for dinner. The Ringenbergs were renting their house at the time from Dr. Andy White, a former SWMC physician who had gone to work in Boston. After supper the Ringenbergs and Schindlers sat on a couch in the back room of the house, and the Schindlers counseled them.

"Look at your strengths," they said. "Which mission would you fit best with?"

Instead of pushing Africa on the Ringenbergs, they tried to help them find God's direction. The two couples shared times of fasting and prayer during the next month.

The Ringenbergs mistakenly believed they could attend candidate orientation for the sponsoring organizations for both Africa and Ecuador, but at the last minute discovered they had to make their decision before going through that process. This was a faith-building exercise.

In February 1985, having decided to sign on with Quito, they traveled to Miami in the middle of a Michigan snowstorm. Marabeth was in her final trimester with their daughter Ruth, who was born on April 10. The Ringenbergs were accepted by their sponsoring organization, HCJB (Heralding Christ Jesus' Blessings) and began the arduous process of seeking support and preparing to move to South America.

The Ringenberg family started language school in Costa Rica in December 1985. In August 1986, they moved to Quito. In March 1987, Dr. Dick Douce came down from SWMC to keynote the first of what would become an annual lecture series.

When Dr. Dick Douce spoke in Quito in 1987, he gave a full week of one-hour evening lectures. He loved what he saw there and began seriously thinking about joining HCJB. SWMC's first infectious disease specialist, Dr. Dick Douce was vital for Lakeland Hospital (formerly Mercy-Memorial Hospital in St. Joseph).

While Dr. Dick Douce and his wife, Marian, were there for the conference, Quito suffered a large earthquake that destroyed the Ecuadorian pipeline and in which several thousand Ecuadorians were killed in a jungle landslide.

At the time of the quake, Dr. Ringenberg was sprawled across his kitchen floor with his plumber's wrench, trying to fix a drain. Suddenly, his pipe wrench slid across the floor and the cupboard doors swung back and forth. Marabeth shouted out when she was thrown onto the floor from their waterbed. They ran out into the street with the Douces to see what was happening. In the next weeks, HCJB spearheaded relief efforts, an incredible testimony to eastern jungles where HCJB had never been able to go in before. The Catholic priests fled the jungle after the quake, while HCJB poured in bringing aid.

Meanwhile, Marian Douce experienced some health problems, and it was a very difficult, crazy week. Dr. Ringenberg worried that he'd not done enough as a host to bolster Dr. Douce's initial enthusiasm for Vozandes Hospital and HCJB. When the Douces left for the states, Dr. Ringenberg felt it unlikely they'd ever return.

But he was too busy to mourn. The next month, he launched the

Family Medicine Residency Program at Vozandes Hospital that trains Latin missionary physicians for worldwide service. Interestingly, Latin physicians are able to work in countries with limited access to North Americans.

Dr. Ringenberg also contacted a team of 12 physicians from Lackland Air Force Base in Texas who were developing a new course they called Advanced Trauma Life Support (ATLS). Because of Dr. Ringenberg's experiences in the ER of Berrien General Hospital, he was keenly interested in bringing this course to his students at Vozandes Hospital. Those physicians helped Dr. Ringenberg develop the ATLS program at Vozandes, and graduates propagated CPR and other techniques throughout Latin America and all over the world.

Even while more Ecuadorian nationals pursued opportunities in medicine at Vozandes Hospital, Vozandes' training programs grew to attract students outside Latin America. HCJB developed online courses as well, for medical missionaries to pursue additional education.

"Some people are saying there's no space for medical missionaries anymore, but I refute that," Dr. Ringenberg says. "Much training is still needed," and bringing top-quality medical training to second and third-world countries is more economical for all, while also encouraging a higher retention of national physicians.

Meanwhile, SWMC supported Dr. Dick and Marian Douce as they prepared to move to Quito through HCJB. SWMC continued to support the Ringenbergs monetarily, through prayer and encouragement. When they returned for furlough in 1989, Dr. Ringenberg signed a contract and formally became part of the clinic that had already transformed his career and his life in so many ways.

Dr. Mike Chupp

Dr. Mike Chupp learned about SWMC while serving at Tenwek Hospital short-term as an intern. Dr. Roland and Kathy Stephens were working at Tenwek for a year on their time off from Karanda Hospital. One day they had Dr. Chupp over for lunch. Kathy leaned toward Dr. Chupp and said, "You're going into surgery. Roland's part of a great group up in Michigan. You ought to check it out. People there are really excited about and support missions."

Dr. Chupp says, "One of my heroes growing up, whose father was pastor of my church, was Roy Ringenberg. I knew he had joined a group up in Michigan — I just didn't know which group. Roy was one of the biggest influences in my life leading me to consider medical missions. Even as a high school student he planned on medical missions, and he was just six years older than I am, so I got to watch him go through school, emerge as a family practice physician and hit the mission field running."

After Dr. Chupp's conversation with the Stephenses, he got a letter from Dr. Ringenberg saying he had joined SWMC.

Despite those ties with SWMC, Dr. Chupp says he might not have joined SWMC without the humble, steady encouragement of Don Gast. Family time was high on the Chupps' priority list in the states. Their families lived in Tennessee and South Carolina. They weren't sure if they could sacrifice so much time away from their families.

In response to the Chupps' concern, Don nodded sympathetically; he understood. But then Don found them a rental house. Don himself put money down on the house and held it for three months in 1993 while Dr. Chupp finished his residency, so they had a home to come to in Michigan.

When Dr. Chupp started in July as a general surgeon in Locations 14 and 18, the Chupps were expecting their first child. During the interview process, the Chupps did not meet many young doctors. They felt mildly out of place as a young couple. By the time the Chupps came in July 1993, they realized they were part of a memorable "massive influx" of new staff.

Dr. Chupp found flexibility to be both a strength and weakness at SWMC. It was a strength in that the clinic says to a young missionary-minded physician, "You do what God has called you to do, and we'll fit you in when you come back."

But it turned out that after 1993-1996, Dr. Chupp did not practice again stateside with the clinic until 2002. In Dr. Chupp's observation, this trend is especially prevalent in the surgery department. For years, Drs. Roy Winslow and Doug Wilson had to carry the heavy load of two consistent on-staff surgeons while all the other surgeons freely came and went from various missions overseas. Dr. Wilson left SWMC in 2009 and has been keenly missed. The department especially needs two or three surgeons like Dr. Winslow. When Dr. Chupp returns to the states ready to put his nose to the ground and practice, he senses the joy and relief among his colleagues.

These are the same colleagues who had two hands involved in Dr. Chupp's departure for Africa in 1996. Under Dr. Bob Schindler and Don

Gast's influence, Dr. Chupp applied for a Project MedSend grant. Project Medsend offers to pay medical school loans for young doctors who want to be missionaries. (Coincidentally, 11 years after Dr. Chupp received his MedSend grant, former SWMC surgeon Dr. Daryl Erickson became the current president and CEO of Project MedSend). Project MedSend released Dr. Chupp from having to stay in the states for years paying off his school loans.

Dr. Bob Schindler, Dr. Bart Comstock, and other seasoned physicians generously mentored Dr. Chupp and his newly-arrived colleagues. Dr. Chupp compares their influence to fathers or big brothers in the workplace. The older physicians likewise enjoyed these relationships, claiming the newbies infused fresh air — energy, new ideas — into the clinic.

Though Dr. Schindler passed away almost a decade ago, Dr. Chupp remembers him on a daily basis. Dr. Schindler embodied the spirit of SWMC — the rare quality of taking joy in building people. Dr. Chupp was a benefactor of some of Dr. Schindler's final years of kindness and encouragement. Though Dr. Schindler was respected nationally and internationally, as well as in the community and the clinic, he freely spent time alongside the young surgeons in his department, offering second opinions, advice, and care. Dr. Chupp tries to emulate those qualities of his late mentor.

Every once in a while, Dr. Chupp considers striking out into new career territory. One reason he stays at SWMC: "I keep getting told, 'Dr. Chupp, when you come back from Tenwek, it's an encouragement for us and helps us keep our priorities straight.'"

He also feels great satisfaction in being a part of something so unique and influential. Other groups of physicians around the U.S. and around the world have been influenced to think about SWMC's model. While no other group has reproduced SWMC, aspects such as a clinic's Christian witness have challenged them. Physicians have met a SWMC physician at a meeting or conference and are inspired. Young doctors interview at SWMC, and even if they have not chosen to work at SWMC, the clinic has influenced the way they practice wherever they do choose to set up camp.

Dr. Chupp asserts that this influence matches SWMC's mission statement. SWMC is a role model in the integration of healthcare and missions at home and abroad. He says, "There's a whole lot more to be done, and I hope that SWMC has not yet seen its best days. Only in heaven will we fully comprehend the influence that SW has had on global health. So many mission organizations are impacted, people impacted — it's a remarkable thing. I think that God is weaving an incredible mosaic of ministry through the clinic."

Dr. Troy Thompson

Dr. Troy Thompson, like Dr. Chupp, found great mentors at SWMC. But like Dr. Johansen, his recruitment and interview left a little to be desired. He flew in for a February 1998 interview at SWMC. Don Gast gave him directions to drive from the airport, and by the grace of God he found the place. Arriving semi-miraculously in the middle of a storm, with all the landmarks covered by falling snow, Dr. Thompson was ready to learn what the Lord might have planned for him.

He attended Monday morning devotions, ready to be blessed. Instead, the familiar face leading devotions jolted him. Dr. Thompson had known the guy in medical school, and he'd always been difficult to get along with. Later, perhaps seeing Dr. Thompson's incredulity, Dr. Ron Baker confided to Dr. Thompson, "God is really working in this guy's life."

All that day, the weather descended into a blizzard. About three feet of snow fell. All the clinics closed. Dr. Thompson couldn't finish his interview. Dr. Chuck Pierson even slept in the office because he couldn't get home.

Many would have been deflated by such an introduction. Not Dr. Thompson. He took it as a positive sign. After three years of living in Tulsa, he exclaimed, "This is home! I'm back! Thank you, Lord!"

Because of the weather, Dr. Thompson's flights were delayed. This gave him a chance for an extended interview during several days. He had lunch with Dr. Ken O'Neill and Dr. Ron Baker and maybe Dr. Schindler and Dr. Atkinson all at once. His impression: Neat guys, all sincere in their faith.

He had an offer for twice as much money in Oklahoma. But he came to SWMC.

It helped that Dr. Thompson had met Dr. Atkinson and Dr. Schindler beforehand and had been highly impressed with them. Dr. Thompson was one of the founding members of an Advanced Life Support and Unplanned Pregnancy (ALSUP) course in Oklahoma, and intrigued and enthusiastic, Dr. Atkinson had come down to check it out. Another time, Dr. Schindler was a guest speaker for an "In His Image" conference focused on spiritual and scientific renewal.

Finding both men at SWMC, Dr. Thompson spent as much time as he could with Dr. Atkinson and Dr. Schindler. He tried to make them take him out for breakfast. He aggressively pursued one-on-one mentorship from both. Dr. Thompson says, "Out of medical school, you believe medicine is 95% science and 5% art. At some point that ratio starts to swing. Maybe at my age it's like 50/50. By the time I met Herb and Bob Schindler, they were pure artists, sharing the love of God wherever they went."

In 2002 Dr. Thompson and his family planned to move to Kazakhstan, where they would spend a year and adopt two of their children. Before Dr. Thompson left for Kazakhstan, he met up with Dr. Schindler and Marian and said, "I won't let go of you until you bless me."

Dr. Schindler was tired, but he prayed for Dr. Thompson anyway.

Dr. Schindler died about five days after the Thompsons left. When Dr. Thompson found out, he was speaking to medical students in Kazakhstan. He spent about an hour talking about his late mentor's character. People on the other side of the world who had never met Dr. Schindler were enthralled. Dr. Schindler was full of joy, never without a smile. His loud, deep voice and large laugh were unforgettable. His retention for folks he met in passing amazed people. He'd run into someone and ask, "Didn't I meet you 25 years ago on a plane in Nigeria?"

Because of Dr. Schindler's example, Dr. Thompson worked on remembering people's names and listening to their life stories. When Dr. Thompson got back to SWMC, he was privileged to hear patients say things like, "You're just like Dr. Schindler."

Dr. Thompson had learned well from his mentor and subconsciously imitated him in the way he saw patients. Young medical professionals across Kazakhstan have learned and put into practice those same methods of relating. The ripple effect has just begun.

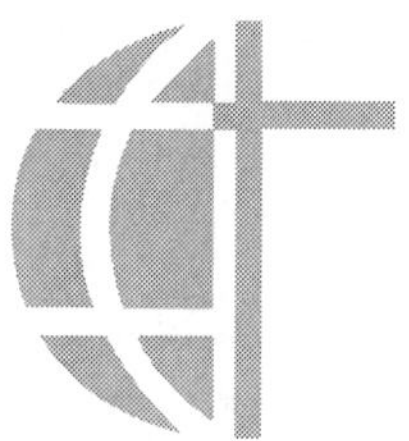

Chapter 28

Under the Radar, into the Global Crowd

Chapter 28

Under the Radar, into the Global Crowd

Some names in this chapter have been changed, and/or locations sometimes generalized or removed for security purposes.

Modern missionaries, like those in previous decades and centuries, are undaunted by threats. They are not fearless automatons, but they are unswerving despite obvious danger. Although they do not face "savages" — these no longer really exist in the world — they face brutal governments and other entities, and these dangers are very real.

One SWMC physician who plans long-term work overseas said he has "broken just about every law" limiting evangelism in one closed country. In fact, on a recent trip, the government raided and arrested people "just one layer away from me. If they'd checked cell phone records, they'd have gotten me." He spent the rest of the trip looking over his shoulder until he boarded the plane.

Dr. Bird (Pseudonym)

Dr. Bird met Dr. Bardin at a medical conference. Already working full time overseas in Asia, Dr. Bird was looking for a place to work short-term on furlough. He'd heard vague references to SWMC back in college through SMDA. Talking with Dr. Bardin, Dr. Bird thought SWMC would be a good place to work.

While Dr. Bird was in the villages in Asia, Don Gast called him on the telephone. He kept saying things you shouldn't say on the phone there. "Are you a missionary doctor?"

"I wouldn't say that," Dr. Bird answered, biting his lip. He prayed that Don would get the hint and that no one was listening in on the phone call.

Thankfully, the only result of Don's phone call was that Dr. Bird was hired at SWMC. He has been a boost to the clinic and an inspiration to many.

Dr. Chris Gordon (Pseudonym)

Dr. Chris Gordon and his future wife, Natasha, both attended Wheaton College. Natasha knew Dr. Dan and Marian Fountain, career missionaries in a primitive bush hospital in Zaire. She spent six months with the Fountains. Dr. Gordon wrote her every day and sent chocolate, and when she came back to the Chicago area, they got married.

Dr. Gordon served a residency in internal medicine at Loyola Hospital. He discovered this was not his calling. He hated the clinic and hospital setting and suffered panic attacks. He took infectious diseases training and dreamed of full time overseas work somewhere outside in the fresh air.

Dr. Fountain, who was not officially part of SWMC but worked as a consultant for five years, kept telling the Gordons great things about the missions-minded clinic. Dr. Gordon called Don Gast several times. Don told Dr. Gordon, "We don't need any infectious disease guys. We already have plenty. We do have an opening for an office-based internal medicine provider in Niles."

Dr. Gordon's hands got sweaty remembering his panic attacks at Loyola. But God loosened Dr. Gordon's tongue, and he took the job. Warren White welcomed him, Don reassured him, and Dr. Gordon went to work every day inside like everyone else. He did not suffer panic attacks, but when Dr. Rick Bardin came 10 months later and wanted an office-based practice, Dr. Gordon's tongue loosened again. He did some fast talking, and they let him start doing inpatient public health and infectious disease work all over Berrien County, just working at Niles one day a week.

The Gordons went overseas full time about two years later. When they came back on furlough, Dr. Froggatt was busy doing five (or maybe 500) things. So, Dr. Gordon got to do more infectious disease work in addition to taking his board exams and reconnecting with western medicine. He also had a great time getting contracts and revenue for SWMC with public health. When Dr. Gordon got ready to leave at the end of the year, Warren White came to have a talk. "You can't leave," he said. "We need you too badly. We can't replace you."

Dr. Gordon reminded Mr. White that when he came to SWMC, he had to beg for a job and squeeze himself into a poor fit. His true calling was elsewhere, on the other side of the world. But he had caught SWMC's vision and believed what it stood for, and he would grieve as he left SWMC behind for another few years.

Dr. Gordon attended Dr. John Ball's (another pseudonym) SWMC recruitment dinner in 2006. Dr. Ball has degrees from Harvard and Columbia Universities, but after 10 years overseas, he couldn't find a practice in the states that wanted to hire him. He networked through to SWMC. At the time, SWMC wanted new doctors to work three years before going overseas full time. But Dr. Ball was honest: "I'm only going to be here one year; then I'm going back to Asia."

SWMC let him sign on. Funny thing: Dr. Ball's wife kept having kids! So, the Balls did stay almost three years before going back to Asia.

When Dr. Gordon left for Asia, Dr. Ball took on his public health job. He worked alongside Dr. Rick Johansen. Dr. Ball also saw patients and set up a smoking cessation program in the Van Buren/Cass County Jail.

On his next furlough Dr. Gordon worked at AL-TACH, the acute hospital in Berrien Springs. It was not a Christian hospital. When Dr. Gordon opened staff meetings, he warned, "Before every meeting I'm going to pray. If my praying is offensive to you, I'm giving you notice to leave the room." No one ever left the room.

Dr. Gordon benefited from the SWMC vision. He was able to take risks and follow God's leading because of what the "grandfathers" in the late 1960s had set up. He's very encouraged that the SWMC board of directors has now made clear that a physician who joins SWMC must go on a short-term overseas mission trip within two years and every four years afterward. SWMC wants all its physicians to catch the vision.

Dr. Holly Sue Tapley

Holly Tapley began her career in medicine as a nurse and loved serving the Lord in medicine. Then God opened doors for her to become a family practice physician. She intended to work in Bangladesh, her adopted sister's country of origin, yet God opened doors for her to serve short-term in another Asian country. When she arrived, she immediately knew this was where God wanted her to work for the rest of her life. Little did she anticipate the arduous journey she would endure, however, to make that mission a full-time reality.

First, she needed experience practicing medicine in the States. In 1999, after completing her residency, Dr. Holly Tapley contacted the Christian Medical and Dental Association for recommendation of a family clinic for her, and they pointed her to Southwestern Medical Clinic. The name rang a bell, and her father, Dr. Dwight Tapley, snapped his fingers in recognition. Living in South Bend, Indiana, they had a peripheral knowledge of SWMC through a family friend. Dr. Holly Tapley joined after meeting with Don Gast.

The dearest memories Dr. Tapley has of SWMC are working in the Bridgman office those first 10 months. She was euphoric about her pending full-time work in Asia, and her colleagues supported her wholeheartedly. Dr. Herb Atkinson, Leslie Tate, and the other staff shared her enthusiasm about leaving soon for Asia. But the prospect of leaving such beloved friends had its bittersweet moments. As the time approached for Dr. Tapley to leave, Leslie joked she'd hang a sign in the office labeled "Asia" so Dr. Tapley would think she was already there and would stay.

In 2000, Dr. Tapley spent a short time on the campus of Wheaton College in suburban Chicago in preparation for the mission field. At about 6 a.m. on June 28, a Jeep Cherokee traveling approximately 35 miles per hour slammed into her blue-and-gold BMX bicycle. Thrown about 60 feet, she landed on pavement.

The accident mangled her so badly, she was not immediately identified. Doctors who spoke to her father, Dr. Dwight Tapley, advised him that she would not likely survive. Diagnoses included severe skull trauma, inner-cranial edema, neck fracture, lower spine fractured twice, dislocated pelvis fractured twice, open fracture of the right leg with significant bone loss resulting from pavement exposure, bruised kidney, collapsed lung, nearly complete laceration of the lower lip, severely fractured jaw, and missing teeth.

She pulled through extensive surgery. Comatose for several days, her prognosis was poor. Doctors were not optimistic about her future as a competent adult, much less one able to practice medicine. In shock, people dropped to their knees. Carol Gonnerman Jewell remembers the dark time at SWMC. "We heard about it right away, and all the drama of her struggle. For days we weren't sure if she'd make it. Sheila Kipp and I would eat lunch together and pray for her. Certainly we didn't think she'd ever practice medicine again."

Several people from SWMC traveled to Central DuPage Hospital in Chicago to visit Dr. Tapley and her family. Although she could not recognize them or remember their visit afterward, hearing of it later both brought great encouragement and provided, in her opinion, a beautiful representation of the caring friendship and personal support linked with the assistance SWMC offers to empower mission service.

The family and SWMC began sending prayer updates to hundreds of people around the world. When Dr. Tapley regained consciousness during a family prayer session, her first words were, "I give it all to Jesus."

Initial neurologist reports were grim. Though Dr. Tapley was able to interact with others, her thought processes remained childlike, with little reasoning ability and no recall. Within the first week after her accident, visitors from her home church in residency, Agape Fellowship, felt a strong impression from the Lord to come in person, anoint her with oil, and pray over her. They procured a small private plane, flew to Chicago from Pennsylvania, and obeyed the Lord's leading. Dr. Tapley believes that this was one of the critical events in an unseen spiritual battle for life that the Lord used to heal her miraculously.

Eight days after the accident she left the ICU. Despite great pain, many more surgeries, and slim odds, she faced her situation with optimism and tenacity. She worked hard during and outside of therapy sessions to regain physical and cognitive skills and memory. Her progress confounded and excited medical personnel in the hospital where she received emergency care. Four weeks after the accident, when she transferred to another hospital for acute rehabilitation, her progress continued to excite medical staff. They called it miraculous. Six months after the accident, extensive neurological tests confirmed her ability to perform the duties of her work as a family practice physician. After an additional surgery two months later, she triumphantly walked back into the office at SWMC.

"How grateful I am to be able to work again!" she said at that time. "I'm certainly more familiar with what it's like to be a patient than I ever cared to be, but I pray this experience will help me become an even better doctor."

For the next year she endured weekly appointments, multiple surgeries and exhausting efforts to resume a reasonable workload. Dr. Tapley returned to work at SWMC less than nine months after the accident. Initially, Dr. Ringenberg shadowed Dr. Tapley, but he found no reasons to be concerned about her professional capabilities.

Two years and four months after the accident, Dr. Tapley was able to leave for full time medical assignment in Asia. She still took Vioxx, an anti-inflammation medicine she began taking after the accident. But Vioxx was not available there. Her parents, coming to visit, could bring some, but one problem loomed. They were unable to procure the amount of medication she needed long-term in Asia.

Dr. Atkinson heard about Dr. Tapley's predicament. He drove around to all the SWMC offices and collected every Vioxx sample he could find. He met her parents halfway and laughed off their thanks. This was the kind of stuff he did every day for people. Nothing special to him. Dr. Holly Tapley, however, will never forget it.

Not a pediatrician, she felt a bit out of her element sometimes, especially in rural settings with a language barrier and no one else to help. Dr. Atkinson tracked down a Harriet Lane Handbook of Pediatrics for her. He also downloaded numerous files of information she could carry around in a Palm Pilot — much handier than lugging an oversized hardcover manual.

Those who warned Dr. Tapley might never walk again now know she regularly traverses some of the most mountainous terrain in the world and easily jogs six miles along Lake Michigan for leisure. Those who predicted she might never work again now attest to her stamina practicing third-world medicine in remote villages. Those who feared she might never awaken from her coma can rejoice as she speaks publicly about her recovery and about the many wonders God has performed through her both in the U.S. and on the other side of the globe.

The Smiths

Dr. Collin P. Smith and his wife, Eleanor, (pseudonyms) met Dr. Herb Atkinson in the early 1980s. Dr. Smith was still doing his surgical residency, and someone recommended they meet Dr. Atkinson, who had spent years in Africa where they were considering working.

The Smiths dropped in on the Atkinsons during an evening rain storm. Not wanting to impose, they checked into a hotel before calling the Atkinsons. Dr. Atkinson immediately offered to come pick them up at the hotel. Instead, the Smiths followed him in their car. Within five minutes of entering his house, they were sitting in the dark watching a slide show about the Congo. Dr. Atkinson and wife Frieda's enthusiasm inspired them. Later, the Smiths worked for eight years in the Democratic Republic of the Congo (DRC), at that time named Zaire. Their jungle experiences mirror the Atkinsons', and like Dr. Atkinson, they do not prefer to talk about the evacuations and tribal killings. They went to the DRC to save lives and be witnesses for Jesus.

The Smiths studied French for a year before moving to a referral hospital in the DRC with their three young children. They were unable to raise their full support after a year of visiting churches. The mission allowed them to go partially supported, as they had some savings they were willing to use. But the accountants who prepared the Smiths' taxes didn't withdraw enough. To pay the government, they drained their savings. They learned an old lesson on a deeper level: the worth of their work does not correspond to how much they earn. "We ate less and lost some weight," Eleanor recalled.

When extra money gifts came from SWMC or individuals, the Smiths felt blessed. After 15 months in the referral hospital, they moved to a district hospital in a town of about 22,000 that desperately needed a surgeon. They finished out their first four-year missionary term at the district hospital, and then returned to the U.S. to join SWMC in 1990. Dr. Smith started in the ER at Berrien General and ran some migrant clinics. Because SWMC had enough surgeons in the clinic, he only occasionally performed surgery while covering for Dr. Bob Schindler.

Returning to the states that first time, Dr. Smith encountered something unexpected: reverse culture shock. He'd prepared for more than a year for the culture transition from the U.S. to Zaire, but was ill-prepared for re-entry into the U.S. Everything felt different. He said, "When I first came back, I was doing things like treating without x-rays and lab work, and the head doctor in the ER took me aside and said, 'This is the U.S., and in the U.S. we do tests.'"

He also confounded his staff by scrawling orders using French abbreviations instead of English. His Congolese French did come in handy, however, when working alongside Dr. Atkinson. The two could talk uninhibited about patients without divulging confidential information to accidental listeners. On subsequent furloughs Dr. Smith found reverse culture shock less troublesome.

At the referral hospital in the DRC, Dr. Smith supervised a two-year residency for general doctors and taught community health in the nursing school. During his own training in Liverpool, even as a general surgeon he had earned the community health medal. "It really irritated some of the general medicine doctors that a surgeon won the award," Dr. Smith recalled with a chuckle.

When they moved to the DRC district hospital, he was the only surgeon. He loved it, and he taught nurses, young doctors, and nursing students. He was principal for one year at the nursing school. However, the area was fraught with tribal conflict. Though never individually targeted in the attacks, the Smiths were evacuated "a number of times." They hid in the jungle once but found it more of an interesting cultural experience than a hardship.

When Dr. Smith returned to the referral hospital to lend a hand, the hospital and town were overrun by hostile militia intent on killing off members of two tribes living in the area. The conflict was not one-sided, as these tribes had militias who raided their opponents' towns. Between one and two thousand villagers were killed in this incident.

Militiamen asked Dr. Smith about the whereabouts of members of the tribe they were out to eliminate. They threatened the local people and demanded money from the missionaries. In the process, some of the militiamen tried to reassure Dr. Smith, telling him they wanted the hospital to keep working, but their words were not very convincing when they were killing his friends and neighbors. In trying to keep as many as possible out of harm's way, Dr. Smith and his national staff sheltered between 50 and 100 villagers, plus their patients, in the orthopedic center. His mission ordered him out of the area after a day and a half. The people hiding in the orthopedic center all later fled the area. Destroying the entire town, the militia looted the hospital and the hospital staff's dwellings down to the roofing material and wiring.

Later in Kenya, Dr. Smith worked in orthopedic rehabilitation at Kijabe Hospital. Eleanor worked as a nurse at the missionary school and also taught French. She filled various positions at the school and hospital and was guest house manager for a year as well.

One time Dr. Smith was called in to treat a Masai man gored by a Cape buffalo and suffering from a sucking chest wound. After stabilizing the patient, he noticed that the patient in the next bed, also a young Masai, was vomiting blood and losing blood from stools. Looking more closely, he saw the man had small areas of bleeding in the lining of his eyelids. He also had a high fever. Dr. Smith suspected a viral hemorrhagic fever, of which Ebola is the most well-known. The CDC sent an investigator.

A few days later Dr. Smith developed cold symptoms. He called in to the hospital as a precautionary measure. The hospital told him, "You'd better get in here. The CDC guy said you're going into isolation."

The hospital lab sent information to Nairobi. Despite efforts to keep the possible outbreak under wraps for obvious panic reasons, Dr. Mike Chupp, also a SWMC surgeon in Kenya, heard about Dr. Smith's isolation. Since the Kenyans were talking about a possible Ebola outbreak, Dr. Chupp became concerned. He told Dr. Mark Harrison, who was at the CMDA national convention. Dr. Harrison sent out some antiviral medication. Word got out that Dr. Smith was dying of Ebola. Prayers were lifted at the national convention and around the world.

"Normally they could call us up [to get the facts], but there was an information blackout," Dr. Smith said. "I didn't know they were calling or had even heard anything about it."

The CDC investigator was unable to establish a diagnosis. But during the next couple of weeks, the hospital admitted seven other young Masai with the same alarming symptoms. Four died, including the man Dr. Smith first admitted with the chest wound.

After two days of boredom in isolation, twiddling his thumbs and reviewing German grammar, Dr. Smith was released. Kijabe returned to hectic normalcy. Not long after, he contacted SWMC about an unrelated issue. The person at the other end of the line gasped and exulted, "You're still alive!" and dropped the phone. Dr. Smith spent several minutes waiting until someone picked up the phone to excitedly finish the call.

"We appreciated the concern and that people would do something," Dr. Smith said. "You can feel you're out there by yourself — that no one knows about what you're doing or is thinking about you. All those prayers were a help to us, even if I wasn't dying of Ebola."

Dr. Smith finds the decision about whether to refer someone to someone else to be easy in the U.S. "because you always have referral." In the Congo he didn't have to weigh whether to refer or not because there were no specialists to refer to. He found Kenya and West Africa difficult because "you sometimes had referral. It depended on whether people had money, their tribe, religious and health beliefs, and where they lived. Sometimes you could refer and sometimes you couldn't. I sent people off for radiation therapy, but they couldn't get it because they had no money. But I sent people out for pacemaker insertion or heart valve replacement and sometimes they could get it. They just had to negotiate with other doctors," he recalled.

By this time the Smiths were rotating four years in Africa, then a year in the states, except for 1999-2001, when they stayed at Southwestern an extra year to allow Dr. Paul Lim to go on a keenly anticipated year-long medical missions trip. If Dr. Smith recalls correctly, the day Dr. Lim returned to the U.S. from that trip, he and his future wife, Susan, were introduced to each other by their mothers. That trip served as a catalyst for additional long-term work for the Lims in Ethiopia, where they have helped open CURE Ethiopia Children's Hospital.

At first the Smiths lived in Bridgman. When Dr. Smith started doing surgery at Lakeland Hospital (formerly Memorial Hospital in St. Joseph) in 1999, hustling up from Bridgman during the first snowfall instigated a move closer to the hospital.

When the Smiths moved to West Africa, that hospital was still being built by a very small church. Dr. Smith was its first surgeon while it was still a clinic. Then he moved them into the new hospital and got things started for them. For a while he served as medical director. The Smiths spent six years working to start up the hospital in this predominantly Muslim country. They are now starting a new hospital in another Muslim country. In the short time they have been there, they have seen at least one miracle.

A boy was brought into the hospital after an auto accident with a broken leg. He was comatose from his head injuries. He had some seizures and vomiting, so the medical staff was worried he might have aspirated. Dr. Smith and another Western physician worked together over the boy, drilling burr holes and looking for bleeding and the reason for his coma. Since they found no blood to drain, they attributed his coma and seizures to brain swelling. In the absence of specialized care, the outlook for the boy was very poor.

The hospital was in an insecure area. The nationals would not let the Western doctors stay the night. They prayed over the child, "but we of little faith, we thought the kid would die in the night," he recalled. "That evening we sat there feeling sorry for ourselves and talking about this kid."

In the morning, not knowing what they would find, Dr. Smith and another doctor went to the boy's bedside. The boy's mother sat with him. He was sitting up in bed, visiting with his mother. Dr. Smith asked the mother how he was doing. She said his leg hurt but other than that he felt fine.

Dr. Smith smiled. He said, "His leg is broken, so it will hurt a little until the bone heals." Then he told her he felt it a miracle the boy was alive, and explained why. The mother was very happy.

"When we excitedly discussed this with local doctors, they were very fatalistic and did not see God's hand in the child's healing," Dr. Smith explained. "We need God's help to be a testimony of His love and compassion."

Blending into the Global Crowd

On Carolyn Philip's desk rests a photo taken at a missions conference in Thailand in 2009. She treasures the photo, depicting several current and recently-past members of SWMC and their families who went to the conference, and in the back row, an older man and his wife whom she's never met. When talking about the photo, Carolyn points this couple out rather reverently and tells the story about how their faces came to appear in the SWMC photo.

Several SWMC physicians attended the international missions conference in Thailand. At the end of one session, an announcement was made for all SWMC physicians and their families to gather outside for a photo. While they gathered, this older man stepped out of the crowd and exclaimed, "I'm a past SWMC doc! Can I be in the photo, too?"

He and his wife quickly introduced themselves. Dr. Wendell Geary worked at Berrien County Hospital from August 1961 to June 1962 before entering the mission field in the rain forest of rural Indonesian Borneo in June 1964. In 1973 he and his wife, Marjorie, "Margie" opened a basic nursing school there. The following year they opened the Bethesda Mission Hospital, which has now grown to a 100-bed facility. The nursing school, now named Bethesda Nursing Academy, graduates 40 to 50 nurses annually. The Gearies retired from full-time service in Borneo in 2005 but continue to return. In 2009, they spent nine months there. The SWMC physicians at the missions conference listened, enthralled and impressed to meet a former colleague most of them had never even heard about.

Dr. Geary and Margie pressed eagerly for information about SWMC and some of the doctors they knew. They smiled for the photo. Then, like the others, they blended back into the conference crowd.

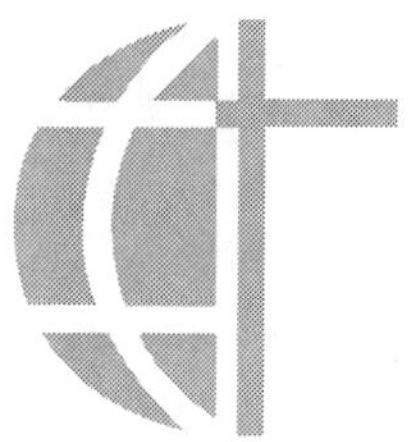

Chapter 29

Testimonies of the Growing Years

Chapter 29

Testimonies of the Growing Years

Dr. Ron Baker

Dr. Ron Baker and his wife, Jane, were full time missionaries from 1974-1990 in Sierra Leone, West Africa. During their first furlough, Dr. Baker was completing continuing medical education in Lexington and met another missionary doctor, Dr. Almarose Cooke Warden, who was Dr. Weldon Cooke's sister. She'd been a missionary in Honduras and then Rhodesia/Zimbabwe. She and Dr. Baker began talking, and she told him about a group in southwest Michigan that did medical missions.

It sounded promising. Dr. Baker contacted Dr. Weldon Cooke. He said, "Look, any time you want to come up here, you have a job."

The Bakers went back to Africa for their second three-year term. Sometime in 1980, looking ahead to furlough in 1981, Dr. Baker wrote a letter to Dr. Weldon Cooke, who wrote back, "See you next year."

Dr. Baker assumed everything was a "go." In late August of 1981, arriving back in the United States, Dr. Baker pulled out SWMC's phone number. Dr. Cooke wasn't there. They transferred his call to Don Gast. "Hello, I'm Dr. Ron Baker letting you know I'm here. When do I start?"

Don asked, "Who are you?"

This was Dr. Baker's first feeling that maybe his position at SWMC was not secure.

"We need to meet you," Don said.

The entire group met Dr. Baker and Jane. The process wasn't traumatic. They let him join, and later they let him serve as chairman of the missions committee. Don helped the Bakers find a house. Dr. Baker filled in at the migrant clinics and the ER and did sports physicals and helped in schools. He worked in the Benton Harbor clinic. He worked at other clinics. After a year he went back to Africa, as planned, and since then his job at SWMC has been secure.

Dr. Thomas Ritter

In the summer of 1983, Dr. Ken O'Neill, Dr. Roy Ringenberg, and Dr. Thomas Ritter all joined SWMC. The corporation had about a dozen doctors stateside at the time. Drs. O'Neill, Ringenberg, and Ritter increased the corporation by about 25%.

The clinic was based by Berrien General Hospital at the time and, in Dr. Cooke's absence, Dr. Schindler was the congenial figurehead. In fact, Dr. Ritter had met Dr. Schindler at a conference at Wheaton College a few years before. Dr. Schindler had regaled him with stories about SWMC and told him to keep the group in mind.

But God had other work for Dr. Ritter, so he hadn't pursued SWMC right after meeting Dr. Schindler. First, he worked with the Indian Health Service in Arizona, and then he filled in at Muttru Hospital in Sierra Leone for a couple of years.

When Dr. Ritter and his wife, Joyce, got to Muttru, Dr. Ron Baker was getting ready to leave on furlough. Early on, Dr. Ritter said to Dr. Baker, "I might look into Southwestern Medical Clinic. Have you heard of it? It might be a great place for you to land for a year in the states."

"That's where I'm going! I've already arranged it," Dr. Baker said. And that whole conversation took on an ironic cast when the mix-up happened to Dr. Baker.

While Dr. Baker got settled into SWMC, the Ritters filled in for the Bakers for a year at Muttru. Then they stayed a second year at Muttru with the Bakers, so it wasn't until 1983 that they came to SWMC. Dr. Ritter had some medical problems, and Dr. Baker sent him to Berrien Springs. They took out Dr. Ritter's kidney stone at old Berrien General Hospital. Almost immediately, Dr. Ritter got out of bed and donned his own white coat. They needed coverage downstairs in the ER.

After much prayer he joined SWMC permanently in September 1983. Dr. Andy White, a family practitioner with Dr. Herb Atkinson and Dr. Helene Johnson, was leaving to go to seminary in New England. They had a busy obstetrics practice. Dr. Ritter was able to step into Dr. White's practice, sometimes traveling to five locations. It was common to work half a day at the Berrien Springs office in the old house by the SDA Spanish church, half a day under the dentist's office in Bridgman, and then moonlight in the Berrien General ER. The next day he might run between the Benton Harbor health department clinic and the Stevensville office. Sometimes to make a delivery, he'd rattle across country roads at 100 miles per hour.

In fact, Dr. Ritter got so busy delivering babies, he decided to get OB/GYN residency training. Dr. Larry Cairns had joined SWMC as an OB/GYN a year before. Sometime during Dr. Ritter's residency on the east coast, Dr. Slater came home and joined Dr. Cairns. When Dr. Ritter returned to SWMC as an OB/GYN in 1990, he worked with Dr. Slater and Dr. Cairns. Dr. Donna Joan Harrison joined shortly thereafter. Then Dr. Slater retired.

Dr. Helene Johnson mounted a memorable poster on the ladies' sleeping room at Berrien General Hospital. The work of Charles Schulz, the poster featured Lucy Van Pelt wearing a hard hat and standing defiantly in the middle of a construction zone. The caption: "One woman can do the work of two men."

Throughout the years Dr. Ritter has remembered that poster as a fitting metaphor for Dr. Johnson's work ethic. Dr. Johnson has delivered three generations of babies. Beyond retirement age, she is still doing two times the deliveries Dr. Ritter does. He says, "When you look at an old guy like me doing more than the average OB/GYN, and she's doing twice that, it's amazing. She's a special member of the corporation who's helped keep us going. She's just quietly and selflessly contributed, working hard for the clinic's success. I don't know if she decided she had to live up to that poster."

Pretty tireless and tenacious himself, Dr. Ritter has worked at almost every SWMC location. As they opened and closed, he moved his practice from place to place. The Center for Women's Health was SWMC's first St. Joseph site, in an old Victorian farmhouse at 3888 Niles Road. That was Dr. Ritter's first foray into Lakeland Hospital. Also, for about nine years in the 1990s, SWMC ran an OB/GYN office on South State Street in St. Joseph in a newly remodeled office building.

For several years Dr. Larry Cairns worked out of both Berrien General Hospital and Lakeland. Eventually, he moved to St. Joseph, where he saw patients at both South State Street and Stevensville. In time, they closed both St. Joseph locations and enlarged the Stevensville office. Dr. Ritter also remembers working with Dr. Donna Harrison and Dr. Cairns out of a double wide in Berrien Springs.

Since 1999, Dr. Ritter and Dr. Helene Johnson practice at a SWMC OB/GYN office near

Lakeland Community Hospital, Niles (formerly Pawating Hospital) on St. Joseph Street. Dr. Karen Zienert and Dr. James Bateman also practice at that location.

Although Dr. Ritter's workplace sometimes felt nomadic, his home was a rock-solid sanctuary in a beautiful setting surrounded by close friends.

For 18 years, beginning in 1991 while they reared their family, the Ritters lived on Rangeline Road in Berrien Springs.

Four doors down from the Ritters lived Dr. Roland Stephens and his family. When Dr. Roland Stephens was in Africa, sometimes his son Dr. Dan Stephens lived there with his growing family when they came home on furlough. Dr. Rick Johansen lived just down the street from the Stephenses. A mile farther down on Concord Circle lived the Pierson and Baker families. The Roach family lived nearby as well.

Many of these men were runners and bicyclists. Dr. Roland Stephens ran several days a week, but Dr. Ritter could never keep up with him. Dr. Roach also ran. Dr. Baker and Dr. Ritter became jogging buddies. They rode bikes too for a while until they had a "little accident" and Dr. Ritter broke his collar bone. They might have been goofing off.

These doctors learned of a Berrien County secret only the Rangeline runners and bikers knew. According to Dr. Ritter, Berrien County's most scenic spot is the dirt road at the end of Lake Chapin Road after crossing the bypass. This may or may not have been the location of the little accident.

On the way home from work, Dr. Baker sometimes dropped by Dr. Ritter's house or vice versa. They compared hunting and fishing notes. In fact, they did a lot of hunting and fishing together. They took their kids to Boundary Waters several times — once with Dr. Roach and Dr. O'Neill.

Dr. Ritter is "Uncle Tom" to the Baker kids; Dr. Baker is "Uncle Ron" to the Ritter kids. "They sort of know we're not blood relatives," Dr. Ritter says. The Pierson's were "Aunt Ruth" and "Uncle Chuck." Their boys all played soccer together.

In Dr. Ritter's mind, in the early 1980s the clinic was seen as a place for missionary doctors to come home to. As it expanded during that decade, it returned more to its original intent as a springboard for younger physicians planning to go overseas. Through thick and thin, all the SWMC doctors had a bedrock commitment to help their friends serving overseas. While none of the medical missionaries received the majority of their monetary support from SWMC or its doctors, all have gotten some financial support from the corporation, as well as from individual SWMC doctors. "That's our primary glue, our common bond," Dr. Ritter has always insisted.

Like his colleagues, Dr. Ritter claims never to have seen a hand come down from the sky passing out hundred dollar bills or tablets of solutions as a guide. Nevertheless, he knows God has an active hand in the clinic. "There were rocky times, but the Lord's blessed us. We're not a bunch of geniuses. It's the Lord's doing. We've always felt the Lord's hand on us. It's his clinic and not ours. If it would survive, it would be his doing."

Likewise, Dr. Ritter has not seen flashy miracles, but he believes that he has witnessed quiet miracles down through the years. "The miracle is that we've stayed together. The Lord's prospered and grown us, which is quite miraculous in our medical culture."

Dr. Bill Wilkinson

Dr. Bill Wilkinson came during the clinic's growing years. When Bill was finishing his residency, his brother-in-law's father, Dr. Ed Manring, called him up. Dr. Manring had worked with Dr. Bob Schindler in Liberia, and although he had never worked at SWMC, he thought the Wilkinsons would fit in. "Call Bob Schindler in Stevensville," he advised.

Dr. Wilkinson looked on a map to find Stevensville. Dr. Schindler put him in touch with Don Gast. Dr. Wilkinson met with Don a couple of times, interviewed, and found him very persuasive but not pushy. SWMC was the only place that interviewed Dr. Wilkinson and did not offer him a contract, only a handshake.

During the interview, Dr. Wilkinson attended a devotion time. Dr. Ron Baker led it that morning. He talked about a SWMC doctor serving over in Asia, Dr. Jones. Their house was raided by police one night. The police confiscated the Joneses' computers and kicked them out of the country. SWMC provided work, counseling, and support until they figured out what God had next for them.

The doctors sat around the table and wrote cards to send to Dr. Jones. Though Dr. Wilkinson had never met him, he found himself writing an encouraging card, too. When he got home, Dr. Bill Wilkinson sat with his wife, Cindy. "Should we take a chance on this?" they asked each other. "It's kind of an unusual thing."

They hesitated because of SWMC's loose structure, low pay, and no contract. But the people they met — Don Gast, Ron Baker, Herb Atkinson — especially impressed them as godly men of high caliber. They thought about it, prayed, and talked again with the Manrings. At one point, Dr. Wilkinson asked Dr. Manring's wife, Nancy, "Does God always want you to do the hardest thing?"

She looked at him without any hesitation and said, "He does."

"That was our answer!" Dr. Wilkinson said. "We were young and inexperienced. She was older and wiser."

They went home and said to each other, "We'll give it a try." They ended up working with SWMC about a dozen years.

When the Wilkinsons came to SWMC in 1993, Don Gast lined them up with a realtor who showed them all around and allowed them to get a mortgage with no money down.

It took them a while to learn about all the missionaries. Every year someone different came back to SWMC on furlough. Dr. Wilkinson heard about Dr. Roy Ringenberg many times before they met.

Every quarter, like the other SWMC members, the Wilkinsons received a bonus check with the expectation that they would give it all to missions of their choice. "It was a lot of fun deciding where to send it," Dr. Wilkinson noted. "At first we didn't know that many people, but over time it was easy. There were always special projects, students going places short-term, plus the long-term regulars. The money was gone in a couple of days, but, boy, did we have a good time seeing it go."

One SWMC physician who encouraged the Wilkinsons as they got started was family practitioner Dr. Baker. A missionary in Sierra Leone who grew up a missionary kid in Africa, he focused on the Lord. He did a lot of surgery and complex procedures in Sierra Leone, including taking out thyroid glands — procedures not normally attempted in the third world. Dr. Baker and Dr. Pierson worked at different hospitals within Sierra Leone.

Dr. Wilkinson started at the Stevensville office. For about a decade he split his time between Stevensville and Benton Harbor. Splitting time between the middle class and the poor was difficult for him. He asked to work full time at Benton Harbor.

While working for SWMC at the Mercy Specialty Clinic in Benton Harbor, Dr. Wilkinson had the opportunity to minister to several different people. One woman came in with stomach problems. She had ingested some harmful things trying to induce an abortion. Dr. Wilkinson evaluated and treated her stomach problems and also prayed with her over her baby. She carried her baby girl to term and later thanked him.

The friendship between Dr. Atkinson and Dr. Schindler was immeasurable. They enjoyed each other and had the same focus. It was contagious to be with them. They weren't moaning and groaning about the pay or the heavy workload. They swapped stories like a pair of fishermen and chuckled about life's ironies. Above all, their focus was on healing in the name of Jesus Christ.

Dr. Atkinson had the gift of being able to work very hard while looking as though he was just having a breezy good time. One time Dr. Wilkinson and Dr. Atkinson were talking about Dr. Wilkinson maybe taking over for Dr. Atkinson as he slowed down. He said, "I only deliver 180 babies a year now," and Dr. Wilkinson tried to keep a deadpan face. Most family doctors deliver 40 or 50 babies a year.

Dr. Schindler's life was focused on missions. For him, missions work was not just relegated to his corner of the world at Elwa Hospital. Wherever he was, that was his mission. That was his personal conviction, and it was also part of his vision for SWMC. Taking care of Medicaid patients — the poor — and having a presence in Benton Harbor was always on his heart. During several conversations, Dr. Schindler impressed his colleagues with the comment, "It doesn't make any cents, and maybe not any sense, but it's what God wants us to do."

One time in 1995 the Wilkinsons sat near the Schindlers at a Lakeland event. Afterward, the Schindlers invited the Wilkinsons out for dessert. The Schindlers suggested going to McDonald's for ice cream. They knew that Benton Harbor had ice cream cones cheaper than the St. Joseph franchise, so they drove out to Benton Harbor. It occurred to the Wilkinsons that the surgeon and his wife certainly could afford the extra dollar, but they were very conscious of how they used their money.

Dr. Wilkinson saw a lot of Dr. Bill Douce. Their paths crossed frequently at work, devotions, meetings, and at church. They struck up a friendship. Both confess to the habit of keeping slips of paper with phone numbers in their wallets — the original Palm Pilot.

Dr. Douce played soccer with the Wilkinson kids — and kept up with them, which was no small feat. He concocted homemade fire crackers. Sometimes they'd be driving down the road and Dr. Douce would suddenly stop the car to chase and catch a butterfly.

Dr. Douce asked the Wilkinsons to come to Ecuador. They took their families for a month. For seven years, the Wilkinsons went to Ecuador for a month, and they ended up adopting one of their sons, Santiago or "Santi," as a result.

When SWMC sold the Benton Harbor office to InterCare, Dr. Wilkinson contracted out through InterCare while still with SWMC. But coming back from Ecuador, he found it hard working for two bosses and liked working with rural clinics. In 2005 he made the difficult decision to leave SWMC and remain with InterCare.

The Wilkinsons treasured interactions with SWMC friends. "You read the books about the martyrs and all those people, and then you hear people like Don Gast or Bill Douce talking about those giants of the faith as friends," Cindy Wilkinson said.

The Wilkinsons maintain friendships they began at SWMC. They thank God for their season at SWMC. In school, the Wilkinsons' goal was to work with the poor in the United States and do overseas missions work. SWMC allowed them to do both. They are very grateful they were able to be part of a group where short-term missions was not an inconvenience but almost expected.

Dr. Chris Harvey

In 2005, around the time Dr. Wilkinson was leaving SWMC, pediatrician Dr. Chris Harvey joined and began working at the Niles office. He had learned of SWMC from a postcard.

Dr. Harvey's father was an Army chaplain, and his wife, Jana, had grown up as a missionary kid in Papua, New Guinea. The Harveys wanted to pursue both short- and long-term missions. Hearing of SWMC's commitment to missions, they anticipated being able to get overseas quickly after joining.

It was more difficult than they imagined. Dr. Harvey joined SWMC's mission committee to work on making it easier for new SWMC physicians to go on short- and long-term missions. By 2010, he and the committee changed some policies so that after physicians had worked at SWMC for two years, they could go on short-term missions for two months every year. The Harveys were subsequently able to go short-term to Kenya and Cameroon.

About a year after he came to SWMC, Dr. Harvey also joined the SWMC Foundation. Since 2000, the foundation has been known mostly for its bi-annual fellowship scholarships supporting medical students and residents who need support for overseas medical missions rotations. A few recipients have come back to join SWMC. Dr. Michele Gray-Ashton,

Dr. Jill Maulding-Wang, and Dr. Callie Bandera (pseudonym) are past scholarship recipients. Of more than 60 recipients since 2000, a handful have also been relatives of SWMC members. These include Eric Snyder; Jeannette Frey; Daniel and Andy Lee; Dan Douce; Sarah E. Schultz; Kimiko Sugimoto; and, most recently, Matthew Cooke, grandson of Dr. Cooke. Dr. Michele Gray-Ashton also served on the foundation board.

Throughout the years, SWMC members such as Dr. Schindler, Dr. Atkinson, Dr. Harvey, Dr. O'Neill, and incoming CEO Warren White conducted interviews of scholarship candidates. The foundation now has a director, Roger Cabe, who participates in the interviews as well.

Retired administrative assistant Stella Wetkowski worked in the Berrien Springs administration office for seven years. Part of Stella's duties was scheduling meetings for the scholarship program. Doctors' schedules were notoriously full. But Drs. Schindler and Atkinson, arguably two of the busiest doctors on staff, told Stella they'd be there whenever she scheduled the meetings. At the time, Dr. Schindler was undergoing chemotherapy, but he never succumbed to discouragement. He remained enthusiastic about serving in any capacity.

Dr. Atkinson and Dr. Sherry O'Donnell were key people in starting up a lay ministry in the doctors' offices. Volunteers now spend time with patients in the waiting rooms, offering prayer and leading some to the Lord. Though Dr. Atkinson has passed away and Dr. O'Donnell has left SWMC to open her own solo practice, this ministry continues.

Dr. Heather Marten

Dr. Heather Marten traveled two different pathways to SWMC. During medical school she attended the Global Health Missions Conference. At one of the hundred booths at the conference, Dr. Jen Powell told her about SWMC.

Dr. Chris Harvey and Dr. Marten did their pediatric residencies together. Dr. Harvey was a year ahead of Dr. Marten. Dr. Harvey joined SWMC, replacing a pediatrician who had passed away, Dr. Rutherford. He told Dr. Marten all about SWMC. Surprised by such enthusiastic ebullience from her normally reserved friend, she asked if SWMC might like another pediatrician the following year. Coincidentally, Dr. Marten replaced Dr. Powell when she left.

In 2006, Dr. Marten may have been one of the last people Don Gast hired before he semi-retired. She wanted to go overseas right away. "I'm coming to leave," she warned. They asked her to stay three years to build a practice first. She thought maybe she could do that, but it would be hard. She'd already waited years to answer her call.

Heather's family and church were missions focused. She felt called to missions at age 12. In an eighth grade essay assignment, she said she wanted to be a missionary when she grew up. She included a photo of India. But she didn't feel called to the ministry, and all the missionaries she'd ever heard about or had met were mission pastors.

When she was 16, she took her first short-term missions trip with AIM (Ambassadors in Missions, an Assemblies of God program) to Venezuela. The experience cemented her call to missions. As a high school senior, Heather decided to be a physician. College professors told her about medical missions. Immediately, she knew that was her calling. She loved children, so pediatrics was a sensible choice.

All through school and residency, Heather took short-term missions trips at every opportunity. She went to Kenya, India, and Sudan. She even looked into joining an HIV clinic start-up in Africa. Although lured by the prospect of a salary rather than having to find her own support, she eventually decided not to sign a contract. She wanted medical missions, not just medical overseas work, because she didn't want to become so absorbed in the medical side she might forget the eternal reason for her calling.

A few months before finishing residency, she discovered a lump on her thyroid. She was very grateful she had not signed the contract with the HIV clinic, because she would've had to break the contract to stay in the U.S. for her own medical treatment. She'd already been hired by SWMC. The future looked bright. Having her thyroid removed was just a minor inconvenience.

Joining SWMC, Dr. Marten planned to take a short-term trip every year to learn where God wanted her to go. Medical missions have hundreds of possibilities. Thus, she faced a daunting search.

Two- and three-week mission trips seemed very insignificant in light of what Dr. Marten believed lay right around the next bend. But "the next bend" began to look farther and farther down the road. Meanwhile, other SWMC physicians found their overseas homes. Drs. Paul and Susan Lim went to Ethiopia. They opened a plastic surgery hospital. Dr. Susan Lim was the only Western-trained pediatrician in the whole country. Needs overseas were overwhelming. Wouldn't God use Dr. Marten, too?

In 2011, Dr. Marten arranged a month-long trip to Zambia. The same day that she landed in Zambia, she was sitting around meeting a dozen missionaries from the area, and one couple looked very familiar. Finally, she asked them, "Have you been missionaries other places?"

They had.

"Were you missionaries in Venezuela before?"

Suddenly, there was happy pandemonium. They'd been missionaries in Venezuela when she had taken her very first missions trip. This was just the beginning of a sort of homecoming she felt several times during the month. That month she traveled "all over Zambia" exploring many long-term mission possibilities. By the end of the second week, she had an idea. She met with the director.

"This is my vision," she said. "You already have a nutrition teaching program. You have nationals talking to their neighbors about nutrition and health. Just six months ago you started the feeding program, giving packets of oil and maize to families of at-risk children who attend an afternoon class. I'd like to build that into a community health evangelism program and a larger teaching program. You already have a farm about an hour outside the city. You're growing maize there right now. I want to raise goats for milk.

Also, I'd like to plant an orchard of moringa trees. Moringas are like multi-vitamins: Vitamin A, C, protein, calcium. You can eat the leaves or dry them, which concentrates their nutrition. You can grind the leaves into a powder to supplement their cornmeal. Moringa seed pods can be eaten like nuts. Best of all, moringas grow in tropical places with poor soil, just like Zambia."

Finally the director got a word in edgewise. "Wait a minute. Let me go get something."

She brought back the formal plan for the farm. The first thing on the plan: goats. The second thing on the plan: moringa trees.

The director asked, "How do you even know about moringa trees?"

In Sudan, a Swiss nurse, very eco-conscious, had talked about moringas. Dr. Marten mentally retained the information for later use.

Dr. Marten and the director looked at each other gleefully. Without a doubt, God had plans for their future together.

Just days later, while volunteering at a government hospital, Dr. Marten befriended a Zambian-trained medical student, a committed Christian who led the choir at his church. A gentle spirit, he felt called to help educate Zambian nurses. He and Dr. Marten were driving along the dirt roads out in the middle of nowhere amid fields of flowers. He turned and asked the American medical expert, the mentor, "What do you do when you pray for someone and that person dies?"

In her half-decade of pediatric experience in America, Dr. Marten had had only two patients die. Both were sad and difficult cases. From those, she gave him her best, very nice answers. Later that day, in the Zambian hospital, two of her patients died. Several more died the next day.

Three days after her car ride with the Zambian medical student, Dr. Marten sat with an old woman while a member of the hospital staff stripped her infected leg of maggots. The poor lady tried to be so brave, but she was miserable. She passed away during the night.

On those days, the fresh and rare "God moment" memories carried her through. Yes, God wanted her in this place, but it did not mean that every patient would be healed.

In America, even in rural southwestern Michigan, expert opinions are only a telephone call away or an hour's drive down the highway. In Zambia, Skype is beginning to bridge the gap. Dr. Marten learned there was another missionary in the area, a neurosurgeon.

While in Zambia, Dr. Marten was asked by the medical director of the residency program to give a lecture. The topic: "What a general pediatrician can do for the health of the world population." With such an open field, Dr. Marten chatted about various things she had learned while in Kenya, Sudan, and India.

Afterward the medical director exclaimed, "Wow, Heather, this is exciting. You've gone a lot of places!"

For Dr. Marten, who'd been chafing to embark on full time mission work and felt that the world was passing her by, this was a wake-up moment. She realized that in five years, she'd been in four different countries and had spent three and a half months overseas. That's not part of a normal U.S. pediatrician's experience. In the regular world, none of her fellow med-school graduates had been anywhere except to Aruba for a medical conference.

Dr. Marten is now back at SWMC building support in preparation for full time service. From this perspective, she can give advice to folks still looking for their calling. She advises finding a few faithful friends who can tolerate listening to your ramblings of euphoria and despair on a weekly basis. Dr. Georg Schultz, a seasoned pediatrician she works alongside at the Stevensville office, fills that need for her. A thoughtful father figure, he has seen dozens of other medical missionaries come and go at SWMC.

Dr. Holly Tapley has been another great friend and mentor. Also a single woman who had bends in the road before embarking on full time medical missions, Dr. Tapley understands.

When Dr. Marten got back from Zambia at the end of May 2011, she gathered friends to show them photos. At some point that evening, she realized how close she was to her lifelong dream. Having a missionary card on somebody's fridge is the missionary equivalent of a Hollywood Walk of Fame star. She turned to Dr. Tapley and said, "I'm this close to having my own missionary card on somebody's fridge! It's like, 'I have arrived!'" And Dr. Tapley laughed; she understood.

Many other SWMC colleagues have encouraged her. Tenwek Hospital has been an open door from the start, and for some reason it's not worked yet for Dr. Marten to go. She believes she'll spend time there. "If you do medical missions in Africa, at some point you'll go to Tenwek," she says. "It's a little strange that I've not been there yet, but maybe that's just as well. Now I'll go to Tenwek sometime with a different perspective of how I can use what they're doing down in Zambia."

SWMC hates to lose Dr. Marten, but it knows this is why she came, and SWMC promises that when she comes back, she'll fit in somewhere. As she does for the other SWMC medical missionaries, credentialing and licensing expert and human resources associate Sheryl Paloucek helps Dr. Marten juggle credentialing and licensing requirements. Because of Sheryl's assistance and for so many other reasons, Dr. Heather Marten considers SWMC a one-of-a-kind blessing.

Dr. Lars Bandera

Dr. Lars Bandera (pseudonym) doesn't exactly remember when he first heard about SWMC. He had been part of the Christian Medical and Dental Society (CMDS) since going into medical school. So it was on his radar for years. He thought SWMC sounded like an interesting place, but he didn't actually consider going there until he started applying for jobs around the time he graduated from medical school in 2001. He saw an ad for SWMC in the CMDS Journal that brought the clinic into sharp focus for him for the first time. He followed up on the ad, and SWMC invited him for an interview.

He was supposed to fly out to SWMC around September 12 or 13, 2001, but because of 9/11, all flights were canceled. His interview was delayed a couple of days. No one knew what was going to happen. Dr. Bandera drove out the next week for the meeting, an exceptionally long interview. During the two days of interviewing, he stayed at Dr. Paul Lim's place a couple of days and then attended a medical student retreat.

He didn't know exactly what to expect. It was his first real interview. He didn't have any particular financial hardship; he didn't need to make much money, so the salary SWMC could offer him didn't bother him. But he took his time making a decision, wanting to consider all career options.

Applying for other jobs, he learned that many practices expect associates to commit to stay long-term to build a practice. He felt pressured to promise to rear his children there — and he wasn't even married. He also thought about working at a walk-in clinic with some friends, but there he felt pressure to make a dollar. He learned he would be encouraged to order tests that might or might not be necessary in order to hit a dollar quota.

Dr. Bandera talked to people at church, and they told him to pray for God's will. Praying about SWMC, Dr. Bandera realized SWMC was exactly what he was looking for: a missions-focused, Christian, ethical clinic.

He joined SWMC in 2001, while projected officially to start in 2002, fitting in a short-term mission trip before the New Year. He started working out of the little Berrien Center office. At that time Tamara Riess and Dr. Ron Baker worked there, and Dr. Van Oosterhout had a little office but did not work there much, and the counseling center operated out of the Berrien Center office. Dr. Sherry O'Donnell had left about a year and a half before. A large portion of her practice was gone by that point, but Dr. Bandera was theoretically taking over her practice.

Another former doctor at the Berrien Center office had built a practice seeing people on the intersection of medical and psychiatric care. Other patients presented various challenges. One patient Dr. Bandera saw had been prescribed 120 Vicodin pills per month. A drug test on him showed no narcotic, which means he'd sold the entire lot of pills. Another man came into the office with a cane, asking for a parking sticker. Dr. Bandera remembers telling him he didn't think the man warranted it. When he left, he actually forgot his cane.

The office was surrounded by farmland. There was a lot of corn, but the corn didn't come into the office for treatment. Dr. Bandera looked around and mused, "It's going to be hard to be commercially successful." Moreover, the patients he served did not necessarily pay their bills. It all left the Berrien Center clinic — and SWMC — in a difficult position. If all the SWMC offices expected support from the other parts of the clinic, SWMC was not viable.

Dr. Bandera worked in that quiet little office shrouded in so much SWMC history for a year and a half. He did talk from time to time to SWMC administrators about his concerns. They discussed options. They decided to close down the internal medicine office in Berrien Center. One idea that resonated with Dr. Bandera was that all internists would set up an office in St. Joseph together. But that idea never matured. Instead, they kicked off the hospitalist program, in which SWMC doctors contracted to work for a hospital. The hospitalist program was not unlike Dr. Weldon Cooke's agreements to staff Berrien General Hospital with SWMC physicians.

SWMC held a meeting to try to figure out how to set up the hospitalist service. At first they ran the same hours as a traditional medical service: Monday through Friday, one weekend on call per month. In order to support his salary, Dr. Bandera had to get business from area surgeons. At the beginning, he saw eight to12 patients per day to support his salary as a hospitalist. It wasn't until a long time afterward that Dr. Bandera realized the commercial value of being a hospitalist.

Another hospitalist group worked at Lakeland Hospital alongside SWMC for several years. The competing groups tried to work side by side as best they could, but there was a lot of underlying tension. Several months after Dr. Bandera started at Lakeland, Dr. Dan Snyder came from Haiti and started with Dr. Bandera at the hospital. Business especially took off. They found themselves working hard, but the salary was set too low to hire another person. Dr. Bandera was itching to go do mission service, but again, his salary was too low to trade money for time. A friend graduated from residency and started out making three or four times Dr. Bandera's hourly wage. He told Dr. Bandera they had openings.

Dr. Bandera didn't want to leave SWMC. But overworked and underpaid, and without the opportunity for missions that he felt called to do, he considered leaving. He set an internal deadline and got some time off for a mission trip. When he came back from the trip, if nothing had changed, he would start looking for another job.

Then Dr. Altressa Drummond came. The other hospitalist group added two doctors as well. Right at Dr. Bandera's internal deadline, Dr. Mark Harrison landed a new hospitalist contract with Lakeland. Not long after, the other hospitalist group disbanded.

Dr. Harrison's appointment as hospitalist manager was pivotal in Dr. Bandera's mind for several reasons. Dr. Harrison knew both internal medicine and infectious control. One of Dr. Harrison's gifts was the ability to see long range. He saw negotiating the hospitalist contract as the first step in negotiating SWMC as a whole, which was half a decade or more down the road. He led the hospitalist group through at least four major contract negotiations before stepping down as manager in 2011. He also had a real knowledge of the commercial value of the hospitalist group. He tracked trends and clued in to what would come next. He figured out ways to get from point A to point B, even if they included point V or Z along the way, and he'd do it 5 to10 years before anybody else did.

Dr. Bandera benefited greatly from the latest contract. Hospitalists work every other week, seven days in a row, 12 hours per day. If they take one week of vacation, they have three weeks off, which would make for a good missions trip.

Dr. Callie Bandera

In medical school, before committing her life to Christ, Dr. Callie Bandera (pseudonym) joined the Christian Medical Student Association, part of the CMDA. CMSA has a chapter on most large university campuses. In 2004, her CMSA hosted a weekend retreat at a camp, and a group of Callie's friends were going, so she went along. Dr. Paul Lim of SWMC was the main speaker. Callie's parents had come to the United States to pursue the American dream. This guy was doing the opposite. What was he thinking?

Not yet a Christian but fascinated by the humanitarian aspects of mission trips, Callie talked further with Dr. Lim during the retreat. At the end of the weekend, Dr. Lim told Callie, "If you have any questions about missions, just email me." During their email correspondence, Dr. Lim told Callie all about SWMC. Her fourth year in medical school, in 2004, when she was considering her first short-term mission trip, he told her about the SWMC Foundation scholarship. She applied for and received that scholarship. She went to Africa. The following year she became a Christian.

Still torn between the worlds of academic medicine, like endocrinology research at a university, and medical missions, she met Dr. Lars Bandera. While they dated for about a year, she asked many tough questions. He'd already been on several missions trips, and he felt called to full time missions. This excited her and scared her at the same time.

It just so happened that a physician at SWMC, where Lars worked, was about to leave for a year at Tenwek Hospital and needed someone to fill in while he was gone. After much thought and prayer, she left her fellowship midway through. Everything fell into place all at once.

The Banderas married in 2008, honeymooned, and she started at SWMC a week later. She stayed on at SWMC for two more years. As of 2011, Dr. Callie Bandera is home full time with their first child. The Banderas continue to take short-term mission trips and are seeking God's will for full time work overseas.

Leading CMSA student retreats seems to be another side assignment for a few SWMC doctors. Dr. Emily McCarty and Dr. Heather Marten are among others who have led several CMSA student retreats. It's a ministry, a way to share with others their passion for medical missions, and a side benefit is recruitment for SWMC.

Dr. John W. Froggatt III

Dr. John Froggatt earned degrees at Vanderbilt University and the University of Miami School of Medicine, and completed his internship and residency in internal medicine at the University of Pittsburgh. He took a fellowship in infectious diseases and hospital epidemiology at the Medical College of Virginia in Richmond and came out running.

That's what's expected — running. It started in residency. He moonlighted and worked insane hours, doing 36-hour shifts and taking every opportunity under the sun. He didn't slow down to consider how this kind of long-term lifestyle would shape him as a person. In fellowship, he prepared to go into academic medicine, training in clinical infectious diseases, hospital epidemiology, and molecular epidemiology, while also moonlighting to support his family.

He went to Boston for a summer course in epidemiology, taking a break from other responsibilities. While there, he felt God convicting him about his priorities.

He came out as an attractive candidate for various positions because of all that he had done. But he felt he was getting warped by the imbalance of overwork. Trying to figure out what God wanted him to do as he started in a position in academic medicine, he clamped his hours, stopped working Sundays, and worked out a plan with his wife, Cathy to continue in the job for five years and then determine if God was leading elsewhere.

Six years went by. The Froggatts felt that God was leading in a new direction. Dr. Froggatt took a clinical job in North Carolina. After another five years, that job morphed away from infectious diseases practice. The Froggatts began praying in earnest again. They set up a three-tier job hunt. Step one was just getting out and looking at the various possibilities. Step two was identifying something interesting and applying. Step three was getting out of his current job.

On the night they changed from step one to step two, they felt especially compelled to pray. Dr. Froggatt talked about his dream of getting into a position somehow involving international missions while maintaining infectious disease work. The very next day he got a letter from SWMC describing an opportunity. It was almost too soon. Head whirling, Dr. Froggatt checked out SWMC's opportunity. Everything fell into place, exactly what he and Cathy wanted.

In retrospect Dr. Froggatt felt that he over-interpreted God's will, with circumstances coming together so smoothly. Soon after the letter from SWMC came, he got another beautiful offer out of the blue to join a private practice in Asheville, North Carolina, the city where they lived. It ruined the image of God opening a single door, which had only to be walked through with a thank-you. Dr. Froggatt took a step back and prayed further.

Looking back, Dr. Froggatt is glad God threw the second golden opportunity into the mix, because it made him really think about SWMC at a deeper level. He interviewed seriously at both places, deliberated and prayed.

As a result, the decision to come to SWMC was more solid than if he'd "just skipped gaily down the path."

The Froggatt family moved to southwestern Michigan in 1999, and Dr. Froggatt took a position in infectious diseases. Dr. Mark Harrison had been the only infectious disease specialist in the county. Weary of the burden, Dr. Harrison diversified into the long-term acute care unit as one of the founding medical directors. Later, he became the founding director of the hospitalist program while Dr. Froggatt served as medical director for infection control at Lakeland Hospital. Dr. Tompkins, also an infectious disease specialist, arrived in Niles — south Berrien County — around that time as well. All three infectious disease specialists, then, could diversify and not feel the weight of a solo operation.

In 2006, Dr. Froggatt was named president of SWMC. As such, he led a multispecialty medical practice that had grown to more than 70 physicians and 25 other providers in specialties such as family medicine, internal medicine, pediatrics, OB/GYN, general surgery, infectious disease, critical care/pulmonary, hospitalist, public health, and physical therapy.

Truly, he can look back and say God directed him to his niche.

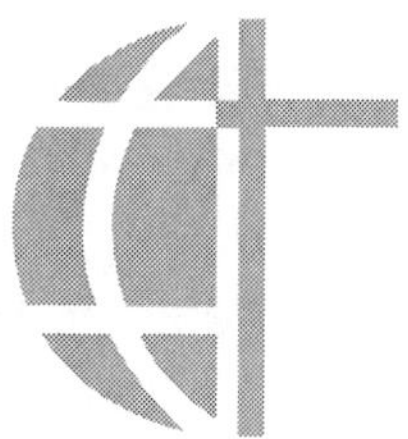

Chapter 30

Transitions

Chapter 30

Transitions

One day in the early 1990s, Don Gast looked around. He said later, "I couldn't take Southwestern any farther. My capacity had run to the end, and we needed someone with more modern expertise. Any one person could only do so much, and I had done enough. The books, finances — I did what I could do. I couldn't expand it any more. I felt for us to thrive, someone else had to expand Southwestern."

A flood of conflicting emotions washed over Don: relief and trepidation, assurance and uncertainty, weariness but a desire to keep coming back. He was sure that God would help him find the right person to take leadership of Southwestern Medical Clinic.

Don held leadership capacities in a number of organizations around the county and the state. MMGMA (Michigan Medical Group Management Association) was one of those associations, and it was there that he became aware of a quiet, unassuming leader — pleasant, always polished in any situation. Don watched him for about a year and thought he could be the right person for SWMC. Warren White made Don's top-three list, but Don waited for God's direction.

In retrospect, the other two people on Don's top-three list were "probably more like myself," he said.

Typically leaders who appoint successors select a junior version of themselves. As many will attest, Don is not a typical leader, nor did he make the selection of his replacement on his own. Continuing to pray over his short list, "I felt eventually things were going to change to meet the need and the times, and Warren would be capable of developing the clinic in a different way." Instead of a directive about hiring a new administrator, God brought Dr. Collin Smith, Dr. Neil F. Martin, Dr. Rob Allen, and Dr. Richard L. Hines in 1990. Dr. John Spriegel came in 1991.

Almost every day during that time, Don, Dr. Bob Schindler, Dr. Herb Atkinson, and Dr. Bob Wesche prayed together by telephone. Their prayers encouraged and inspired each other as well as glorifying God. In prayer, Drs. Schindler and Wesche often focused on missions. Dr. Atkinson prayed for the staff. Don prayed for the big picture of SWMC and asked the Lord for strength for everyone to do God's will. Inwardly, he continued to pray for the Lord's provision of the next administrator.

In March of 1992, Warren White called Don. He'd heard about SWMC not just from Don but others. Working in a Lansing hospital at the time, he just wanted to visit SWMC and see what the Christian group was all about.

Warren remembers Don being more than cordial — he was thrilled to have Warren visit. He spent the day with Warren, took him around and introduced him to a few people. It was exciting. Warren's respect for Don and the organization's tenacity for Christian service and international medical excellence grew. He found himself beaming at those he met, thoroughly enjoying the visit.

At the end of the day, Don dropped a bombshell. "You ought to think about joining us," he told Warren.

"What do you mean?" Warren managed to ask. "In what capacity?"

"I'm looking for someone to replace me," Don said. "Would you think about that?"

Floored, Warren returned to Lansing. Don's invitation to join SWMC was completely unexpected. Warren thought about his wife happily teaching, his young kids settled in East Lansing schools. He prayed for a year.

As he prayed, these concerns came to mind: "'Working with like-minded physicians committed to Christ, what can I bring to the group in terms of leadership?' I saw my role would be to formalize the organization, to create leadership and a functioning board of directors, implement written policies, and move SWMC along the organizational structure."

Meanwhile, God saw fit to fill SWMC's roster with physicians. In 1992, Dr. David Grellmann joined, and Dr. Gary C. Prechter came around that time as well. In the first six months of 1993, no fewer than nine physicians came: Drs. Mark and Donna Joan Harrison, Dr. Keith Van Oosterhout, Dr. Gregory Crabill, Dr. Daniel Hayward, Dr. William "Bill" Wilkinson, Dr. Douglas Wilson, Dr. John R. Slater, and Dr. Mike Chupp.

At the time Warren called Don Gast back and showed interest in seriously investigating the possibilities involved in joining, SWMC was flooded with new physicians. Warren came in July 1993, a new face to lead a sea of new faces.

Through the spring, before he officially came aboard, Warren familiarized himself with SWMC's halls and offices. He spent time with the O'Neills. He talked with Don and his family to figure out what the place was like and to identify opportunities and limitations. Warren found this unusually challenging.

Vagueness, a cultural norm at SWMC for decades, exasperated Warren the exacting calculator. He tried to wheedle specifics from Don and everyone else. His opportunities and his role were not defined, nor was compensation for that matter. At one point he turned to Don and said point blank, "What are the terms of the offer? Are you even making an offer?"

They were sitting in Don's car. Don whipped out a yellow pad. He wrote a number down, scribbled some benefits and handed the torn-off paper to Warren. It was so unlike anything Warren had ever experienced, he could not respond. Stepping out of the car, holding the side of his face, he thought, This is it? This is their job offer?

Eventually, Dr. Bart Comstock, president of SWMC at the time, sent Warren a letter with a few more details. Warren sensed the wild risk he had to take. It was also an exciting opportunity. Things weren't defined? Well, he had the opportunity to define them.

SWMC created a new title for Don: Senior Vice President of External Affairs. A plethora of honors and awards have been given to this quiet, unassuming gentleman throughout his career. One award seems especially appropriate. In May 1995, for his volunteering community spirit, a local counseling center honored Don with its "Samaritan of the Year" award.

Unbeknownst to him, he won a contest through the South Bend Tribune in 1986. SWMC staff nominated him. They were supposed to describe their boss in 50 or fewer words. They couldn't meet the tight word count, but convinced the newspaper that he was the best nominee. Don keeps a framed, signed copy of the nomination letter, which was presented to him at the staff Christmas party that year. He felt very honored by all of this, which was great, but he kept in mind, "It's not what I did to the clinic, it's what the staff did. They made it great. I didn't do anything. The staff did everything."

Not officially retired, on January 16, 2010, Don was feted with a special tribute at Santaniello's Restaurant on Glenlord Road in Stevensville. Several hundred SWMC friends attended — as many as could fit into the place. They showered him with toasts and presented him a supersized scrapbook commemorating his SWMC career.

Never one for a long, flowery speech, Don sums up his career and SWMC's future with a prophet's viewpoint: "Things change. You have to change. You can't stay still."

Because Don remained, the transition of having people learn who's in charge could have been a bit tricky. Don moved out of his administrative office, and that was a signal to people. Warren compared the situation to a pastor who retires and stays within his congregation. Don took an office next door to Warren's, and Warren was happy to let people rely on Don for certain things. Whereas Don had always been highly accessible to all the staff, Warren knew he would be unable to fulfill the heavy administrative responsibilities as SWMC grew and changed if he tried to duplicate Don's gregarious open-door policy. Don was more than happy to continue in that role.

For his part, Don made sure his presence was not limiting to Warren. He allowed Warren to lead, even when he didn't agree. He'd nod his head slowly, settle his hand on the table, and quietly say, "Warren, you're in charge. Do things that you think need to be done."

Don was gone a lot in 1993 and for the next few years. He was involved in things external to the clinic, in organizations, with local charities and groups, perhaps some military involvement. His SWMC office would be vacant for days at a time. Warren quickly found go-to people who could fill in for Don and do some of the hands-on tasks he had always done so well. If a receptionist at any location was sick, they'd called Don and he'd find someone to fill in. Missionaries relied on Don tremendously to manage their home lives while they were gone: get their homes rented, their grass mowed, important documents parlayed, and so on. For a small group, the administrator could do that. But Warren came in, and he had a different role.

Hiring nine new physicians to a roster of 25 full time physicians in the U.S. was a huge amount of growth. Add an additional administrator and the bottom line gets shaky. Warren says, "I'm always looking for a challenge, and change is not uncomfortable for me, but we could've done it in a more structured way. We experienced a lot of financial stress. God provided through those hard times and we learned, and some was the organization becoming more formal. In one year, that is a huge amount of growth."

Updating billing systems and technology helped. Creating organizational and management structures and defining roles streamlined the mechanism of day-to-day operations as well.

One mark of these changes was physicians' workdays. In 1993, doctors traveled to two or three offices a week. They weren't making money driving from one end of the county to the other. Lab reports and records showed up in odd places. Duplicated paperwork, marked on and passed around, confused everybody. Limiting physicians to one location improved efficiency in many ways.

The plan was to meet the needs of the community, and that necessitated growth and consolidation. In a building project, the Stevensville office doubled. Bridgman moved to its larger office. SWMC doubled the size of the Niles facility. Administration moved to a larger building and Berrien Springs clinical offices closed.

Board meetings started at 7 a.m. and at one point they met every other morning at 6:30 for group prayer. Through most of the 1990s SWMC scheduled optional prayer and fasting one day a month. Also, to everyone who wanted one, SWMC sent out a prayer memo.

Regular "State of the Practice" meetings pulled physicians and staff together. On the backside of SWMC's in-house September 28 "Brainwaves" newsletter, topics included a profit-sharing update, future plans, mission trips, and expansions.

SWMC threw open its doors through the rest of the 1990s for like-minded physicians. They poured in. In 1994, Dr. Jonathan Saxe came. That was the quiet year after so many new faces in 1993. In 1995, they migrated in flocks. Dr. Christopher Harvey, Mary Beth Good, PA, and Dr. Susan Davis joined in May. In August, Dr. Marilyn Hunter and Dr. K. Suzanne Hayward joined. Dr. Barbara S. Carlson arrived in September, and Drs. Annelise and Robert Spees came at the end of October 1995.

The physicians hoped more doctors meant a better bottom line. Because of so many uninsured and indigent patients, that wasn't necessarily the case. But doctors kept coming. In 1996, Janet Nightingale, CNM and Dr. Daniel Mitchell came in March; physicians assistant William Makovic came in April; Dr. Ernesto Chioco in July; Brandy Feikema, CNM in August; Kathryn Ross, PA in September; and Dr. Lois Lello joined that year as well.

In 1997, Dr. Dale I. Carroll, Dr. Roy Winslow, Dr. Stephen R. Clingman, Dr. Paul Lim, and Dr. Daniel Joyce joined. The next year brought Dr. Troy Thompson and Dr. Sherry O'Donnell, and also

Dr. Wayne Carlson under contract. By the end of 1999, Dr. Holly Tapley, Dr. Delbert G. Huelskoetter, Dr. Stephen Hempel, and Dr. John Froggatt were part of the group.

Dr. Tami Fisk was a physician who joined SWMC looking to land temporarily before going to the mission field. She worked for SWMC for a short time with a vision to go to China. Inexplicably, she was diagnosed with cancer; treatment failed her, and she died in her 30s. "She touched our lives and inspired us," Warren White said. "We want to support people like that, but financially it became harder and harder."

Pat Meyer

Pat Meyer was happily working for another company when he met Dr. Dan Hayward of SWMC at Sawyer Highlands Baptist Church around 1994. The two became friends, and the families grew close after Drs. Dan and Suzanne Hayward married.

Two years later, the company Pat Meyer worked for was going out of business. Dr. Dan Hayward introduced him to Warren White. Pat joined SWMC as financial controller on August 1, 1996. He remembers the date well. He and his wife were foster parents. On that first day of work, their household grew from six to nine kids.

With doctors constantly coming and going, keeping books was like simultaneously wrestling several families of alligators. Pat came away from the first board meetings thinking, I wonder when I'll begin to feel better prepared. Soon, surely, I'll get a better handle on it all.

The accounting alligators never metamorphosed into marching rows of ants or anything else. Board meetings never eased into comfortable recitation of acceptable figures. During weekly financial meetings in crisis times and regular monthly board meetings, they always wrestled with the same three items on the agenda: reduce cost, increase efficiency, try to save money. Every year, Pat and the board wrangled with numbers that just wouldn't settle down well onto pages. Together, they muscled line by line and sweated their way to the bottom line, which never felt good enough. Pat learned these challenges were a way of life, or rather, survival. Pat's consternation had nothing to do with his abilities and everything to do with the unique dichotomies of running a revolving-door, multispecialty physicians group which also happens to try to exist like a charitable organization. More than meeting the challenges, Pat rose to head accountant and eventually moved into the position of Chief Financial Officer.

The physicians were willing to work outrageous hours for much less than market rate and, according to Pat, that's the only reason SWMC stayed open. They ran double-sided copies to save paper. They emptied their trash and vacuumed their own offices to slash cleaning costs. To further reduce expenses, SWMC closed two offices in Berrien Springs, closed Berrien Center, and merged the St. Joseph location with Stevensville.

The words rang clearly to physicians: see more patients. Target to see 25 patients per day, per doctor. Expenses continued to rise: labor, property, supplies, insurance — it all kept inching up. Medicare and Medicaid froze reimbursement, and when they finally resumed, they actually cut their already impossibly low reimbursement. Everyone at SWMC shouldered the grindstone, desperate year after year to make SWMC work. They hired more physicians to grow clientele and increase revenue.

Warren White and Sheila Kipp recruited and hired most of the new physicians, later supplemented by Don Gast's son-in-law, John Newcomer. Susan Newcomer, the Gasts' oldest daughter, has worked at SWMC for years as a Registered Nurse, and her sister, Nancy, has worked for years as a receptionist in the Stevensville office. Sadly, John passed away after working at SWMC only about a year.

SWMC birthed itself by recruiting young, energetic, and idealistic physicians out of medical school who didn't mind working for peanuts in exchange for working alongside seasoned missionary physicians and being enthusiastically assisted in launching their own missionary careers.

Throughout Pat Meyer's 15 years at SWMC, he saw that the physicians they were recruiting were coming out of medical school with more and more student debt. The cost of medical school increased tremendously. Some young doctors clearly wanted to practice SWMC's kind of medicine. But if they had $200,000 of debt, and SWMC could offer a $60,000 per year starting salary, it just wasn't possible for them. Recruiting, always a challenge from Dr. Cooke's first frantic years at Berrien General Hospital, turned into a time-consuming and heartbreaking series of brick walls.

To make matters more heartbreaking, adding physicians did not guarantee more revenue. The clinic prided itself in taking high levels of needy patients: patients on Medicaid or the uninsured. An average clinic in Michigan sees about 1 to 2% Medicaid patients to stay afloat. A conservative business average for the clinic was 25% Medicaid, which pays roughly 25 cents on the dollar. Insurance pays 80 to 85 cents on the dollar. Plus (or minus), physicians were forever giving free care, writing off bills. They felt called to do it. The board tried to put through policies to limit these practices, but the doctors continued anyway. Knowing the fundamental beliefs of the clinic, who could fault the doctors?

Another way Pat saw the spirit of the physicians was by the number of prayer meetings they scheduled. Quietly behind closed doors, they cried out to God to bring in money for the next payroll; they pleaded with Him to provide in ways they could not predict. God did provide. He did keep SWMC open for Berrien County residents and for many others around the world.

The Lord did not operate by sending a splashy epiphany or breakthrough or a huge sum of cash. It was just little good things that would happen. At the last minute, some contracts would come through to help SWMC keep going another year. Dr. Andy Rutherford and Dr. Helene Johnson, two of SWMC's highest revenue generators, got them through tough scrapes. Through it all, there was always a sense that the Lord was leading the group.

In 1998, following a calling, Pat Meyer and his family moved to central Romania. SWMC allowed Pat to do his job from Romania! He got an office there and worked online via computer for SWMC during the day, then served the church after hours and on weekends. Especially back in the 1990s, Pat is certain no other clinic would allow a key employee to pack up and move halfway around the world.

One way it worked: SWMC had a remarkable asset in Carol Gonnerman Jewell, head of finance. She was Pat's hands and feet while he was in Romania. But when Carol announced plans to retire in 2001, and another giant financial crunch loomed over the clinic, the Meyer family reluctantly moved back to Michigan. They moved back in August, just weeks before the 9/11 attacks.

SWMC looks disaster in the face. They organized several emergency employee mission trips during the years to places like Rwanda and Haiti. Following disasters, these trips were organized very quickly with specific staff in mind to meet desperate needs and aid in disaster relief. Other times, overseas SWMC physicians have faced unplanned crises.

Pat Meyer has also faced crises. During his 15 years at SWMC up to the present, he and financial disaster stared eye-to-eye regularly. Projections were perennially gloomy, and many old-timers had gotten accustomed to hearing it. Pat's eyes never glazed over — he felt panic every time.

In a way, he felt personally responsible to find a financial solution where there wasn't one. Some people had a sunny perspective that electronic health records would be the answer. SWMC bought and adopted an electronic health system that put additional financial pressures on the clinic. Many in the clinic thought the return on that investment was going to be better than it was. In some aspect, because it was a significant cost that didn't provide a sufficient rate of return, that inevitable purchase triggered SWMC's next in-your-face financial crisis requiring major changes.

Of course electronic records were inevitable. The world was going that way. Electronic records alone didn't cause SWMC's financial meltdown. The overall economic environment was toxic for a physician's group that had struggled financially from day one.

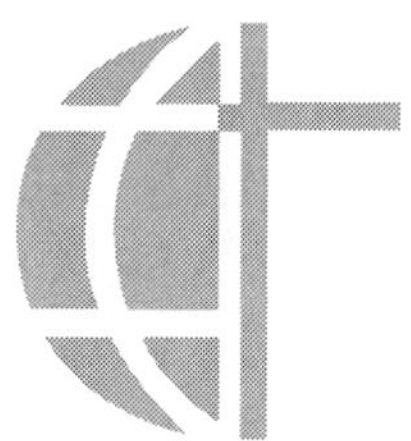

Chapter 31

The Upper Room, the Fate of SWMC's Birthplace, and Other Late Turning Points

Chapter 31

The Upper Room, the Fate of SWMC's Birthplace, and Other Late Turning Points

SWMC members attended an infinity of meetings at which Topic #1 to discuss was Medicaid reimbursement (or the lack thereof) vs. financial survival. Sometimes these meetings became a bit emotional and lasted late into the night. The corporation had always run a tight ship, so saving pennies here and there by cutting housekeeping or recycling tin cans had already been done.

There were never any easy solutions. The feeling, especially of the older physicians, remained, "If God wants to keep us around, we just need to be faithful and do what is right." Most people agreed.

One of these meetings stands out in SWMC history, sometimes referred to as "The Upper Room." The Upper Room took place in the new administrative offices purchased a few months earlier in August 1998, on Old U.S. 31 just northwest of Berrien Springs. The upstairs room was going to be renovated into office space. It was disheveled at the time of the meeting. Doctors didn't assemble around one big table; they sat helter-skelter where they could fit around the boxes and debris, in a rough oval shape.

As always, they opened with a prayer. Quickly, the meeting came to its point. SWMC was in serious financial jeopardy. There was not enough income to support the expenses.

Warren White presented a word picture that Dr. Winslow recalls now with irony. "Imagine a few years from now, you're a missionary returning from Africa," Warren White said. "You land in South Bend and you drive up through Niles. You pass the office that used to be SWMC, and now its sign reads, 'Lakeland Healthcare.' SWMC is no longer in business."

At the time of that meeting, the possibility of being intergrated with Lakeland Healthcare was a real concern. Considering that very real possibility brought worry into the room.

The old refrain was sung once more: "How can we sustain ourselves?"

The physicians promised to see more patients per day. They'd lower thermostats again. Staples would be re-bent and re-used, if necessary.

Anything to avoid going out of business.

Everyone said what they'd always said, that they didn't come for a salary, they came for the mission. But, honestly, without appropriate income, SWMC's mission was apt to die.

Two key decisions were made that night. First, SWMC pledged to continue to accept Medicaid patients and would share the financial burden of caring for them. Second, individual primary care physicians (pediatrics, family practice, and internal medicine) would be accountable for making sure that their practice was financially successful. For the first time, SWMC reduced the base pay of primary care physicians (family practitioners, pediatricians and such) if their productivity was too low. But would this be enough? What was in store for SWMC?

Fervent prayers were lifted. No lightning bolt zapped down from the sky. A million dollars didn't drop into anyone's lap. But God worked in hearts around the room. Faith grew almost tangibly that night. And when the meeting finally adjourned, although no great solutions had surfaced, the SWMC members left feeling certain that God would sustain the clinic.

Some of the doctors credit prayers lifted outside the upper room as much as their own deep intercessions. On their own accord, while their husbands sweated through The Upper Room, wives had gathered for a spontaneous prayer meeting of their own at the O'Neills' house.

As Cindy O'Neill remembers it, Joyce Ritter called Cindy. Joyce was burdened for SWMC and felt led to call some of the other wives. When she suggested the wives gather to pray, Cindy invited them all to her house. About a dozen gathered. Some of the wives there that night were: Jane Baker, Elaine Metzger, Ruth Pierson, Marian Schindler, and Bev Winslow. Joyce led the women in a time of praise and confession. Each wife prayed aloud for her husband. Then they prayed for the corporation as a whole.

Many of the women in the circle had been with SWMC for a long period of time. They could look around the O'Neills' living room and say, "Remember 15 years ago when we were having a similar huge crisis? God met us then, so He can do it again now."

This meeting was iconic for doctors such as Dr. Roy Winslow. "It was touching to me and reassuring that our spouses were saying, 'This isn't a financial matter, but a spiritual one,'" he said years later. "Their example served as a challenge to all of us to be more prayerful."

Not that the doctors weren't praying before, during, and after the meeting. And not that the prayers removed all future fears or difficulties from SWMC's path. On the contrary, within a few years after The Upper Room, an event everyone had worked so hard to avoid for decades would rock SWMC from its moorings as never before. This cataclysmic event would also foretell another much-dreaded turning point.

The Fate of SWMC's Birthplace

Dr. Helene Johnson had delivered the first baby born in The BirthPlace at Berrien General Hospital in 1984. She also delivered the last baby born at the renamed Lakeland Medical Center, Berrien Center, on May 1, 1999, at 6:26 p.m. This birth, so uncomplicated in every other way, made the front page of The Journal Era newspaper.

After decades of quality service to Berrien Springs and the surrounding tri-county area, the little hospital in the cornfields was seeing the end of its days of service. Bravely, the doctors and staff of SWMC had paved the way into the future as far as they could take it. Now the hospital had been sold to Lakeland Regional Medical Center, and looking at the financial bottom line, Lakeland was closing most departments of the hospital.

In a somber ceremony sponsored by the auxiliary, former Berrien General Hospital chief of staff Dr. Herbert Atkinson, Lakeland Hospital president and CEO Joseph Wasserman, and others lauded the great work of all who served at Berrien General Hospital.

Dr. Atkinson spoke about the three-point legacy Berrien General workers built: technical excellence; dedication and discipline; and warmth and caring. He said that during Bronson Hospital reviews of Berrien General, they praised thorough documentation in the charts and sharing of valuable information between the two facilities, which led to better care of patients who transferred from one to the other. Dr. Atkinson also thanked staff for creating a family atmosphere that made patients feel at home and led to better communication and care hospital-wide.

Former chief of staff Dr. Johnson and several members of the obstetrics and surgical staff were honored for their dedication to their patients and contributions to Berrien County medicine.

On June 1, 1999, Berrien General Hospital officially became Lakeland Specialty Hospital. As such, the hospital closed its OB/GYN and childbirth services, ER, and OR. Instead, Lakeland chose to focus the campus as a complex long-term medical care facility.

Dr. Johnson, who had been in practice in Berrien Center since June 1972 and had delivered more than 10,000 babies at Berrien General, was moving her practice south. She opened a new obstetrics office on 60 North St. Joseph Avenue, Niles, with childbirth services at Lakeland Community Hospital, Niles (formerly Pawating Hospital).

The Journal Era article stated, "During Dr. Johnson's career at Berrien General, the obstetrics unit was formed and later became BirthPlace, a name synonymous with exceptional care."

Further, the article quoted the eloquent words of Kathy Montague, Vice President of Corporate Development for Lakeland Regional Health System:

> *How can I talk about what she has meant to the facility except to say that she has been a dedicated pioneer for women's health issues and she has tirelessly served her patients. She has created a practice that is designed to meet the needs of her patients in every single way, and that approach was adopted in the Berrien Center facility and it was extremely successful, leading it to be the preferred obstetrics facility in Berrien County for many years.*

Dr. Johnson read the following poem at the farewell ceremony:

Gone, but not Forgotten
A county poor farm was the start
The corn so tall and free
Gave way to brand new ways to birth:
Lamaze, Leboyer, and C

Many years have come and gone
And many babies, too
Many friendships came to pass
We made a motley crew

The merger joined the medical staffs
And time condensed the rest

Nothing's left to call our own
So we will move the best
It's off to Niles to start afresh
We all feel pretty rotten
We sadly leave our imprint here
It's over, but not forgotten

Joseph Wasserman, President and Chief Executive Officer at Lakeland Regional Health System, had these words of praise:

> *Over the past 30 years you have created a legacy of care. That legacy meant that when you came to this facility, you would receive top quality care and an unsurpassable level of compassion. As Lakeland moves into the future, it is important for us to remember where we have been. Our vision and goals for the years to come are only possible because of the standards and precedence you all have helped to create in your respective departments here at Berrien….*

Thus ended SWMC's birthplace. Berrien General Hospital was where it had all begun with Dr. Cooke and his team in the 1950s and 1960s. To be sure, SWMC doctors have remained at Lakeland Specialty Hospital and its Long-Term Acute Care Hospital (LTACH) up to this writing, but on a much smaller scale. The future-sighted administration of Don Gast, Warren White, and the presidents and board of SWMC had already broadened SWMC beyond Berrien General years before the hospital's closure.

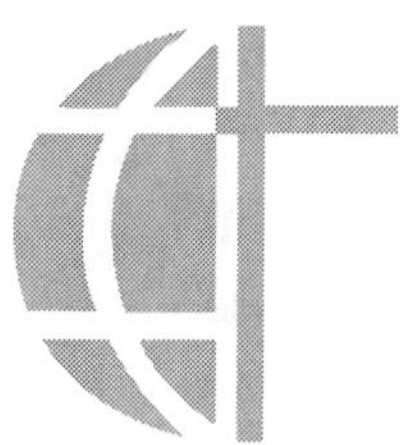

Chapter 32

Dr. Harrison and the Hospitalist Program

Chapter 32

Dr. Harrison and the Hospitalist Program

One major propellant of SWMC's expansion beyond Berrien General Hospital was Dr. Mark Harrison.

The Harrisons arrived in 1993 along with nine other new physicians who had interviewed in 1991 and 1992 during a SWMC "morale slump." Dr. Harrison saw that SWMC had been actively praying for a visionary renewal and for healthy growth. But nine new physicians coming all at once changed the clinic in ways no one had predicted. Adding nine to 18 was a big addition. Several years later, another similar-sized crop of new physicians came.

From Dr. Harrison's point of view "the older guys weren't ready for us, all the new young doctors in higher echelons of medicine. I think they were reeling. It was a challenge to fit us all into the system," Dr. Harrison said. SWMC's growth exceeded the need at tiny Berrien General Hospital.

All who interviewed — some who came and some who did not come — looked at Berrien General and believed, "This hospital's going to be dead in five years. It's just too small to support the kind of care you need to do with CT scans, MRIs, and laparoscopic surgeries, while being able to attain and maintain the technology." In the age of technology, a small hospital just couldn't afford to be state of the art anymore.

SWMC was, in Dr. Harrison's words, outgrowing its britches. It was a hard time. SWMC was understandably attached to Berrien General Hospital: that was where all of its history was. They'd hired most of Berrien General's employees, and didn't want to think about losing them. But Dr. Harrison looked around. Dr. O'Neill, the senior internist, was driving to Mercy-Memorial Hospital in St. Joseph to do consults and care. "It was becoming clear what new pair of pants SWMC needed to put on, Dr. Harrison said."

As SWMC continued to grow both in numbers and in quality of specialty fields, it expanded their Mercy-Memorial Hospital (what would become Lakeland) presence. As a natural result, SWMC became involved in leadership there, recruited physicians, and built practices. SWMC physicians acquired large numbers of patients out of Mercy-Memorial, but as at Berrien General, a lot didn't pay anything.

Around 1996, Dr. Harrison was elected onto SWMC's board of directors. Dr. Ken O'Neill was president. When Dr. Harrison was on the board sorting things out, he discovered the clinic wrote off $2 to $3 million dollars a year, coming directly out of the physicians' salaries. SWMC doctors were already making financial sacrifices, working for half or less the salaries they'd be making elsewhere, and all the write-offs made their incomes even tighter.

At the same time SWMC was giving away another million to the mission field. Dr. Harrison put his head in his hands, mulling over the numbers. The clinic's annual revenue was $12 to $15 million dollars. It was giving a huge percentage of time, energies, and money away.

Looking at the figures, Warren White and the doctors on the board put their heads together around the table. Despite their growing pains, they realized they had to grow the group further. The clinic needed more revenue to support its ministries both overseas and at home in southwestern Michigan.

All this led directly to the clinic's next phase: aggressive growth to survive. The administration aggressively recruited and consciously built programs as opportunities arose. At this same time, Berrien General Hospital was going through the same financial crisis as SWMC. The hospital's write-offs were a huge drain on the county. Eventually, the county commissioners finally said, "Enough is enough."

Lakeland Specialty Hospital

There was a proposal to bulldoze Berrien General. Lakeland HealthCare stepped in and bought it, seeing a need for doing something else with the building. At the time long-term care facilities (LTCs) were supported by the federal government. Berrien General Hospital had for years run a successful nursing home wing staffed by Dr. Edling and others. It turned out that by expanding this, Berrien General could serve as an LTC and be financially feasible, while bringing in a new aspect of care the community was not yet getting.

As this was all being ironed out, a question came to Dr. Harrison's mind: Who would direct the LTC? Physicians were obliged to provide care if they were available. At that time Dr. Harrison lived in Berrien Springs. He looked around and noted that he was SWMC's closest doctor to Berrien General. He knew he was doomed.

He went to the Lakeland vice president Dr. Dave O'Connor, who was infamous at that time for wanting SWMC to cease to exist. Part of Dr. O'Connor's responsibilities was establishing the LTC. Dr. Harrison figured, "If I'm going to be stuck with this job, I want to be paid for it."

So he told Dr. O'Connor, "I'll take it on. It's down the road from me." Though his heart wasn't in it, he negotiated Lakeland up. Midway through negotiations, Dr. Harrison got cold feet. With a growing family, he was going to be on call all the time. It was going to be miserable. He backed out of the deal.

Dr. O'Connor also knew who to talk to in a pinch: Dr. Schindler. Dr. Schindler was a strong advocate for the underdog. Dr. O'Connor said to him, "The people working at Berrien General now will all lose their jobs unless there is an LTC."

An incredibly affable man, Dr. Schindler knew everyone at Berrien General by name. Dr. O'Connor's words resonated. Dr. Schindler was on the board with Dr. Harrison. He went to Dr. Harrison said, "Mark, you're going to do it."

In 1998, one year before the ER and BirthPlace closed, Dr. Harrison was appointed medical director. The briefly renamed Berrien Specialty Hospital was a successful experiment, but Lakeland and SWMC saw more potential. Dr. Schindler, Dr. Harrison, and others dialogued with Dr. O'Connor and others at Lakeland about opening a Long-Term Acute Care (LTAC) unit.

The LTAC could provide a more intense hospital-type care to patients who didn't meet strict hospital criteria but who were a little too ill for a nursing home. It would be unique in the area and save a lot of jobs, as well as bring Lakeland Healthcare System and SWMC new revenue. The proposal was well-received and solved the problem of how to make the Berrien Center location viable.

In 1999 the hospital was renamed Lakeland Specialty Hospital, Berrien Center. The Mattix Center (LTC nursing home) was renamed Lakeland Continuing Care Center and remodeling was completed to open the new Long-term Acute Care unit.

Hospice

Back in 1993, SWMC physician Dr. Keith VanOosterhout (Dr. VanO) had taken on the leadership role of medical director for the nursing home, then called the Mattix Center at Berrien General Hospital. As medical director of the Continuing Care Centers at Lakeland HealthCare, Dr. VanO found himself on an impressive list. Throughout the years his predecessors as medical director of the nursing home included Dr. Edling, Dr. Atkinson, Dr. Schindler, Dr. Pierson, Dr. Roach, and Dr. Baker. Dr. Al Snyder served as interim medical director as well before Dr. VanO came.

Dr. VanO saw that the nursing home, soon designated an LTC, had established a well-defined care model. Beyond medical care, the nursing home focused on activities, special events — including regular community involvement with school groups — and socialization. Also, ahead of the trend, they offered choices in things such as menus. Everything ran smoothly. So he looked beyond the specialty hospital. He wanted to improve medical relations along various avenues across the county. His first interest outside the LTC was for appropriate geriatric care in the hospital setting, to better prepare pre-patients and to follow up on residents who were sent out to the hospital.

Dr. VanOosterhout was instrumental in bringing Hospice at Home into the nursing home. The Hospice team was invaluable to the nursing home staff during a resident's last months, weeks, and days before death. Focusing on that one patient, the Hospice at Home team provided respite for the nursing home staff who had to focus on many patients.

In 1995 Hospice at Home administrator Steve Townsend approached Dr. VanOosterhout with an interesting proposition. He needed a medical director for one of his teams. At the time, Hospice at Home provided services in three locations: South Haven, St. Joseph, and Niles-Buchanan. Dr. VanO considered the opportunity. He saw Hospice at Home as an extension of what he did at Lakeland Specialty Hospital — relieving the pain and stress of the dying process and helping unite the family during those last times.

Dr. VanOosterhout led each of the three Hospice at Home teams at one time or another until 2007, when Lakeland Healthcare asked him to head their Hospice program. Dr. VanO received the 2009 community service award from the Region IV Area Agency on Aging. He served as Lakeland's Hospice medical director until December 31, 2011, when the two program merged. He was a pivotal figure in the integration of Hospice at Home with Lakeland Healthcare.

In the capable hands of Dr. VanO, the Continuing Care Centers at Lakeland HealthCare expanded its quality services to the elderly. In this way, that historic landmark's doors remain open, providing a needed medical niche to Berrien County into the foreseeable future.

Dr. Harrison, Dr. VanO, and other SWMC physicians and medical staff helped ease that transition from Berrien General ownership to Lakeland Healthcare ownership. Dr. Harrison would further serve as a catalyst between Lakeland and SWMC.

The Hospitalist Program

SWMC's next phase was a natural outcome of another need in the community. When Drs. Mark and Donna were going through medical school in the late 1980s and early 1990s, training was downright brutal. Movies made at the time depicting medical training were right. It was horrible. The chairman of the Harrisons' school's internal medicine department went on to be famous and infamous later for saying, "The only problem with being on call every other night is that you miss half the good cases."

Dr. Donna Harrison wanted to be a surgeon but chose OB/GYN instead, because at that time, during the first two years of surgical internship the intern was on call every night. That was standard. If anyone could live through it and wasn't divorced or stark raving mad, he or she could go on to be a general surgeon.

This was doubly horrible because it was unnecessary. It was true in the old days that when a surgeon was on call, he or she was the only one. If a patient needed surgery, the surgeon went in because it was life or death for the patient. In 1960 that was true. By 1970 it was less true. By the 1990s, ERs were everywhere and a plethora of well-trained doctors and staff shifted around the clock, so it was no longer true.

At Berrien General, Dr. Harrison had an office practice in addition to being on call in the ER. If one of his patients came into the ER in crisis, Dr. Harrison was awakened. Jolted out of slumber, he'd answer the phone and have to tell the hospital staff what to do. A few hours later, he'd get up and do his morning rounds at one or two or three hospitals, then rush to the office. If any of his patients were admitted during the day, he'd go back to a hospital in the evening. This was the story for all the surgeons and internists. Supper went cold on the table, the wives were screaming, and that was the normal day. On the weekends the doctors signed out. One guy, the guy on call for the weekend, would take everybody's cases.

A couple of weekends in a row, Dr. Harrison saw 40 patients in a day — almost third-world numbers. It wasn't safe, but that was what was expected. Internists took everything that came through the door, frequently in Berrien General and Mercy-Memorial Hospital both.

Young internists and surgeons began to see the unnecessary burden of that lifestyle. They began agitating for division of labor like a real job with eight-hour shifts. They thought it only reasonable that staff only call surgeons at 2 a.m. in a true emergency. While everyone began to see this, it really took financial incentives for hospitals to make it happen.

On the local scene, this process created a lot of frayed nerves both for surgeons and hospital leadership. At the same time, while most groups turned away Medicaid and nonpaying patients, SWMC doctors were taking reduced income and served at 2 a.m. the patient they knew would never pay them.

Warren White, Dr. Ken O'Neill, Dr. Rick Johansen, and Dr. Mark Harrison and the others on the board and off it — they saw the need to have increasing manpower to strategically grow revenue. Whereas they did hire people who stayed, it was painful the number of people who didn't stay during those tough growing years. The clinic lost some good people because of the highly demanding work and reduced income.

Eventually, SWMC had the largest internal medicine and family practice presence in the community. The clinic grew to 60 to 70 stateside providers. Cedarwood Medical Clinic, the next largest, had 30, with very little primary care.

As growth occurred, the SWMC presence had an impact on inpatient statistics at the hospitals in St. Joseph, Niles and Berrien Center. In all those venues of care, SWMC populated or largely populated the physicians.

Enter the era of Quality Medicine. In the mid-1990s, the government and insurance companies started demanding quality. (In their definition, quality really meant quantity and streamlined costs.) They began asking, rightly, "Why does it cost you $7,000 to cure your pneumonia cases when the guy down the street can do it for $3,000?"

SWMC did well early on because so many had been trained to work in the jungle. These physicians could save someone with very little, compared to the academic physician who needed numerous tests and x-rays and second opinions. SWMC's no-nonsense care made sense. That caught Lakeland's eye and some insurers' eyes.

Dr. Mark Harrison and Dr. Rob Allen had met in the early '90s before Dr. Allen took intensive care training. When Dr. Allen came back to SWMC, he and Dr. Harrison were the last two internists at Berrien General. The two ran the ICU together. They saw the writing on the wall and came to the conclusion that, in the end, though everyone hated to see it happen, the community would benefit in several ways from a centralized ICU in St. Joseph.

First, St. Joseph was a bigger house to provide the kind of ICU care that was emerging in medicine. Second, the old style of managing critically ill patients was too fragmented. One general internist managed one set of patients, another internist worked with other patients, and a specialist came in and did something else — none communicating with each other. Dr. Allen, a newly trained specialist, could do things that the general internist couldn't. As soon as he came on board, he outperformed all the Cedarwood doctors. He was so good at what he did, the county's mortality dropped, the cost per patient dropped, and Lakeland administration was noticing. Now was the time to recruit a critical care team.

But there was a problem. Dr. Allen was by himself. He was burning out. Dr. Mark Harrison, chief of staff at Lakeland at the time, remembers Dr. Allen and his wife saying, "This is too much. We've got to leave."

Dr. Harrison fast-talked him. They talked about the vision of a critical care team; but the talk wasn't going anywhere, and Dr. Allen found another great opportunity. He sold his home. He was literally ready to leave. Dr. Harrison went again to Lakeland vice president Dr. Dave O'Connor. He said, "You have a great asset. Things will go downhill if you let him slip through your fingers. You must make this critical care team happen now! He's getting ready to leave! You know how good he is, and how vital critical care is here. I want that kind of care for my family and the rest of my patients. If you don't see that, maybe I'll leave too."

Somehow Dr. O'Connor got Lakeland President and CEO Joe Wasserman's permission to offer Dr. Allen a salaried position, with reasonable hours, and promised Lakeland would recruit three other critical care specialists if Dr. Allen would stay. That was the beginning of the employed staff (hospitalist) position in southwest Michigan.

Around this time, Cedarwood Medical Clinic had started to dissolve.

More internists started to displace retiring family doctors, and the internists naturally began to create their own little hospitalist services. "Hey, you're at Mercy-Memorial, see my patients for me. Next week I'll be half-time in the office so I'll see everyone's patients."

By the late 1990s, that had become the trend: one internist just worked in the hospital, while his buddy worked just in the office. They cared for each other's patients. It was such a relief. In 2000, non-SWMC physician Dr. George L. Heenan, who was on the Lakeland board of directors, started saying, "Hospitalists are where it's at. We're tired of being up all night." He started lobbying and pressing Lakeland formally to develop a hospitalist service.

Dr. Harrison became hospitalist director for Lakeland Regional Medical Center, St. Joseph. He saw Dr. Lars Bandera (pseudonym), a good new internist, floundering out in the boodocks in the Berrien Center office. He moved Dr. Bandera to the hospital. Then SWMC recruited Dr. Susan Dilan-Szanto, and Dr. Dan Snyder came home from Haiti around that time. Dr. Steve Hempel was recruited, and Dr. Chuck G. Nwakanma, and a few PRNs (Pro Re Nata – Latin – who fill in as needed). They built the team, and it was like turning a switch on. Quality care increased.

Infectious disease specialists tend to be systemic thinkers. They see things by whole systems, communities of care, from a quality and delivery standpoint. It was a no-brainer then to have them leading quality improvement at Lakeland. Lakeland noted that SWMC's involvement in general improved quality medicine and Dr. Steve Hempel and Dr. Rob Allen's interventions in critical care topped the list.

At the same time, the state of Michigan began sponsoring a quality program, called the Keystone Initiative. Joe Wasserman read it and gave it to the quality improvement team. The quality improvement team studied the world's literature on quality improvement and gave a report to Lakeland. "We're doing over half of this stuff already, spontaneously. But look, these giant hospitals do it this way so much better and cheaper. Could we implement these practices?"

It was the first time Lakeland HealthCare looked around and compared themselves seriously to some of the larger hospitals in the state. Joe Wasserman implemented many of the changes the team requested. At the end of the Keystone Initiative, little Lakeland scored in the top three of hospitals nationwide.

The Keystone Initiative put Lakeland on the map, and because the doctors were all SWMC members, it put SWMC on the map as well. In 2006 and again in 2007, Lakeland HealthCare was awarded the Premier CareScience Select Practice National Quality Award for superior patient outcomes in both quality and efficiency, an award given to only the top 1% of acute inpatient facilities in the United States. SWMC could deliver quality, negotiate through sometimes reticent administration, and deliver great care. The process gave SWMC name and presence at Lakeland and national acclaim.

Looking back, the hospitalist service brought about a contract relationship with Lakeland HealthCare that saved money for both sides, improved quality, and earned medical fame for both. In five years of hospitalist service, the program went from three anchors to 18 doctors. That built a huge SWMC presence in the hospital and created a working relationship with Lakeland. In the old Berrien General days in 1970s and 1980s, hospitals were competitively minded. It's no secret that Mercy-Memorial Hospital administrators did not like Berrien General Hospital and basically wanted to put it out of business.

The irony of that is, for years Berrien General saved Mercy-Memorial money. Berrien General absorbed a large number of nonpaying patients and Lakeland didn't get stuck with the bill, for the county indirectly paid it. That's why the county commissioners said to SWMC back in 1968, "Fine, you come and share some of this financial burden." In that way and in many ways, SWMC rescued Berrien General.

As SWMC migrated from Berrien General, expanding surgeons and primary care and internists up into St. Joseph and Niles, it took a few years for Lakeland finally to recognize SWMC as an asset. It was an epiphany: "SWMC really is a partner. If they didn't exist, we'd be in deep trouble. These doctors are driven and conscientious, care passionately for their patients, are quality-minded, and they have a sales point that will draw quality doctors who want to go overseas to our community. These guys have a Christian ethic to care about people and treat them right. What a valuable business partner."

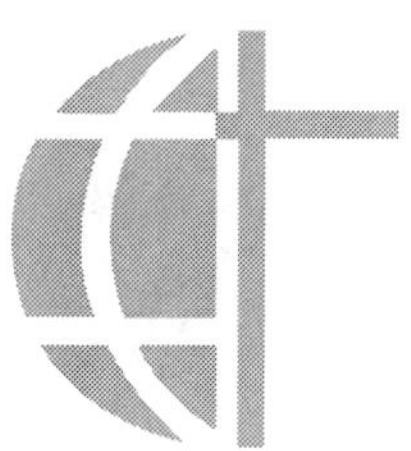

Chapter 33

What Had to Change and What Had to Stay the Same — the Integration

Chapter 33

What Had to Change and What Had to Stay the Same — the Integration

Increasingly through the 1990s, and by the turn of the millennium, a "coopetition" formed between SWMC and Lakeland. No longer antagonistically eyeballing each other, SWMC and Lakeland began collaborating to solve staffing issues, quality issues, and myriad other details that often arise when working side by side in a healthy community.

The leadership capital within the SWMC community became critically important to Lakeland. SWMC physicians were highly respected overall, and some rose to staff leadership positions. SWMC produced Lakeland's go-to intensive care physician and three successive chiefs of staff.

Amid all of this professional affirmation, SWMC's financial situation headed for the cliff. Reimbursement for services nosedived; operating costs climbed; and across the nation it became clear that the independent practice business model was struggling for survival.

Lakeland CEO Joe Wasserman and other Lakeland leaders weren't blind to SWMC's struggles. They began to see SWMC's tenuous position as a risk for the community and its projected failure as an irreplaceable loss.

When Dr. Froggatt became SWMC board president in 2006, like everyone else, he did not anticipate integration. It wasn't on the radar. In hindsight, he remembered Warren White tossing out the possibility. Warren had pointed out integration was happening elsewhere and was something the board should discuss. At the time, nobody had the heart to think it through.

In 2004 or 2005, seeking expert navigation through the group's options for the future, the SWMC board of directors had hired strategic planner Dale LeFever. He encouraged SWMC CFO Pat Meyer and the board to draw trajectory graphs projecting the clinic's future finances in light of reimbursement, client trends, and other factors. The pictures prophesied in black ink what doomsayers had ranted for years: the clinic simply couldn't go on forever. On paper the end loomed formidably close.

Half an inch to the right of this month's figures towered the brick wall. For years the clinic's energy had been focused on new markets, new ventures to sustain itself short-term or beyond. It had done a thorough exploration of expansion options: counseling, bone densitometry, clinical research, physical therapy, laser therapies, women's health, and even spa-type services. These venues were a little tape on a mortal wound. Looking at the projections, no one could ignore the obvious, short-range juncture.

In August 2008, desperate for cash flow, SWMC's executive committee approached Joe Wasserman and the hospital leadership and offered SWMC's ancillaries for sale. Joe said quietly, "Are you sure that's really going to be enough?"

Before SWMC's directors really had time to shake their heads, just as the light dimmed in their eyes, Joe continued, "We've had a healthy collaboration of sorts now for several years. We don't want you to go under. If we were to talk about some kind of integration, what would be your non-negotiables?"

SWMC doctors asked each other, "What would prevent us from integration?"

During the next few months, Warren White and the board developed a specific list of non-negotiables. The mission statement and what it stood for was key. No matter what else got muddled on the table, they knew they must protect the leverage to maintain and enhance SWMC's ability to achieve its mission both locally and internationally.

Dr. Ken O'Neill and a committee prayerfully revisited SWMC's mission statement:

"SWMC, by God's grace and following the example of Jesus Christ, strives to be a distinctive role model and leader in the integration of medical care, Christian witness, and missions. Medical care: to provide for our community compassionate, quality, accessible health care for the whole person. Witness: to proclaim Jesus Christ by word and example. Missions: to serve and support foreign and domestic medical missions."

The committee also affirmed a statement of faith that is read aloud and signed by all SWMC providers present at the first corporate meeting of the year:

> *"In keeping with our goal of being a Christ-centered, missionary-minded group of providers, the acceptance of a statement of faith by our providers is essential. We believe in one God in three persons: God the Father, God the Son, and God the Holy Spirit. We believe that the Bible*

is our sole authority in faith and conduct. In addition, we believe in a personal faith in Jesus Christ and His death on the cross and resurrection from the dead as our only means of eternal salvation. Further, we believe in a commitment to Christ as Lord of our lives, as all things were created by Him and for Him. (He is our Head, that in all things He may have the ultimate glory.)

From this commitment to Christ will come a personal commitment to build each other up in our faith and unity, to the end that our missionary outreach, both at home and abroad, might be enhanced. (By this shall all men know that we are His disciples, if we have love one for another. John 13:35.)"

Refocusing on these key beliefs of the clinic helped to crystallize priorities during the exploration of integration. Many things might feel in flux, but these core beliefs were solid.

A letter of intent to explore integration — just to investigate the idea — was passed by the SWMC board in November 2008, and by Lakeland's board in December 2008.

In January 2009 SWMC and Lakeland jointly hired a Medical Group Management Association consultant, Nick Fabrizio and an attorney, Bruce Johnson of Faegre and Benson, LLP in Denver, to negotiate a possible integration. Through the spring and summer of 2009 Nick and Bruce further deciphered both sides' non-negotiable lists, and Dale LeFever helped SWMC's board work through the practical implications and strategy of integration. Rather than asking what many at SWMC whispered ("Can SWMC survive integration?"), Dale asked, "How do we make integration advance and improve SWMC?"

One aspect that took several years to take shape was the culture-sharing potential involved. Amid all the discussions between Warren White and the SWMC board, and then-Lakeland CEO Joe Wasserman and incoming Lakeland CEO Loren Hamel and the Lakeland board, the concept of valuing and retaining SWMC's unique culture kept coming up.

As the talks developed, Lakeland began to appreciate SWMC's insistence on maintaining its culture. Further, Lakeland wanted to learn of SWMC's culture and absorb some of it into its own culture.

Instead of the dreaded merger, the two worked out details of a healthy integration. An integration is different from buying out a dying company and pillaging its revenue stream and working assets. It's a sharing of cultures, knowledge, and experience and an allowance for both entities to function together and independently. If some sort of a merger was no longer a choice, an integration was a sunny possibility. The SWMC board met at Lakeland's table after much prayer with renewed, if wary, optimism.

SWMC and Lakeland negotiated for months with only a couple of impasses. Both parties broke off talks and took some needed space, then came back to the table. They were ultimately able to see through those seeming impasses.

In October 2009, both boards walked out of the meetings satisfied with the agreement. The integration was passed by SWMC's board of directors and Lakeland's board of directors in separate meetings in November 2009.

As Dr. Ken O'Neill says, "Joe Wasserman was able to tackle the tough questions, and Loren had the flexibility to make it happen."

Dr. Froggatt says, "I think we really felt God's hand in it (the integration concept) in that it was such a counter intuitive idea initially that all of our board members really had to seek God in an intentional way to try to understand how it could work. Everyone initially felt leery. We could hardly even think about it at first… Yet the way it came about was remarkably peaceful."

Once SWMC's board grew unified with the idea of integration, it presented the hard facts and the best options to the corporation members. The corporate viewpoint had shifted; now it was necessary to change individual hearts and minds, an entirely different process.

Locally, SWMC was certainly not the first organization to consider integration. Hospital mergers actually took place as early as 1977, when Mercy Hospital of Benton Harbor and Memorial Hospital of St. Joseph combined to create Mercy-Memorial Medical Center. SWMC took notice. In 1992, Mercy-Memorial integrated with Niles' Pawating Hospital, forming Lakeland Regional Health System. With doctors practicing at Pawating, SWMC experienced this transition. Two years later Berrien General Hospital merged into Lakeland Regional Health System, a painful precedent for SWMC. Since the 1990s, this phenomenon has trickled down to clinics nationwide.

SWMC members talked to their colleagues on the east coast, west coast, and everywhere in-between, and they found SWMC's plight was not unique. Clinics all over the U.S. were exploring integration. SWMC members investigated the big picture and they asked about colleagues' own integration experiences. "What kind of deals are you getting? What literature are you reading? What are the pros and cons?"

As they compiled answers, they also gathered reassurance. This brick wall might not mark the end of SWMC; it might be just a sharp turn in the road.

God also clarified His will, not with celestial marquees, but in quiet, personal ways that spoke to each individual. Each month that passed while Lakeland HealthCare and the SWMC board worked through the details of integration, Pat Meyer watched SWMC's financial figures get worse and worse. As each month-end report added up, he realized on a deeper level that the deal had to get done, and that God was in it.

At this same time, Pat watched clinics folding into healthcare systems across the country, and he began to see benefits as viewed by a top governmental level. From the top, it makes sense to integrate healthcare under one system. Pat acknowledged that records permeated throughout the whole system can go anywhere, and everybody would have access to those same records. In that way, collaboration made sense to him.

Knowing that didn't make Pat feel any happier about hitting the financial brick wall. He still wrestled with bittersweet emotions: "I'm the financial guy. I should've been able to prevent it (the integration)."

After both the SWMC board and Lakeland board approved and signed the integration agreement in November 2009, a special SWMC shareholders' meeting was held at 6:30 p.m. on Tuesday, December 1, 2009. The corporation overwhelmingly voted in favor of integration. Thirty-five shareholders voted in favor of integration; three opposed; and 14 members were absent, most out of the area on long-term missions. Monumental in its core, the meeting moved forward with dignity and order.

SWMC surgeon and former board member Dr. Roy Winslow recalled later the consternation he and many of his colleagues experienced regarding the desire to be independent as a missions-minded, physician-led organization. The idea of being subservient to a larger corporation that did not share those goals was tough. They wondered how such an affiliation would affect their core beliefs and their very identity.

According to Dr. Winslow, it all boiled down to trusting SWMC's leadership. While he never seriously planned to leave, he and his wife, Bev, talked about other career possibilities. They felt that to stay they must be able to support the board's decision entirely. Like many others, the Winslows prayed a long time before signing the contract with Lakeland.

Affiliation with Lakeland felt risky, but it allowed SWMC to exist — to provide its unique mission to medical missionaries and to the communities in Berrien County and around the world benefiting from the medical missionaries' care. Signing the contract required trusting SWMC's leadership to preserve its core beliefs and identity, so that they would be able to serve Christ and maintain the mission they came to SWMC to be part of.

Although deeply involved in the integration process, SWMC president Dr. John Froggatt also experienced consternation as he signed the contract. He felt a loss of control and wondered about the reactions of his 50-odd colleagues as they stared at the same paperwork. But pen in hand, Dr. Froggatt also pondered the very different way the process could have developed.

Thinking from a conventional worldly view, a horrific, contentious, bitter struggle could have blown the whole thing apart. Instead, with God's hand in the midst of it, the process up to and including the special corporation meeting was remarkably peaceful. No one ever yelled or shouted. Deliberations proceeded calmly, purposefully. There was very good discussion, an appropriate level of concern and even grief. Dr. Froggatt could state afterward that God provided above what they could never have imagined in a vast array of details from the facilitator Dale LeFever's specific gifts to the non-coincidental verbiage during numerous meetings to the reinvestment of everyone into the clinic's vision and mission. In his mind, the process went incredibly well.

Dr. Froggatt felt it was God rewarding SWMC for its faithfulness through the years up to the present day. The board continually prayed, "Show us, God. Lead us through. We have fears. If you don't want this integration to go forward, shut it down."

In Dr. Froggatt's experience, "God loves it so much when you make even simple steps of faith and take your hands off the controls. He rewards you above your effort, disproportionally to the measure of the faith you exert. He's so pleased by simple faith, and in the prayer you feel His pleasure and you are able to take a few more steps forward. [Because of that], it (the smooth integration process) went really beyond my expectations. Not easily, not pie in the sky. But in the exploring and debating and working through the details, I felt His hand."

At the time of the integration, SWMC's services included x-ray, mammography, bone densitometry, clinical laboratory, ultrasound, and counseling. Fifty-seven physicians and 18 mid-level providers served at eight SWMC clinical sites in Berrien County and Lakeland HealthCare facilities.

In the integration process, the SWMC physicians signed contracts with Lakeland HealthCare. The support staff became Lakeland employees.

During several years following the integration date, Lakeland closed ancillaries that duplicated services, including the laboratory.

But Lakeland brokered mutual respect as the business partners integrated. This respect revealed itself in the retention of a high percentage of SWMC's staff. Lakeland also appointed Warren White as vice president of Lakeland Physician Practices. Dr. John Froggatt was named medical director of Lakeland's Hospitalist Services. And Dr. Ken O'Neill became medical director for Lakeland Medical Practices.

In a further gesture of mutual goodwill, Lakeland created a physician board to which SWMC assigns a portion of members, Lakeland Physician Care Network assigns a portion of members, and Lakeland HealthCare appoints three members. Dr. Ken O'Neill was asked to join the physician board not as a SWMC representative, but as one of Lakeland's three members.

Dr. O'Neill updated the SWMC physicians' manual around the time of the integration. In it he documented several other areas of expertise that Lakeland values in SWMC. The manual states:

> *"The SWMCP providers look forward to providing valuable services to the people of Southwestern Michigan as part of the Lakeland Healthcare System. Lakeland brings to the integration stability and strength. SWMCP brings a multispecialty medical practice with experience in managing outpatient practices and EHR (electronic health record)."*

Lakeland's support of SWMC's vision and mission became tangible in February 2010 when it actively encouraged SWMC physicians to keep their annual pilgrimage to Tenwek Hospital. As plans for the trip developed and commenced, Lakeland came into contact with SWMC's international influence. "People all over the world in medical missions know all about Southwestern," a person in Lakeland administration gleefully commented to Warren White.

SWMC signed the paperwork February 26 with March 1, 2010, the effective date. "We didn't sell the company," Dr. O'Neill clarifies. "The old SWMC still exists, still winding itself down over several more years as it collects government moneys and promised future payments for things such as computer conversions.... We sold hard assets: ancillaries, chairs, medical records, and transferred operations to Lakeland Medical Practices."

Meanwhile, a new non-profit company, Southwestern Medical Clinic Physicians, Incorporated (SWMCP), was created effective March 1, 2010, to continue the history and values of SWMC.

When the documents were signed, Pat Meyer and many of his colleagues did not feel the doom they had anticipated. As the inevitable integration happened, they were glad to have a place to work and were relieved SWMC didn't just go under and fade away. The integration was a relief in tough times. Essentially, God kept the ship afloat for 15 years beyond what SWMC's bottom line had predicted, and with the integration He provided a new and exciting way for SWMC to keep working together — and to broaden its community and worldwide influence — for His glory.

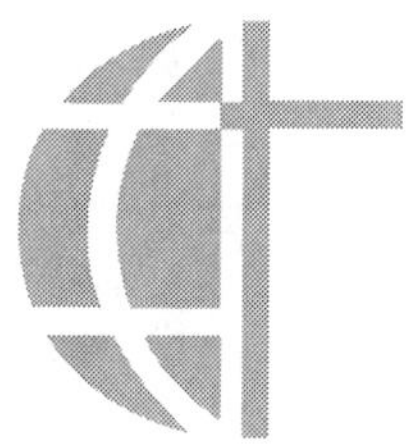

Chapter 34

Why It Began and Why It Will Never End — SWMC'S Legacy

Chapter 34

Why It Began and Why It Will Never End — SWMC'S Legacy

Through the hand of God, SWMC was born in a hospital. When Dr. Weldon Cooke hired his first two medical missionary physicians in the late 1950s, they were employees of Berrien County Hospital. There was no clinic. The papers of incorporation were signed almost a decade later. Dr. Weldon Cooke, Dr. Charlie Patton, and Dr. Almarose Cooke were hospitalists.

Even after SWMC incorporated, Berrien General Hospital hired SWMC's physicians. They had a hospital that needed to be staffed, and SWMC provided that service. As Dr. Mark Harrison pointed out, for decades Berrien General Hospital told Dr. Cooke and his physicians, "Show up for these shifts, do this work, and we'll pay you and spring, you to go overseas for a month." A quarter of a century later, that was exactly how the hospitalist program developed with Lakeland in the 1990s. In a way, SWMC's story came full circle with its integration with Lakeland HealthCare.

Beyond the structural repetition, the continuity of mission and values permeates SWMC's timeline and culture. To Dr. O'Neill, this continuity that relies on faith was critical to the successful integration transition process.

Lakeland HealthCare is a community-based hospital system, not a faith-based organization. Remarkably to Dr. Mike Chupp and others, simultaneous to the integration, a number of Seventh-Day Adventists joined Lakeland leadership. Lakeland's Christian awareness and sympathy ramped up, even outside of SWMC's influence.

Only God could have prepared Lakeland for SWMC, and SWMC for Lakeland. The awakening spiritual climate at Lakeland just at the time when SWMC was preparing to integrate, the growing mutual admiration between SWMC and Lakeland – these factors were beyond Warren White and Dr. Froggatt's control. God orchestrated these factors.

Will this sympathetic climate continue at Lakeland? As Dr. Chupp said, "It's all going to come down to the people and the leadership," both at Lakeland and at SWMC.

"Leadership at Southwestern now is as solid as it's ever been in its history," Dr. Chupp continued. "People like Warren White, [Drs.] O'Neill and Froggatt, Pat Meyer — that group of four had to have been [God-ordained]. To pull off this integration and still keep the vision, those are the folks I would trust."

Dr. Chupp compared the integration with the situation SWMC faced when it hired him and nine other physicians. "When you hire nine or 10 new physicians…the fresh blood will make things more or less Christian. There's a potential with the merger [for SWMC] to have either more or less [Christian] influence."

SWMC Administrator Warren White spoke of these same concerns. "We'd been through changes before. The integration with Lakeland is another identity change. People have been asking, 'Can we integrate and maintain our identity?' It's painful, but, so far, yes, we can." He pointed out that not many physicians left as a result of the integration, and, in fact, SWMC was able to retain physicians and staff it wouldn't have been able to retain otherwise.

Dr. Froggatt experienced a mixture of trust in God and concern for the clinic. "One thing you have to do is get to the point where you realize the clinic is, after all, God's. We don't have a charter from God guaranteeing that Southwestern will exist in perpetuity. Whatever His pleasure is, that's what we want. If we needed to exist for a period of time and then not exist anymore, we don't have a say in that."

While Dr. Froggatt continues to trust in God for the future of the clinic, he does fear one thing. He fears the human factor, the old self that can stray:

> *"You see many institutions that began as Christian institutions and then changed their leadership or affiliation and ceased to be Christian at some point. If God is working in us to accomplish a change, I'm okay with that, but if we're doing something neglectful that leads to a bad outcome for the clinic, then obviously that would be [failing on every level]. God is not limited by any subset of us. He can work around that. I want to make sure we're good stewards, that whatever happens to the clinic is a result of us walking through things with Him, not of us turning from Him."*

Integration has opened up new areas of impact and ministry that SWMC would not have been able to access before. Because of its formal affiliation with Lakeland, SWMC is discovering the ability to bring a broader audience to some of the things that SWMC does. For example, physician futurist and award-winning writer and educator Dr. Richard Swenson spoke at a conference, invited by SWMC. Instead of just speaking to SWMC, because of the integration, he spoke to Lakeland, a much broader invitation.

Additionally, when SWMC goes on mission trips, it now has opportunities to enlist participants from all of Lakeland. Lakeland employees are, indeed, becoming involved.

If Lakeland HealthCare integrates into a larger system down the road, of course no one knows how that will impact SWMC's ability to carry out its vision. But, optimistically, Dr. Froggatt would ask:

> *"Is God moving us into a position where we now have an entirely new opening to expand our mission/vision into a larger population? A lot of interesting things, I think, may end up happening long range from this. We have a nice model within the integration to maintain our mission and vision, and Lakeland values what we bring from that. The challenge to us is, how do we leverage where God is leading us, how he's equipped us, into maintaining that value for the community and Lakeland so that our role not only continues, but thrives and grows into new ways we didn't even anticipate?"*

In the two years since the integration, God has revealed the opportunities the integration has allowed for His work to be glorified, and even in part carried out by an ever-widening circle of community. Truly, Lakeland HealthCare is involved and identifying with SWMC's mission and vision.

For years Lakeland has reached out to provide donated items to hospitals around the world. Since the integration, donations have ramped up to a new level because of the hospital's increased awareness of need. Lakeland donated a shipping container of old gurneys to Tenwek Hospital's ER.

When Dr. Mike Chupp came home in the fall of 2011, he didn't make a specific speaking itinerary. He waited for God's lead. Pronto, an unforeseen opportunity arose. Lakeland management called him. "Can you give a talk in 10 minutes to the Lakeland management team?" Dr. Chupp hustled to the meeting, delighted to share his story to more than 100 people across all levels of the hospital, who normally wouldn't know anything about Tenwek or missions. His fascinated audience, now colleagues, contained a few future members of a short-term mission team to Tenwek.

February 2012, marked another annual, official SWMC trip to Tenwek to cover for Tenwek's doctors going to their medical missions conference. SWMC physicians have enabled medical missionaries to attend mission conferences since the beginning. Dr. Rick Johansen, part of the team to Tenwek in February 2012, covered at Elwa Hospital during the original Breckenhurst Missions Conference in the 1970s so that Dr. Bob and Marion Schindler could go. Most years since, SWMC physicians have filled in somewhere during the conference. Before the integration, several SWMC doctors quietly took a month's leave, and no one else in Berrien County would be aware of it. In 2012, a Catholic and two Seventh-Day Adventist doctors, Lakeland but not SWMC staff, joined the Tenwek team. The annual Tenwek trip has become an outreach on new levels.

The Tenwek team had to return to the States by February 25 to launch Lakeland HealthCare's new electronic health records system. All the training for the new computer system and the logistics of key personnel being gone in February opened up natural avenues of discussion. Dr. Susan Hayward expected antagonism about their departure at every corner. But Lakeland was accommodating, open, and interested.

Another unexpected benefit of the integration has come to light. At SWMC corporate and leadership meetings a perennial item on the agenda that sometimes consumed most of the meeting was billing and managing office staff. The meetings were about survival, about running a business in addition to the mission. Now integration has taken away the burden of billing and management, allowing meeting agendas to refocus on the mission and vision. Leadership retreats can focus on the core values of SWMC, not a four-hour seminar on how to bill better. Ironically, the integration with a community hospital has allowed a new focus to SWMC that many feared might be lost.

In another irony, the integration freed up SWMC finances for a flip that missions-minded physicians had sought for years. Before integration when a new doctor joined the group, it was a $150,000 cost to the clinic to get him or her up and running. Because it took several years for cash-strapped SWMC to recoup that money, the new doctors couldn't take off and go on a mission. For those called overseas, it felt restrictive. But no one could figure out how to do anything to change the financial necessity of having them stay until they reached their even mark. Now SWMC has actually passed a requirement that new SWMC physicians go on a short-term mission trip within their first two years — a complete flip!

Years ago, SWMC physicians' salaries were low — 60% at best of market salary. It was difficult to recruit young ,missions-minded physicians. They had student loans and couldn't financially swing the low salary even if they endorsed the mission. SWMC knew its new members endorsed the mission because it was such a sacrifice financially to join.

Now as a Lakeland-affiliated brand, SWMC physicians do make market salary. New doctors joining SWMC must now read and endorse SWMC's written vision and mission statement. If doctors come along to interview who don't think they can in good faith sign that vision, then they can work directly with Lakeland HealthCare. Salaries are the same.

Along with signing the vision and mission statement, SWMC physicians agree to donate three percent of their salary to the SWMC Foundation. Additionally, 10 percent of their salary is set aside as missions-giving money. Quarterly, SWMC doctors receive that money to dispense to missions of their choice. Missions money can be spent on the physician's own missions trips. So, SWMC as a corporation supports medical missions, and each of its physicians individually commits to support missions.

New doors are opening for SWMC physicians to share their medical missions experiences. For example, Lakeland hosts medical education. Drs. Dan and Sue Hayward spoke to Michigan State University medical students who visited Lakeland and were able to alert students who were part of their Christian Medical and Dental Society chapter about the opportunities at SWMC.

Dr. Froggatt also looks to the next generation for clues about SWMC's future. "How are we doing with the younger generation we're trying to bring into the clinic? Are we transmitting the vision and mission in a way that God is matching up their passions with what He has for the future? If so, we're building a lot of intriguing, exciting scenarios for the future."

Meanwhile, healthcare worldwide is evolving rapidly. Even insiders have few concrete pictures to illustrate what the healthcare system in this county is going to be like in five years, let alone 20. Warren White believes SWMC is not finished with identity or format changes.

But if the future can at all be predicted by analyzing the past, SWMC will write more chapters of its history. As Warren said, the clinic's story has been, is, and must continue to be about "God working through this organization, and individuals trusting God to lead us through the turbulent times."

Only God Himself could have pulled together so many mavericks, herded them along through the years, and enabled them to help each other pursue their separate callings. God Himself illuminated the way when things became desperate.

The future of the clinic remains bright, according to the Douces and so many others, but only if God remains the center of it. Prayer, petition, and dedication to Him and His work, living and pursuing all for His glory – these are the methods, above all others, that will guarantee continued success.

God's hand at work has been evident to all. God has revealed Himself in and through the clinic from its earliest moments as an idea in Dr. Cooke's mind to the present time and into the future as far as anyone can see. Invariably, every interviewee for this book, from Virginia Stover and Sheila Kipp to Dr. Cooke and Don Gast and Warren White, has emphasized God's hand at work in the clinic.

Because of God's hand, Southwestern Medical Clinic rose out of a cornfield in rural Berrien County, Michigan. Doctors at a hospital that might otherwise have been closed and razed saved thousands of lives and assisted thousands more lives into the world. In the process, they shared God's love and His story to their patients and the community. Some doctors worked with SWMC for a year, others for decades, but each made a difference because of God's hand.

By God's grace, Southwestern Medical Clinic has left an indelible mark on medical missions worldwide. This mark has been made through dozens of SWMC physicians' stellar careers abroad: from New Guinea to Ecuador to Kenya to Kazakhstan, and myriad other places both written and unmentioned. This mark has also been made through organizational leadership, such as Dr. Robert Schindler's coordination at the Christian Medical and Dental Society and Dr. Donna Joan Harrison's work in helping governments and individuals choose life.

SWMC's story is not finished. With God's help, SWMC and its physicians and staff will continue to glorify Him as He leads. The future is God's. SWMC is God's. May His will be done.

SWMC Foundation

The SWMC Foundation mobilizes resources and people who integrate medical care and Christian witness worldwide.

Our goal as a Foundation is to proclaim the Gospel of Jesus Christ through:

- Supporting foreign and domestic medical missions projects and organizations
- Supporting short and long term medical missionaries
- Providing scholarships for student participation in medical missions
- Providing support service in medical settings

If you know someone who could benefit from our services of if you desire to read current stories, or view missionary videos, visit us at, www.swmcf.org, our Foundation website. There is also a place on our HOME PAGE for you to support our international efforts. Just click on the "DONATE TODAY" button in the top right corner, our send your gifts to the address listed below.

We affirm the statement that one of our African associate hospitals proclaims… "We treat, JESUS HEALS." Thank you for your continual prayers and encouragement.

Southwestern Medical Clinic Foundation
2550 Meadowbrook Road
Benton Harbor, MI 49022
www.swmcf.org

Bibliography Chapter 1:

1. Emails, Dr. Roland Stephens, 11 September 2010, 25 October 2010, 11 November 2010.
2. Emails, Dr. Weldon Cooke, 28 September 2010, 1 October 2010, 5 October 2010, 16 October 2010, 20 October 2010, 23 December 2010.
3. Emails, Mrs. Margie Shealy of Christian Medical and Dental Society, 11 November 2010, 15 November 2010.
4. Brochure, "Reflections," mailed bulk rate by Berrien General Hospital, 1250 Deans Hill Road, Berrien Center, Mich. 49102, ca. 1980.
5. Interview, Mrs. Elaine Chaudoir, 9 November 2010.
6. Interview, Dr. Bob Wesche, 26 February 2010.
7. Interview, Dr. Dan Stephens, 25 June 2010.
8. Berrien General Hospital Tour, given by Virginia Stover and Diane Demler, 15 October, 2010.
9. "News in General," monthly staff and volunteer newsletter of Berrien General Hospital, Vol. 10 No. 3, December 1977, page 16, article "Richard Chaudoir, Registered Pharmacist," written by Pam Frank and Julie Odiorne.
10. *A History of Berrien General Hospital, 1832-1982*, by Katherine A. Cornelius, prepared under Berrien General Hospital Purchase Order 6007, October 1982.
11. Website, Tyndale House Publishers, www.tyndale.com/50_Company/dr_taylor_story.php
12. Document, Providers PAST & PRESENT, 2009, compiled by Carolyn Philip.
13. Article, St. Joseph *News-Palladium*, 20 May 1964.
14. Article online, *The New York Times Business Day*, "Wilson Greatbatch, Inventor of Implantable Pacemaker, Dies at 92," by Barnaby Feder, 28 September 2011.
15. Other various internet websites, for general historical information.

Bibliography Chapter 2:

1. Berrien General Hospital Annual Report, 1966.
2. Berrien General Hospital Annual Report, 1967.
3. Tour of Berrien General Hospital, 14 October 2010.
4. Telephone interview, Dr. Robert Wesche, 26 February 2010.
5. Emails, Dr. Roland Stephens, 11 September 2010, 25 October 2010, 11 November 2010.
6. Interviews and telephone conversations, Virginia Stover, ca. 2010-2012.
7. Copy of the incorporation papers, 28 June 1968.
8. Tenwek Hospital website
9. Interview, Beverly Stover, 14 October 2010.
10. Berrien Center Bible Church directory photo, undated, ca. 1978.
11. Interview, Bev Stover and retired SWMC women Virginia Stover, Betty Christner, Lou Bergey Ellis and Bonnie Howe, 5 November 2010.
12. Interview, Ken O'Neill, 2 September 2010.
13. Interview, Don Gast, 14 April 2011.
14. Interview, Dr. Janet Frey, 7 October 2010.
15. "The News in General," Berrien General Hospital's bulletin, vol. 1 no. 3, August 25, 1965, page 2: "Drs. Wesche and Patton Join Staff," from an archived collection of Elaine Chaudoir.
16. Brief article welcoming Dr. James L. Wierman, "The News in General," a monthly newsletter for the staff of Berrien General Hospital, page 3, vol. 1. No. 2, July 15, 1965.
17. Email from Dr. Roland Stephens, 24 January 2011.
18. Email from Dr. Dan Stephens, 25 February 2012.

Bibliography Chapter 3:

1. DVD, "Dr. Herbert Andrew Atkinson," 17 April (2009?)
2. Interview, Frieda Atkinson, 26 October 2010.
3. Christmas Letter 1977, Dr. Weldon Cooke.
4. The Living Bible

Bibliography Chapter 4:

1. Interview, Don Gast and Virginia Stover, 25 February 2010.
2. Interview, Carol Jewell, 10 January 2011.
3. Interview, Elaine Chaudoir and Virginia Stover, 9 November 2010.
4. Letter written by Donald Gast, 3 July 1973.
5. Letter typed by Donald Gast 1 July 1981.
6. DVD, Dr. Herbert Atkinson, 7 April (2009?).
7. Interview, Lou Ellis, Bonnie Howe, Betty Christner, Bev Stover and Virginia Stover, 5 November 2010.
8. Berrien General Hospital General Report 1964.
9. Christmas Letter, by Dr. Weldon Cooke, 1975.
10. Interview Mindie Sirk, 14 October 2010.
11. Interview Debbie Crane, 14 October 2010.
12. Article, "Voters Pass School Millage," *The Journal-Era*, 12 June 1974.
13. Article, "Berrien General Appoints Administrator," *The Journal-Era*, 5 November, 1974.
14. Brochure, "Reflections," published by Berrien General Hospital, Berrien Center, MI, ca. 1980.
15. SWMC Newsletter "Brainwaves," 11 May 1995, brief article regarding Don Gast's Samaritan of the Year award.

16. Telephone interview, Dr. Janet Frey, 7 October 2010.
17. Interview, Don Gast, 26 April 2011.
18. Interview, Don Gast, 14 April 2011.

Bibliography Chapter 6:

1. *Following the Great Physician: The First 70 Years of the Christian Medical and Dental Associations*, by Dr. Bob and Marian Schindler, 2002, Central Plains Book Manufacturing, Winfield, Kansas.
2. *Niles Daily Star*, undated clipped resource circa January 1-5, 1972, written by Pat Gallagher, staff writer.
3. Undated *Herald-Palladium* newspaper article written by Ginger Hanchey.
4. Dr. Cooke's 1977 Christmas letter.
5. Brainwaves newsletter 6 July, 1995.
6. Eulogy given by Kenneth Y. Best in the *Liberian Observer*, ca. August 2002.
7. Interview, Virginia Stover, 25 February 2010.
8. Gup, Ted. *The Book of Honor: The Secret Lives and Deaths of CIA Operatives*. 2001: Anchor Books.
9. From a tribute written by Dr. Dave and Ruth Van Reken, who served with the Schindlers, read at Marian Schindler's funeral in April 2010.
10. Emailed eulogy April 8, 2010, 5:21 p.m., by fellow missionary Mrs. Clarice Miller, at the time of Marian Schindler's death www.elwa-mausa.org/archives/2010/04/tributes-to-marian-schindler.html
11. ELWA Hospital's Website, www.elwaministries.org
12. Interview, Carol Jewell, January 2011.
13. *Mission Possible*, by Dr. Robert and Marian Schindler.
14. Obituary published online at http://hosting-20864.tributes.com/show/355021

Bibliography Chapter 7:

1. Brochure published by Men For Missions International, Box A, Greenwood, IN 46142, April 1993.
2. Interview, Dr. Bill and Ilene Douce, 23 March 2010.
3. Email, Dr. Hal Kime, 1 October 2010.
4. Email, Dr. Weldon Cooke, ca. October 2010.
5. "Destination Ecuador: Living a Legacy," pp. 12-13, OMS Outreach, May-August 2006, written by Rev. Roger Skinner, Executive Director of OMS/USA.
6. Article in *The Chapel Free Press*, ca. 28 March 2010.
7. Email, Dr. Bill Douce, 2 March 2011.
8. Telephone interview, Dr. Dick Douce, calling from Quito.

Bibliography Chapter 8:

1. Telephone interview, Dr. Edling and his daughter Nancy, 15 November 2010.
2. Telephone interview, Dr. Norbert Anderson, 11 January 2011.
3. Telephone interview, Dr. Charles Pierson, 27 October 2010
4. Dr. Cooke's 1977 Christmas letter.
5. Email, Dr. Weldon Cooke, ca. 2011.
6. Article in *The Herald-Palladium*, ca. 1979 about Dr. Silvernale returning.
7. Article in *The Journal-Era*, 7 March 1973 about the TB treatment program.
8. Various websites for fact and spelling checks.

Bibliography Chapter 9:

1. Emails, Dr. Helene Johnson, 7 and 8 March 2011.
2. DVD, Dr. Herb Atkinson, 7 April (2009?).
3. Telephone interview, Dr. Chuck Rhodes, 27 October 2010.
4. Telephone interview, Dr. Bob Patton, 13 July 2010.
5. Interview, Virginia Stover and Elaine Chaudoir, 9 November 2010.
6. Interview, Lou Ellis, Bonnie Howe and Bev Stover, 5 November 2010.
7. Conversation, Dr. Rick Johansen, 26 February 2010.
8. Cassette-tape-recorded interview, Don Gast and Virginia Stover, 25 February 2010.
9. *Journal-Era* article and photos 2 January 1974 "Annual Staff Christmas Party at Berrien General"
10. *Journal-Era* article 5 November 1974 "Berrien General Appoints Administrator."
11. *Journal-Era* article 26 December 1973 "New Chief of Staff at Berrien General."
12. *Journal-Era* article 19 July 1973 "Southwestern Medical Clinic Will Open Offices in Berrien Springs."
13. *Journal-Era* article 23 April 1975 "Open New Addition at Berrien General."
14. *Journal-Era* article 14 February 1973 "Seek to Lease Land at Berrien General."
15. *Journal-Era* photo and caption 7 May 1975 "First Birth in New Obstetrics Wing."
16. Document, "Providers PAST & PRESENT 2009," compiled by Carolyn Philip.

Bibliography Chapter 10:

1. Interview, Dr. Helene Johnson, 27 October 2010.
2. Interview, Betsy Zech, 27 January 2011.
3. Emails, Dr. Helene Johnson, 2 November 2010, 7 and 8 March 2011.
4. "*Reflections*," Berrien General Hospital Annual Report, ca. 1980.
5. DVD, Dr. Herbert Atkinson, 7 April (2009?).
6. *The Journal Era*, 20 June 1984, special section devoted to Berrien General Hospital. "Berrien General Hospital: Hospital of Choice. Berrien General Hospital's Birthplace."
7. *Dowagiac Daily News* article ca. June 1984, "Berrien Opens Birthing Facility" by Sue Knopka, (Dowagiac) Daily News Editor
8. *Herald-Palladium* article 13 March 1985 about the new women's specialty house on Niles Rd.
9. *Herald-Palladium* article by Debra Haight, "Labor of Love: Southwestern Medical Clinic Doctor has delivered 10,000 Southwest Michigan babies."
10. Numerous archived undated, uncredited local newspaper articles in the scrapbooks of Betsy Zech.

Bibliography Chapter 11:

1. SWMC News Brief, 1/20/1982: "Meet Your Staff at 300 W. Ferry (New Location of Berrien Springs Family Service Clinic)."
2. Interview, Don Gast and Virginia Stover, 25 February 2010.
3. Interview, Carol Gonnerman Jewel, 10 January 2011.
4. Telephone interview, Dr. Janet Frey, 7 October 2010.
5. *Journal-Era* article, 3 December 1979, regarding the new Berrien Springs clinic.

6. *Journal-Era* article, 23 August 1982, announcing the new Stevensville clinic.
7. Document, Providers PAST & PRESENT, compiled by Carolyn Philip.
8. Article, *The Benton Spirit*, "The Evolution of Lakeland Healthcare in the Twin Cities, 1899-2010," 22 July 2010.
9. Email, Bev Stover, ca. 2010-2011.
10. Interview, Marilyn Hurrle, 11 Nov. 2010.
11. Interview, Dr. Rick Johansen, recorded to DVD, 24 August 2010.

Bibliography Chapter 12:

1. Article, *The Journal-Era*, "Two Doctors Join Berrien General Staff," 16 September 1981.
2. Article, *Dowagiac Daily News*, 28 June 1982, written by John Eby, Daily News Editor.
3. Letter written by Dr. Slater, 7 November 1982.
4. Letter written by Dr. Slater, 19 December 1982.
5. Letter written by Dr. Slater, 22 January 1987.
6. Document, Providers PAST & PRESENT, compiled by Carolyn Philip.
7. Conversation with Carolyn Philip, ca. January 2011.
8. Website, http://cehguinea.org/slater-dwight
9. Interview, Don Gast and Virginia Stover, 25 February 2010.
10. Website document dated 2009, www.oasishospital.org/news/50/81/Oasis-Hospital-Dedicates-the-New-Surgical-Suite/
11. Website page archive of a blog of Dr. Dwight E. Slater: http://archive.constantcontact.com/fs044/1103024749229/archive/1107079999357.html

Bibliography Chapter 13:

1. Telephone interview with Dr. Bob Patton, 13 July 2010.
2. Christmas letter written by Dr. Weldon Cooke, 1977.
3. Article, *The Herald-Palladium*, 1 December 1982, regarding the new Sawyer office.
4. Article, *The Journal-Era*, undated, regarding the new Stevensville office.

Bibliography Chapter 14:

1. Telephone interview, Dr. Janet Frey, 7 October 2010.
2. Interview and Berrien General/Berrien Center SWMC tour with Virginia Stover, 14 October 2010.
3. DVD, Dr. Herbert Atkinson, 17 April (2009?)
4. "News in General" brochure printed by Berrien General Hospital, December 1980, note regarding the Advanced Cardiac Life Support course.
5. Christmas 1977 letter written by Dr. Weldon Cooke.
6. Telephone interviews with Dr. Charles and Mrs. Yvonne Bruerd, 10 November 2010.
7. Letter written by Dr. Bruerd kept in SWMC archives ca. July 1982
8. Letter written by Dr. Bruerd kept in SWMC archives dated 10 October 1982
9. Letter written by Dr. Bruerd kept in SWMC archives ca. October 1982
10. Email, Dr. Helene Johnson regarding caliber of SWMC physicians, [date]
11. SWMC newsletters archived, 1981-1983.

Bibliography Chapter 15:

1. Interview of Dr. Rick Johansen, recorded to DVD, 24 August 2010.
2. July 2006 *Herald-Palladium* Health Monthly article.
3. Interview, Dr. Weldon Cooke, 10 August 2010.

Bibliography Chapter 16:

1. Interview, Dr. Weldon Cooke, 10 August 2010.
2. Email, Dr. Weldon Cooke, 11 May 2011.
3. Email, Dr. Weldon Cooke, 26 December 2010.
4. Email, Dr. Ken O'Neill, 30 June 2011.
5. Unpublished historical document, "A History of Berrien General Hospital: 1832-1982," by Katherine A. Cornelius, conducted under the auspices of the Berrien County Historical Association, Inc., Berrien Springs, Jan H. House, Director; Robert C. Myers, Administrative Assistant, October 1982. 68 pp.
6. Website, http://earlyaviators.com/ecooke/htm
7. Interview, Dr. Weldon and Mary Cooke, 8 February 2012.

Bibliography Chapter 17:

1. Interviews, Dr. Kenneth O'Neill, 3 August and 2 September 2011.
2. SWMC website, www.swmc.org.
3. Email from Dr. O'Neill, 24 August 2010.
4. Interview with Sheila Kipp, 26 July 2010.
5. Interview with Carol Gonnerman Jewell, 10 January 2011.

Bibliography Chapter 18:

1. Telephone interview, Dr. Richard Roach, 1 February 2011.
2. Email, Dr. Richard Roach, 1 February 2011.
3. Email, Dr. Ken O'Neill, 30 June 2011.

Bibliography Chapter 19:

1. Undated article published by *The Herald-Palladium*, in the archives of Don Gast: "New Family Care Clinic is Opening in Bridgman."
2. Interview, Cathy Erickson, R.N., 10 February 2012.
3. Interview, Dr. Osburn, 10 February 2012.
4. Interview, Mary Beth Good, P.A., 10 February 2012.
5. Interview, Dr. Kroeze, 10 February 2012.
6. Telephone conversation, Nancy Labis, 22 February 2012.
7. Brochure, "Christian Counseling and Psychological Services: Directory of Services and Information Referral Guide," published by Southwestern Medical Clinic, P.C.

Bibliography Chapter 20:

1. Interview, Marilyn Hurrle, 11 November 2010.
2. Telephone interview, Dr. Georg Schultz, ca. 9 May 2011.
3. Email, Marilyn Hurrle, 4 May 2011.
4. Emails, Dr. Ken O'Neill and Carolyn Philip, 13 December 2011.
5. Telephone interview, Dr. Richard Hines, 2 February 2012.
6. Email, Carolyn Philip, ca. 2011.
7. Brief history of SWMC as documented by Dr. Ken O'Neill in the SWMCP physicians' manual, 2010.

Bibliography Chapter 21:

1. Interview, Joyce Bailey, 20 December 2011.
2. Annual SWMC year-end reports archived by Joyce Bailey.
3. Interview, Dr. Bird, 20 December 2011.
4. Interview, Dr. Chris Gordon, 20 December 2011.
5. Interview, Sandy Criswell, 20 December 2011.
6. Website, www.urmccf.org/events/fountain_bio.htm, about Dr. Dan Fountain.
7. Online document, www.onlineopinion.com.au/ author.asp? id=4137 *On Line Opinion: Australia's E-Journal of Social and Political Debate* (bio of Dr. Donna Joan Harrison).
8. Interview, Dr. Mark Harrison, 18 November 2010.
9. Email, Carolyn Philip, regarding Dr. Mark Harrison's leadership at SWMC and Lakeland.
10. Email, Sally Hanson and Diane Baker, 13 February 2012.

Bibliography Chapter 22:

1. Interview, Ruth Rutherford, 17 November 2010.
2. Interview, Dr. Dan and Elaine Metzger, 17 November 2010.
3. Interview, Joyce Bailey, 20 December 2011.
4. Website, www.teamworld.org

Bibliography Chapter 23:

1. Interview, Dr. Dan Stephens, 25 June 2010.
2. Blog: www.teamworld.org/medical/KarandaHospital
3. Blog: http://mcquilleninternational.blogspot.com/2010
4. Website: www.zimhydroceph.com
5. Website: www.karanda.org
6. Website: www.good-sam.com
7. Emails, Dr. Dan Stephens, 25, 28 and 29 February 2012.

Bibliography Chapter 24:

1. Website, www.wgm.org
2. Website, www.wikipedia.org/wiki/world_gospel_mission
3. Blog, Carol Spears, http://cckmissions.wordpress.com/2007/06/20/update-from-carol-spears-in-Africa/
4. Website, www.azcentral.com/community/surprise/articles/0326
5. Website, www.africanbrains.net/2011/09/20/toshiba
6. SWMC Brainwaves newsletter, ca. fall 1991.
7. Email, Dr. John Spriegel, 25 May 2011.

8. Lewis, Gregg. *Miracle at Tenwek*: The Life of Dr. Ernie Steury. Grand Rapids, MI: Discovery House Publishers, 2007.

9. Interview, Drs. Dan and Suzanne Hayward, 29 January 2012.

10. Email, Dr. Mike Chupp, 11 February 2012.

11. Telephone interview, Dr. Mike Chupp, 14 February 2012.

Bibliography Chapter 25:

1. Email from Dr. Janet Frey, ca. 2011.

2. Snyder, C. Albert. *On a Hill Far Away: Journal of a Missionary Doctor in Rwanda*, Life and Light Communications, Indianapolis, 1995.

3. Interview, Dr. Roy and Bev Winslow, 27 January 2011.

4. Chandler, Lila. "A Return Trip to Rwanda: St. Joseph Surgeon and His Wife to Make 11th Trip to African Nation Since 1979." *The Herald-Palladium*, 2 January 2009.

5. Letter written by Dr. Roy Winslow via e-mail, ca. 2010.

Bibliography Chapter 26:

1. Telephone interview, Dr. Dick Douce, Quito, Ecuador, 29 January 2011.

2. HCJB website (about Rev. Graham visiting) http://www.hcjb.org/HCJB-Global-News/quito-enthusiastically-embraces-franklin-graham-festival.html

3. Email letters sent to supporters from Dr. Dick and Marian Douce, dated between 2008-2011. Email from Marian Douce 4 February 2010 summarized Jornadas Medicas.

4. Telephone interview, Dr. Chuck Pierson, 27 October 2010.

5. Interview, Dr. Dan and Dee Ann Snyder, at their home, 14 December 2010.

Bibliography Chapter 27:

1. Telephone interview, Dr. Roy Ringenberg, 12 August 2010.
2. Telephone interview, Dr. Mike Chupp, 22 June 2010.
3. Telephone interview, Dr. Troy Thompson, 3 October 2010.
4. SWMC Brainwaves newsletter, July 1993.
5. Newsletter, "Project Medsend News Special Edition 2008," www.medsend.org
6. Telephone interview, Dr. Mike Chupp, 14 February 2012.

Bibliography Chapter 28:

1. Interview, Dr. Holly Tapley, 16 July 2010.
2. Interview, Carol Gonnerman Jewell, 10 January 2010.
3. Heflin, Bryant and Cindy. *Experiencing the Great I AM*: 40 Faith-Building Stories from Contemporary Christians. Google e-Book by Kregel Publications, 2005.
4. Interview, Dr. and Mrs. Smith, Lakeland Hospital, 2 May 2011.
5. Interview, Carolyn Philip, ca. 2011.
6. Email. Dr. Holly Tapley, 18 October 2011.
7. Emails, Dr. Wendell Geary, 9 November 2010.
8. Interview, Dr. Bird, 20 December 2011.
9. Interview, Dr. Chris Gordon, 20 December 2011.

Bibliography Chapter 29:

1. Telephone interview, Dr. Ron Baker, 27 October 2010.
2. Telephone interview, Dr. Thomas Ritter, 6 December 2010.
3. Interview, Dr. Bill and Cindy Wilkinson, 12 October 2010.
4. Interview, Dr. Chris and Jana Harvey, 11 January 2011.
5. Interview, Dr. Heather Marten, 29 January 2012.
6. Telephone interview, Drs. Lars and Callie Bandera, ca. March 2011.
7. Interview, Dr. John Froggatt, 22 February 2011.
8. Website, swmc.org
9. Lakeland HealthCare 2009 Annual Report, page 5.
10. Email, Dr. Chris Harvey, 31 January 2012.
11. Email, Carolyn Philip, 31 January 2012.

Bibliography Chapter 30:

1. Interview with Warren White, 9 November 2010.
2. Interview with Pat Meyer, 16 November 2010.
3. Brainwaves newsletter, Sept. 28, 1995.Email from Carolyn Philip late 2010.
4. Email from Carolyn Philip 28 October 2011.
5. *Benton Spirit*, front page, 27 April 2011.
6. Wilder-Smith, Annelies and Einar. *Grasping Heaven: Tami L. Fisk, A Young Doctor's Journey to China and Beyond*. Sisters, Oregon: Deep River Books, 2010.

Bibliography Chapter 31:

1. Email, Cindy O'Neill, 27 October 2011, regarding women's prayer time.
2. Photo and caption of Dr. Helene Johnson and the last baby born at the former Berrien General Hospital, *The Journal-Era*, 5 May 1999, page 1.
3. "Obstetrics, Surgical Staff Leave behind Legacy of Care, Compassion," *The Journal-Era*, 5 May 1999, page 1 and 22, article with photos.
4. Interview, Dr. Helene Johnson, 27 October 2010.
5. Email, Dr. Helene Johnson, 2 November 2010.
6. Interview, Betsy Zech, 27 January 2011.
7. Interview, Dr. John Froggatt, 22 February 2011.
8. Interview, Dr. Roy and Bev Winslow, 27 January 2011.
9. Interview, Dr. Bill and Cindy Wilkinson, 12 October 2010.
10. Email, Carolyn Philip, 25 January 2012 citing a lease agreement for the administration building.
11. Email, Dr. Ken O'Neill, 31 January 2012.
12. Interview, Dr. Keith VanOosterhout, 14 February 2012.
13. Email, Cindy O'Neill, 17 February 2012.

Bibliography Chapter 32:

1. Interview, Dr. Mark Harrison, 18 November 2010.
2. Telephone interview, Drs. Lars and Callie Bandera, ca. March 2011.
3. Bock, William C., MD, and Carter, John H., MD. *The History of Lakeland HealthCare: Celebrating the History of Healthcare in Southwest Michigan*. Lakeland HealthCare Marketing Department, St. Joseph, MI, 2011.
4. Website, www.lakelandhealth.org
5. Telephone conversation and email, Diann Demler, 16 February 2012.

Bibliography Chapter 33:

1. Interview, Pat Meyer, 16 November 2010.
2. Interview, Warren White, 9 November 2010.
3. Interviews, Dr. Ken O'Neill, 3 August 2010 and 2 September 2010.
4. Interview, Dr. John Froggatt, 22 February 2011.
5. Interview, Dr. Roy and Bev Winslow, 27 February 2011.
6. SWMCP physicians' manual updated by Dr. Ken O'Neill, 2010.
7. Lakeland HealthCare physicians' News Brief, "Lakeland HealthCare and Southwestern Medical Clinic, P.C., Announce Integration," February 2010.
8. Interview, Dr. Ken O'Neill, 9 August 2012.
9. Minutes of the SWMC Board of Directors.

Bibliography Chapter 34:

1. Interviews, Dr. Kenneth O'Neill, 3 August and 2 September 2010.
2. Interview, Warren White, 9 November 2010.
3. Interview, Dr. John Froggatt, 22 February 2011.
4. Interview, Drs. Dan and Suzanne Hayward, 29 January 2012.
5. Interview, Dr. Bill and Ilene Douce, 23 March 2010.
6. Interview, Pat Meyer, 16 November 2010.
7. Interview, Dr. Roy Winslow, 27 February 2011.
8. Telephone interviews, Dr. Mike Chupp, 22 June 2010 and 14 February 2012.
9. Interview, Dr. Mark Harrison, 18 November 2010.